Diversity Issues in Substance Abuse Treatment and Research

Diversity Issues in Substance Abuse Treatment and Research

Sana Loue
Case Western Reserve University
Cleveland, Ohio

Kluwer Academic / Plenum Publishers
New York   Boston   Dortrecht   London   Moscow

Library of Congress Cataloging-in-Publication Data

Loue, Sana.
  Diversity issues in substance abuse treatment and research / Sana Loue.
    p.   cm.
  Includes bibliographical references and index.
  ISBN 0-306-47775-0
  1. Minorities—Drug use—United States.   2. Women—Drug use—United States.
3. Gays—Drug use—United States.   4. Lesbians—Drug use—United States.   5. Drug
abuse—Treatment—Social aspects—United States.   6. Substance abuse—Treatment—Social
aspects—United States.   7. Drug abuse—Research—United States.   I. Title.

HV5824.E85L68   2003
362.29′1561′080973–dc21   2003051311

ISBN: 0-306-47775-0

© 2003 Kluwer Academic/Plenum Publishers, New York
233 Spring Street, New York, New York 10013

http://www.wkap.nl/

10 9 8 7 6 5 4 3 2 1

A C.I.P. record for this book is available from the Library of Congress

Permission for books published in Europe: permissions@wkap.nl
Permission for books published in the United States of America: permissions@wkap.com

Printed in the United States of America.

Preface

Although the term "diversity" is widely used, there is often no agreement as to its meaning or how attention to diversity should be operationalized within the context of programming or research. This text provides a foundation for the examination of such issues, with suggestions for the integration of various approaches into substance use treatment programs and research. The impetus for this work derived from multiple interactions over a period of several years with colleagues, students, research participants, and community-based providers, who noted the frequent inattention paid to such concerns in the context of treatment and research, often despite an acknowledgment of a group's particular historical legacy in the United States and the impact of that history on the initiation and prolongation of substance use within a specified community, or the barriers to treatment that may have resulted.

Chapter 1 defines what is meant by diversity through an examination of related terms, such as "culture," "ethnicity" "race," "sex," "gender," and "sexual orientation." Clearly, this discussion does not and cannot reflect all possible permutations of human existence that reflect diversity. For instance, although the text does make mention of considerations related to religious differences and cognitive capacity, neither is highlighted as a separate topic. Additionally, the emphasis on specified groups is not meant to imply that other groups, such as Euro-Americans or heterosexual men, do not have concerns that may differ from those of other communities and that deserve consideration in the development and implementation of programs and research endeavors. However trite it may seem, one text cannot do it all.

Chapter 2 begins with an examination of the concepts of addiction and dependence and continues with a review of what we know today about the effects of alcohol, tobacco, marijuana, cocaine and crack, hallucino-gens, and heroin. These particular substances were selected for discussion for several reasons. First, each substance mentioned is now or has been legal for general use during some period of time in United States history. Second, this listing reflects the position of these drugs along a spectrum of legality, ranging from alcohol and tobacco, which are legally available with some restrictions; to marijuana, whose legality varies depending on the lo-cale; to cocaine and heroin, which are currently illegal for use. Chapter 3 focuses on the development of policy over time with respect to each of these substances, with special emphasis on the relationship of that policy to the attributed characteristics of the groups who were perceived to be the most fervent users of the substances. The characterization of behavior as sub-stance use or dependence, or of an individual as being dependent, and our approach to that condition are necessarily a function of various assump-tions and decisions: our definitions of substance use and dependence; our choices regarding the (il)legality of specified substances; and our percep-tions of the cause(s) of this condition, the individuals believed to reflect the condition at issue, and the appropriateness of various responses to both the causes and the individuals. One writer has explained:

Both miracle or dangerous drugs are made, not born, and borne largely from cultural and political circumstances. A teleological or Whig view of drug control regimes—that they progressively emerged as we became enlightened about the relative health risks of certain substances—is unrealistic. Chemistry and biology are at work, but make risky guides for deducing drug history and its moral outcomes. Definitions of harm to individuals or societies are rarely resolved in the "pharmacocentric" or medical sphere, as testified by our current cultural struggles to reassess (or even invert) the roles of tobacco and marijuana. Drugs are protean and relational things, and cultural magnets for charged meanings. The line between today's licit and socially ingrained drugs and taboo ones was historically drawn. Clearly, constructionist perspectives are apt for looking at transformations in the status of drugs and at the erection of control regimes (Gootenberg, 1999: 7).

Chapters 4 and 5 focus on the history of specified groups in the United States and the relationship of that history to substance use, access to care, and health issues related to substance use. These groups include African-Americans, Asians and Pacific Islanders, Hispanics/Latinos, and various communities defined by sex, gender, and/or sexual orientation. Chapters 6 and 7 provide guidelines for the integration of diversity considerations into treatment programs for and research procedures with these communities.

Acknowledgments

The impetus for this work derived from multiple interactions with colleagues, students, research participants, and community-based providers over a period of several years. These individuals are too numerous to mention but, nevertheless, deserve to be recognized for their insightful comments relating to diversity and the lack of attention to such issues in the context of treatment and research.

Several people deserve special mention for their assistance with the development of this text. Nancy Mendez, a student and a colleague, provided me with invaluable feedback on earlier drafts of this book. Gary Edmunds, Jenice Contreras, and Ingrid Vargas provided me with invaluable research assistance. Mariclaire Cloutier of Kluwer Academic deserves accolades, as always, for her editorial support and encouragement.

Contents

Chapter 1

Diversity

Theory and Meaning

M any of us have heard or seen commentaries regarding the increasingly diverse nature of the United States' population and of the need for cultural competence and cultural sensitivity. All, too often, however, attempts to address complex issues that may fall within this rubric are reduced to "laundry lists" of "do's" and "don'ts," to an inventory of characteristics supposedly attributable to particular groups or populations, or to a series of edicts for the management of a "diverse" workforce and clientele. Too often, well-intentioned efforts to address what is meant by diversity and multiculturalism fail to reach beyond a recitation of that which is deemed to be politically correct at that time. And, even though well-meaning, attempts to generalize group characteristics to all individuals within those groups may result in the unfortunate perpetuation of stereotypes rather than the enhancement of understanding.

But why, one might ask, is it even necessary to address diversity? At least three reasons are immediately discernible: (1) a recognition of demographic changes in the population, in general, as well as changes in the client populations among providers, which may be related to the general population changes; (2) a desire to reduce insensitivity borne of cultural ignorance, bias, or myopia, and its deleterious consequences; and (3) the need to comply with local, state, and/or federal provisions that mandate a recognition of diversity in its various forms (Anderson, McPhee, and Gowan, 2000), such as the Americans with Disabilities Act and protections against sexual harassment. Additionally, depending upon one's perspective and values, a recognition of and attention to issues of diversity may facilitate the fulfillment of various goals, such as the promotion of social justice and

1

equal opportunity, the equitable distribution of wealth and power, and the provision of alternative life choices (Sleeter and Grant, 1987). This chapter provides, first, a theoretical framework for the discussion of diversity, drawing on readings from a wide range of disciplines, including education, anthropology, and management. This discussion is followed by an examination of how identity is formed and the meaning of diversity in the context of race, ethnicity, sex, gender, and sexual orientation. The validity of various classifications is also addressed. The chapter concludes with a brief examination of barriers to addressing diversity.

DIVERSITY DEFINED

Definitions of "diversity" vary widely, as they are often dependent upon the discipline from which they arise. The following definition draws extensively from management literature:

> [T]he attitudes, beliefs, and hence, behaviors, of individuals are socially constructed within a context of group and intergroup relations and . . . people act through social, political, and economic institutions that create, embed, and reproduce the inequality among people which we then call diversity. Diversity is then acted out in the practices of everyday life and interpreted through lenses of moral and ethical reasoning that, when unexamined, legitimate both unearned privilege and unearned disadvantage. The origin of diversity, however, is not in the reactions to differences in daily interaction . . . but rather diversity is created and perpetuated in the historical, institutional, cultural, and hence, moral, construction of difference and is reinforced by the structures of opportunity, resources, and power. While there may be "real" differences rooted in biology, we would argue that the dimensions of such differences are unknowable, given the filtering and conditioning that occurs through interaction with culture, history, and social institutions (DiTomaso and Hooijberg, 1996: 164–165).

Other writers, however, have defined diversity in the context of multiculturalism:

> Multiculturalism . . . refers to the doctrine that cultural diversity should be recognized as a permanent and valuable part of political societies (Tempelman, 1999: 17).

> [Multiculturalism] is the mastered knowledge and skills needed to feel comfortable and to communicate effectively with people of all cultures and in all cross-cultural situations (Onyekwuluje, 2000: 69).

A multicultural perspective has been said to be founded on collective interactions, abstract problem solving, and acceptance of all people, a recognition of a global community, and the attribution of value to multiple perspectives (Onyekwuluje, 2000). Significant disagreement exists, however, as to whether multiculturalism rests on the assumption that all persons are fundamentally the same (Onyekwuluje, 2000), or whether the focus of multiculturalism is more appropriately directed towards a recognition of shared similarties, the identification of those differences that are critical and those that are unimportant, and the development and maintenance of a supportive environment in which to pursue this examination (Sengstock, 2000).

These definitions, in turn, demand an explanation of "culture":

> [Culture is] a complex and global variable that represents the beliefs, language, rules, values and knowledge held in common by members of a society (Matthews, 1997: 35).

> [Cultures are] powerful human creations, affording their members a shared identity, a cohesive framework for selecting, constructing, and interpreting perceptions, and for assigning value and meaning in consistent fashion. The complex systems of thought and behavior that people create and perpetuate in and for association are subtle and profound, forged as to be endowed by their bearers with the attributes of universal truth: Things that fit into their cultural framework are given labels 'human nature,' 'instinct,' 'common sense,' 'logic.' Things that don't fit are different and therefore either illegal, immoral, nonsensical, or the result of a naïve and inferior stage of development of human nature (Galloway, 1992: 88).

Hogan-Garcia (2003: 11–23) has offered a detailed explanation of culture:

> Culture is both subjective and objective. Subjectively, culture is comprised of a meaning system. Objectively, culture dictates how and why we behave in certain ways. The subjective aspect, beliefs, values, and explanatory cognitive frameworks that are communicated both verbally and nonverbally are learned through social interactions in the family and in the general social milieu...Culture operates on several levels simultaneously...Culture exists at the micro level of the individual—that is, in a person's assumptions, values, beliefs, explanatory systems, and behaviors, which are learned in the family and other basic social groups. At the same time, culture exists, at the meso and macro levels in organizations and institutions. *Culture in general*...[refers] to the customary ways in which humans live,...diet, family forms and processes, social organizations, and religions...the term ethnic group...refers to the cultural heritage, or aspects of culture, that a group shares and attempts to hand down from one generation to the next through learning (italics in original).

Hogan-Garcia (2003) has also enumerated 12 features deemed to be essential to culture: history, social status, points of interaction within and between social groups, value orientations, verbal and nonverbal language and communication processes, family life processes, healing beliefs and practices, religion and religious practices, art and other forms of expression, dietary preferences and practices, recreational forms, and manner and style of dress.

CONSTRUCTING DIVERSITY

Theories of Individual and Collective Identity Construction

Identification with a particular culture, then, implies the formulation of specific individual and collective identities. In the context of a collective identity, this involves the demarcation of boundaries that determine who and what are to be included in and who and what are to be excluded from a particular group (Tempelman, 1999). Diversity, then, can be said to be a reflection or function of these various groups, as the groups are defined by their memberships and by those outside of these groups. Diversity also reflects the multiple identities that individuals may simultaneously have of themselves.

Various mechanisms for the construction of a collective identity have been postulated. In other words, how do we construct the differences that are "seen" between various groups of people? The formulation of what is known as primordial identity rests on the identification of characteristics that are deemed to be immutable and that are presumably "natural" and shared by all members of a group. Accordingly, those outside of the group are perceived as unalterably different, without the ability to be educated into the group or understood by the group (Eisenstadt and Geisen, 1995). One example of this construction is that of race, which is often perceived to be an immutable characteristic, notwithstanding the nonexistence of a biological basis for such an assertion. (The concept of race is discussed more fully below, together with the concept of "ethnicity." "Race" is also addressed further in chapter 4.)

In contrast, the civic construction of collective identity views the core of that identity as the composite of historically developed rules, routines, and institutional arrangements. As such, boundaries are vague and vary over time. The acquisition of a familiarity with these rules and routines permits outsiders to become insiders, albeit somewhat removed from those who are bearers of these traditions. That being said, the authority of such practices is subject to open and continuing debate (Parekh, 1995). Such debates acknowledge both the variability that exists within communities and overlapping characteristics between communities (Tempelman, 1999).

The third mechanism for the construction of a collective identity is that of the universal mode. Membership in a collectivity is premised on the shared acceptance of and belief in a central core. Outsiders may become insiders upon acceptance of that which is deemed to be sacred; they remain outsiders only as a result of their unwillingness to accept the basic precept(s). The universal mode demands that one's principles be defended against all others (Tempelman, 1999). An example of such a formulation might be a religious group that ascribed to a core tenet and believes that those individuals who fail to accept and ascribe to this tenet are mistaken and must be converted in their belief.

It is an oversimplification, however, to believe that individuals maintain a singular identity over time and place and ascribe to membership in a single collective. In fact, individuals may maintain multiple memberships at any given point in time (Turner, Hogg, Oakes, Reicher, and Wetherell, 1987). Consider, for instance, a United States-born middle-aged woman, married, with several children, trained as a physician, and raised by a Mexico-born Jewish father and a United States-born Catholic mother. She simultaneously maintains memberships in various collectives: middle-aged persons, women, mothers, and so on.

Additionally, how individuals self-identify may be intimately associated with changes in the shared environment, and with the emotions and experiences that individuals associate with their various memberships (Tajfel and Turner, 1986; Tajfel, 1974). For instance, this same woman may not have self-identified as a Latina in her youth but, as a result of the numerous political and social changes that have occurred during the intervening years, has developed a self-awareness and identity as a Latina. Essentially, then, identity is the product of a process that permits the integration and acceptance of new elements into one's identity.

The complexities of the development of individual and collective identities militate against simplistic attempts to address diversity. One cannot attribute to an individual, for instance, characteristics, behaviors, or attitudes that may be present among some members of a specific collective merely as a function of the individual's self-identified or attributed membership in that collective. For instance, all women do not experience harassment in the same way (Nast and Pulido, 2000). Similarly, the attribution of specific characteristics to a specific collective may serve to reinforce pre-existing stereotypes (Anderson, McPhee, and Govan, 2000) and/or to create erroneous expectations with respect to individuals' behaviors or reactions. An examination of the construction of race and racial categories across time and place illustrates the process by which collective identity may be defined in the larger social and political context and the interplay of this identity with individuals' self-categorization.

Diversity and the Construction of Racial and Ethnic Identities

Defining Race

The concept of race has been used to explain differences in appearance and in behavior across individuals and groups of individuals (Gaines, 1994). A variety of criteria have been used to define race, including region or geographical area of origin (King and Stansfield, 1990), nationality (Taylor, 1988), language, skin color, and religion (Gaines, 1994). These distinctions have provided the foundation for numerous suppositions about race in the United States: (1) the existence of a fixed number of distinct races (Segen, 1992; Campbell, 1981), (2) some of which are superior to others and (3) each of which is characterized by distinct mental, physical, or behavioral attributes (4) that are reproduced over time (Gould, 1981; Montagu, 1964a; Boas 1940). As an example, consider the following "scientific" distinctions drawn between black and white individuals on the basis of skin color, made by a physician in 1851 in the context of examining disease:

> Before going into the peculiarities of these diseases, it is necessary to glance at the anatomical and physiological differences between the Negro and the white man; otherwise their diseases cannot be understood. It is commonly taken for granted, that the color of the skin constitutes the main and essential difference between the black and white race; but there are other differences more deep, durable and inedible in their anatomy and physiology, than that of mere color. It is not only in the skin that a difference in color exists between the Negro and the white man, but in the membranes, the muscles, the tendons, and in all the fluids and secretions. Even the negro's brains and nerves, the chyle and all the humors, are tinctured with a shade of the pervading darkness. His bile is of a deeper color, and his blood is blacker than the white man's (Cartwright, 1851).

With respect to the reproducibility of such characteristics, consider the statements of the scientist Nott (1843), who argued against the intermarriage of the races based on his observation that (1) mulattoes live shorter lives in comparison with other classes of humans; (2) mulatto women are more likely to suffer from chronic diseases and inability to reproduce than are other women; and (3) the children of mulatto women are more likely to die at a young age. (Nott obviously failed to consider that mulattoes' relatively darker skin color might have affected their ability to obtain care which, in turn, have impacted on their morbidity and mortality.)

The conceptualization of "black" identity has varied over time, place, and purpose of designation (Gaines, 1994; LaVeist, 1994; Osborne and Feit, 1992). The United States alone has used a multitude of definitions and terms in its attempts to distinguish "whites" from "nonwhites" (Davis, 1991). For instance, the censuses of 1840, 1850, and 1860 counted mulattoes, but failed to explain the term's meaning. The 1870 and 1880 censuses specifically defined "mulattoes" as "quadroons, octoroons, and all persons having any perceptible trace of African blood" (Davis, 1991). The 1890 census required that the enumerators record the exact proportion of "African blood," while the 1900 census required that "pure Negroes" be distinguished from mulattoes, defined as persons "with some trace of black blood" (Davis, 1991). The scientist Lawrence (1819, 1823) had earlier devised an informal test for use in the West Indies to detect the "blackness" of any such individuals who may have become indistinguishably white through the successive intermarriages of previous generations:

> Europeans and Tercerons produce Querterons or Quadroons (ochavones, octavones, or alvinos), which are not to be distinguished from whites; but they are not entitled, in Jamaica at least, to the same privileges as the Europeans or the white Creoles, because there is still contamination of dark blood, although no longer visible. It is said to betray itself sometimes in a relic of the peculiar strong smell of the great-grandmother.

As of the 1930 census, "black" was defined as an individual with any black blood. In 1960, the basis for enumeration changed again, to permit the head of each household, rather than the enumerator, to identify the race of its members (Davis, 1991). This system of designating race was embedded in the protocol used for the assignment of race on birth certificates prior to 1989: a child was considered to be "white" only if both parents were considered "white" (LaVeist, 1994). An individual with one "white" parent and one "black" parent, then, would have been classifiable as a mulatto in 1900 and as a black in 1930. The 1990 census requested that each respondent report his or her racial classification as the one that he or she most closely identified with, but failed to provide a definition of race, resulting in confusion and "misreporting" (McKenney and Bennett, 1994).

Designation of an individual's race has been shown to vary by place as well. Even among the various states, the racial classification of an individual could differ. For instance, the "privileges of whites" were extended to a "quadroon" female by the Supreme Court of Ohio in 1831 due to "the difficulty of . . . ascertaining the degree of duskiness which renders a person liable to such disabilities" (*Gray v. Ohio*, 1831). By contrast, the Supreme Court of California construed the word "white" as excluding "black, yellow, and all other colors . . . The term 'black person' is to be construed as including everyone who is not of white blood" (*People v. Hall*, 1854). The black/mulatto child born in the United States would be classified as a mulatto in Brazil, and further categorized by the degree of darkness or lightness of the skin color as a *preto* (black), *preto retinto* (dark black), *cabra* (slightly less black), *escuro* (lighter), *mulato esuro* (dark mulatto), *mulato claro* (light mulatto), *sarara, moreno, blanco de terra,* or *blanco* (LaVeist, 1994). Prior to 1989 in the United States, a child born to a "white" father and a Japanese mother was classified as Japanese on his or her birth certificate. The same child would have been classified as white on his or her birth certificate in pre-1985 Japan (LaVeist, 1994).

The purpose or process of racial designation may also impact the ultimate classification of an individual. For instance, a child's race on his or her birth certificate is designated by the infant's mother, whereas the assignment of race at death is often made by the funeral director for completion of the death certificate. It is not inconceivable that an individual classified as a member of one race at birth will be classified as a member of another race at death (Hahn, 1992). Self-reported race/ethnicity has been shown to vary significantly from that recorded on birth certificates. A study of the validity of racial/ethnic information on California birth certificates found that although the sensitivity of the classification of race/ethnicity on birth certificates was very high for African-Americans, Asians and Pacific Islanders, Europeans, Hispanics, and those of Middle Eastern descent, the sensitivity for classification for Native Americans was only. 54 (Baumeister, Marchi, Pearl, Williams, and Braveman, 2000). Misclassification has been noted, as well, in data collected by the Health Care Financing Administration relating to elderly Medicare enrollees (Lauderdale and Goldberg, 1996). Finally, shifting perceptions of self-identity may result in inconsistent self-designation across time and circumstance (Snipp, 1986; Siegel and Passel, 1979; Johnson, 1974).

These classification schema and the discrepancies they create underscore the difficulty of applying the concept of race, however it is defined. They also lend credence to the observation that "race is a societally constructed taxonomy that reflects the intersection of particular historical conditions with economic, political, legal, social, and cultural factors, as well as racism" (Williams, LaVizzo-Mourey, and Warren, 1994).

Ethnicity

"Racial" identity is often confused with "ethnic identity," and the two terms have often been used interchangeably. Consider, for example, the following definitions of ethnicity. The first correlates with the previously noted definitions of "culture," whereas the others refer to "race" in defining "ethnicity" or "ethnicity" in defining "race."

> [An ethnic group is] a segment of a larger society whose members are thought, by themselves or others, to have a common origin and to share important segments of a common culture and who, in addition, participate in shared activities in which the common origin and culture are significant ingredients (Yinger, 1994: 3).

> An ethnic group represents one of a number of populations, comprising the single species of Homosapiens, which individually maintain their differences, physical and cultural, by means of isolating mechanisms such as geographic and social barriers. These differences will vary as the power of the geographic and social barriers acting upon the original genetic difference varies (Montagu, 1964b).

> It [an ethnic group] is a vast family of human beings, generally of common blood and language, always of common history, traditions, and impulses, who are both voluntarily and involuntarily striving together for the accomplishment of certain more or less vividly conceived ideals of life (DuBois, 1897: 7).

> [Race] 1. an ethnic stock, or division in mankind; in a narrower sense, a national or tribal stock; in a still narrower sense, a genealogic line of descent; a class of persons of common lineage. In genetics, races are considered as populations having different distributions of gene frequencies. 2. a class or breed of animals; a group of individuals having certain characteristics in common, owing to a common inheritance; a subspecies (Taylor, 1988).

> [Ethnicity is] the relevant form of raciation among a species where cultural differentiation predominates (Cooper, 1994).

Not surprisingly, this lack of demarcation between "race" and "ethnicity" has been noted:

> In practice, the distinction between a racial and an ethnic group is sometimes blurred by several facts. Cultural traits are often regarded as genetic and inherited (e.g., body odor, which is a function of diet, cosmetics, and other cultural items); physical appearance can be culturally changed (by scarification, surgery, and cosmetics); and the sensory perception of physical differences is affected by cultural perceptions of race (e.g. a rich Negro may be seen as lighter than an equally dark poor Negro, as suggested by the Brazilian proverb: 'Money bleaches') (van den Berghe, 1967: 9).

As an example of our oversimplification of diversity, consider the currently common practice in the United States of categorizing all individuals as either "black" or "white," and their subsequent classification as Hispanic or non-Hispanic. Such a classification scheme fails to account for the vast differences between individuals who originated from and have ties to communities in Africa, the Caribbean, and the South Bronx in New York.

Diversity in Sex, Gender, and Sexual Orientation

It is generally assumed that sex and gender are sexually dimorphic, meaning that there exists a phylogenetically inherited structure of two types, male and female (Herdt, 1994). Lillie's (1939) thoughts represent an early explanation of such sexual dimorphism:

> What exists in nature is a dimorphism within species into male and female individuals, which differ with respect to contrasting characters, for each of which in any given species we recognize a male form and a female form, whether these characters be classed as of the biological, or psychological, or social orders. Sex is not a force that produces these contrasts; it is merely a name for our total impression of the differences...In the strictly historical sense of these words, a male is to be defined as an individual that produces spermatozoa; a female one that produces ova; or individuals at least having the characters associated with these functions.

The identification of an individual as a biological male or female rests on an evaluation of one or more of the following elements: chromosomal sex, gonadal sex, morphological sex and secondary sex traits, and psychosocial sex or gender identity (Herdt, 1994). In general, it has been assumed that biological sex, determined by one or more of the first three elements, is inextricably linked with gender identity, as well as with gender role/social identity and sexual orientation (Bolin, 1994). Because we have so often accepted these assumptions without question, we often do not conceive of diversity in sex and in gender. However, these assumptions merit critical scrutiny.

Biological Sex

This general overview of the development of biological sex presumes a basic knowledge of anatomy and human reproduction. Individuals wishing further details are urged to consult Moore and Persaud (1993).

The chromosomal sex of an embryo depends on whether the fertilization of the ovum occurs by an X-bearing or Y-bearing sperm. Fertilization by an X-bearing sperm results in an XX zygote, which will normally develop into a female. Fertilization by a Y-bearing sperm will produce an XY zygote, which normally develops into a male (Moore and Persaud, 1993). However, the gonads of both males and females are identical in appearance prior to the seventh week of the embryo's development; during this period, they are referred to as indifferent or undifferentiated gonads.

Hermaphroditism or intersexuality occurs when there appears to be a discrepancy between the morphology of the gonads (testes or ovaries) and the appearance of the external genitalia. (For a discussion of the development of the testes and ovaries, see Moore and Persaud, 1993). True hermaphroditism is extremely rare and occurs only when both testicular and ovarian tissue are present. However, these tissues are generally nonfunctional (Krob, Braun, and Kuhnle, 1994; Moore and Persaud, 1993; Talerman, Verp, Senekjian, Gilewski, and Vogelzang, 1990).

Gender Identity and Gender Role

Stoller (1968: viii–ix) distinguished between sex as a function of biology and gender as a function of culture:

> Dictionaries stress that the major connotation of sex is a biological one as, for example, in the phrases *sexual relations* or *the male sex* . . . It is for some of these psychological phenomena [behavior, feelings, thoughts, fantasies] that the term *gender* will be used: one can speak of the male sex or the female sex, but one can also talk about masculinity and femininity and not necessarily be implying anything about anatomy or physiology.

Gender has been defined as

> a multidimensional category of personhood encompassing a distinct pattern of social and cultural differences. Gender categories often draw on perceptions of anatomical and physiological differences between bodies, but those perceptions are always mediated by cultural categories and meanings . . . Gender categories are not only "models of" difference . . . but also "models for" difference. They convey gender-specific social expectations for behavior and temperament, sexuality, kinship and interpersonal roles, occupation, religious roles and other social patterns. Gender categories are "total social phenomena" . . . ; a wide range of institutions and beliefs find simultaneous expression through them, a characteristic that distinguishes gender from other social statuses (Roscoe, 1994: 341).

Despite this distinction, (biological) sex has often been considered synonymous with or predictive of gender (social role). The following excerpt illustrates how biological sex was determinative of social function:

> Thus it was claimed that women's low brain weights and deficient brain structures were analogous to those of lower races, and their inferior intellectualities explained on this basis. Women, it was observed, shared with Negroes a narrow, childlike, and delicate skull, so different from the more

robust and rounded heads characteristic of males of 'superior' races. Similarly, women of higher races tended to have slightly protruding jaws, analogous to, if not as exaggerated as, the apelike jutting jaws of lower races. *Women and lower races were called innately impulsive, emotional, imitative rather than original, and incapable of the abstract reasoning found in white men* (Stepan, 1990: 39–40) (emphasis added).

Gender identity and gender role are distinct. Nanda's (1994: 395–396) explanation is instructive:

> Gender identity has been defined as the private experience of gender role: the experience of one's sameness, unity and the persistence of one's individuality as male, female, or androgynous, expressed in both self-awareness and in behavior. Gender role is everything that a person says and does to indicate to others or to the self the degree to which one is either male, female or androgynous. Gender role would thus include public presentations of self in dress and verbal and nonverbal communication; the economic and family roles one plays; the sexual feelings (desires) one has and the persons to whom such feelings are directed; the sexual role one plays and emotions one experiences and displays; and the experiencing of one's body, as it is defined as masculine or feminine in any particular society. Gender identity and gender role are said to have a unity, like two sides of a coin.

Stoller's conceptualization of gender identity and gender role similarly distinguish between the private and the public experiences:

> I am using the word *identity* to mean one's own awareness (whether one is conscious of it or not) of one's existence or purpose in this world or, put a bit differently, the organization of those psychic components that are to preserve one's awareness of existing (Stoller, 1968: x).

Gender identity is to be further distinguished from "core gender identity," a "person's unquestioning certainty that he belongs to one of only two sexes" (Stoller, 1968: 39). Stoller elaborated as follows:

> This essentially unalterable core of gender identity [I am a male] is to be distinguished from the related but different belief, *I am manly* (or masculine). The latter attitude is a more subtle and complicated development. It emerges only after the child has learned how his parents expect him to express masculinity (Stoller, 1968: 40).

This, too, can be contrasted with gender role. "Core gender identity" signifies the feeling of "I am a male" or "I am a female," whereas "gender role" represents "a masculine or feminine way of behaving" (Walinder, 1967: 4).

Gender identity is to be distinguished, as well, from sexual identity:

The term "gender identity" [is] used . . . rather than various other terms which have been employed in this regard, such as the term "sexual identity." "Sexual identity" is ambiguous, since it may refer to one's sexual activities or fantasies, etc. . . . Thus, of a patient who says "I am not a very masculine man," it is possible to say that his gender identity is male although he recognizes his lack of so-called masculinity (Stoller, 1964: 220).

Sexual Orientation

We have come to equate the choice of one's sexual partner—male or female—with one's sexual orientation. It is clear, though, that homosexual behavior is not synonymous with homosexuality. For instance, a recent study of male sexual behavior in the United States found that 2% of the respondents aged 20 to 39 reported having had any same sex sexual activity during the previous 10 years, but only 1 percent reported exclusively same sex sexual activity for the same time period (Billy, Tanfer, Grady, and Keplinger, 1993). Identical sexual acts, including the choice of the sexual partner, may vary in meaning and significance, depending on their cultural and historical context (Vance, 1995). As illustrated by the following examples taken from both history and current events, we see that the biological sex of one's sexual partner may have as much or more to do with power, economic relations, and the availability of alternative partners as with sexual desire or orientation.

In a number of societies, sexual relations between younger and older men were structured by age (Greenberg, 1988). The older male often assumed the active role in the relationship, while the younger male assumed the passive role. The sexual act could include masturbation, anal intercourse, and/or fellatio. The motivation for these relationships varied depending on the culture, but could include the sexual transmission of special healing powers from the older male to the younger disciple; the belief that a boy must have semen implanted in his body by an adult in order to mature physically; a fear that heterosexual intercourse would deplete men's vitality; a scarcity of women; and a belief that heterosexual intercourse would harm men because of women's polluting qualities (Greenberg, 1988).

Homosexual behavior—as distinct from homosexuality—may also reflect a differential in power between the sexual partners. This includes, for example, the use of one's body rather than money to deter violence, a situation that may arise both on the street (Scacco, 1982), in prisons, and during war (Greenberg, 1988; Trexler, 1995).

The status of berdache and hijra both exemplify relations that might be termed homosexual based on only a superficial understanding of sexual behavior but, in fact, signify something quite different. Williams (1992: 2) defined a berdache as "a morphological male who does not fit society's standard man's role, who has a nonmasculine character." Native Americans often referred to berdaches as "halfmen-halfwomen," although they were neither hermaphrodites nor transsexuals (Williams, 1992). Berdaches, who are now known as "two-spirit people" (Lang, 1996), existed within various Native American tribes, including the Cheyenne, Creek, Klamath, Mohave, Navaho, Pima, Sioux, and Zuni (Greenberg, 1988; Roscoe, 1991; Williams, 1992). Rather than being termed effeminate, two-spirit people are more accurately described as androgynous. They are not perceived as either men or women, but rather as an alternative gender. Often, two-spirit persons combined the behavior, social roles, and dress of both men and women. Although some assumed the passive role in a sexual relationship with another man, the sexual relationship was a secondary component of status as a berdache (Callender and Kochems, 1986; Williams, 1992). Homosexual behavior was not synonymous with status as a berdache (Williams, 1992). Similarly, some "two-spirit" women adopted some male roles and dress and had sexual relations with women (Schaeffer, 1965).

As a result of missionary efforts and United States government agents, the berdache tradition has declined. Younger Native Americans may have rejected the role of the berdache in favor of a self-identity as a gay male (Williams, 1992).

The hijras of India have been characterized as "neither man nor woman and woman and man" (Nanda, 1990; Nanda, 1994). Based on that status, hijras play a religious role, derived from Hinduism, by blessing newborn male children and performing at marriages (Nanda, 1990). Hijras are defined as such by their lack of desire for and sexual impotence with women, rather than by their sexual relations with men. Their impotence with women is attributed to a defective or absent male sexual organ, which is lacking due to an accident of birth or to intentional emasculation, the surgical removal of the male genitals (Nanda, 1990). In defining themselves, hijras collapse sex and gender into one category, defining themselves as "not men" because of their impotence with women and as "not women" because of their inability to bear children. They simultaneously incorporate aspects of the female role, such as dress, gendered erotic fantasies, desire for male sexual partners, and a gender identity of a woman or hijra, with those of a male role, such as coarse speech and the use of the hookah for smoking (Nanda, 1994). Clearly, despite their sexual relations with men, hijras are not defined and do not define themselves as homosexuals.

Homosexuality has been variously conceived of as an innate, relatively stable condition (Murray, 1987); a congenital, but not hereditary condition (Heller, 1981); a form of congenital degeneracy (Gindorf, 1977); an earlier evolutionary form of the human race, *i.e.*, bisexual or hermaphroditic (Krafft-Ebing, 1965); a perverse and immature orientation resulting from family interactions during childhood development (Dynes, 1987; Freud, 1920); and the result of psychological processes similar to those that lead to heterosexuality, modifiable through various forms of therapy (Akers, 1977). It was not until 1973 that the American Psychiatric Association removed homosexuality as a mental illness from the *Diagnostic and Statistical Manual of Mental Disorders* (Greenberg, 1988).

Transsexuality

Transsexuals have been defined as "individuals with a cross-sex identity," regardless of their surgical status (Bolin, 1992: 14), while transsexuality has been classified as a gender identity disorder resulting in "clinically significant distress or impairment in social, occupational, or other important areas of functioning" (Reid and Wise, 1995: 241). Whether transsexuality per se constitutes a disorder, which then necessitates treatment, is subject to considerable dispute (Loue, 1996). Diagnosis rests on the presence of "a strong and persistent cross-gender identification" and "a persistent discomfort with one's sex or a sense of inappropriateness in the gender role of that sex (Reid and Wise, 1995: 241). Diagnosis requires that the condition be distinguished from hermaphroditism, a desire to change sex in order to gain a cultural or social advantage, and a desire to change sex due to nonconformity with prescribed sex roles (Reid and Wise, 1995: 240).

Researchers have estimated that approximately 1 out of every 11,900 men (male to female) and approximately 1 out of every 30,400 women (female to male) are transsexuals (Bakker, van Kesteren, Gooren, and Bezemer, 1993). Estimates of the sex ratio have varied widely, from 2.5 men to 1 woman in the Netherlands to 5.5 women to 1 man in Poland (Bakker et al., 1993; Godlewski, 1988; Pauley, 1968).

Treatment for transsexualism has included long-term hormonal therapy and sex change surgery. Genital reassignment surgery from female to male is complex and extensive and, consequently, must generally be performed in several stages (Hage, Bouman, de Graaf, and Bloem, 1993). Phalloplasty is used to construct a penis in a female-to-male transsexual (Hage, Bloem, and Suliman, 1993). In addition to the surgery, female-to-male transsexuals must often adhere to a long-term regimen of androgen administration (Sapino, Pietribiasi, Godano, and Busolati, 1992). Potential adverse effects include necrosis, hernia, venous congestion, and phallic shaft fistulas (Hage, Bloem, and Suliman, 1993). Male-to-female transsexuals may also undergo extensive surgery (Eldh, 1993) and hormonal treatment (Valenta, Elias, and Domurat, 1992). Potential adverse effects include the lack of a sensate clitoris (Eldh, 1993), vaginal stenosis (Crichton, 1992; Stein, Tiefer, and Melman, 1990), and pain during sexual intercourse (Stein, Tiefer, and Melman, 1990). Many transsexuals may ultimately decide to forgo the surgery due to its high cost, the lack of health insurance coverage for the surgery (Gordon, 1991; Stein, Tiefer, and Melman, 1990), and the fear of an unsatisfactory surgical outcome (Crichton, 1992; Hage, Bout, Bloem, and Megens, 1993).

Transgenderism

The word "transgender" has several meanings. First, it can encompass all those who "challenge the boundaries of sex and gender" (Feinberg, 1996: x). Alternatively, it refers to those who reassign the sex they were labeled at birth, and those whose expressed gender is considered inappropriate for their apparent sex (Feinberg, 1996). A distinction is often made between transsexuals, who change or attempt to change the sex that they were assigned at birth, and transgender individuals, who "blur the boundar[ies] of the *gender expression*" traditionally associated with the biological sexes (Feinberg, 1996: x).

Such blurring may take the form of cross-dressing (Garber, 1992). Cross-dressing, *i.e.*, wearing the clothing that is most often associated with the opposite sex, may occur for various reasons and in numerous contexts. Women may assume an "imitation man look" in an attempt to be more successful in business (Molloy, 1977). Men, some homosexual and some heterosexual, may perform as female impersonators. Gay men may dress in drag as a means of self-assertion or activism (Garber, 1992). Cross-dressing has been central in theater (Baker, Burton, and Smith, 1995; Heriot, 1975) and, to some degree, in religion (Barrett, 1931; Garber, 1992; Warner, 1982). It is important to recognize that not all of these are associated with being a transgendered individual.

BARRIERS TO ADDRESSING DIFFERENCE

Numerous barriers to addressing difference have been identified at the individual and organizational/systemic levels. At the level of the individual, these include language; style and content of nonverbal communication; the existence of prejudice, arising from various attitudes and beliefs;

the existence of stereotypes and biases; and stress. The attitudes or beliefs of an individual are often related to the stereotypes that they hold. An attitude expresses favor or disfavor; it becomes a belief when it is generalized (Allport, 1979). A stereotype represents "an exaggerated belief associated with a category. Its function is to justify (rationalize) our conduct in relation to that category" (Alport, 1979: 191). For instance, an individual may disfavor individuals of a specific ethnic group and believe that "they have no sense of responsibility." That stereotype may then be used as a means of rationalizing a desire to avoid enrolling an individual of that group into a specific treatment program or research study. Barriers at the individual level are made known and are reinforced in any number of ways, including verbal rejection through antagonistic language, gossip, or humor; through segregation, including avoidance; and through physical attack (Allport, 1979).

At the organization or systemic level, these same barriers may be formalized through the promulgation and establishment of verbalized and nonverbalized norms, policies, procedures, and programs that undermine efforts to address difference effectively. Additionally, many individuals and organizations in the United States may operate from one or more of the following assumptions, further enhancing the difficulties involved in addressing difference adequately: (1) All individuals in the United States are equal and our system functions on the basis of merit. (2) "Americans" don't have a culture. (3) Anything that is different is, by its very definition, wrong. (4) Discussions about cultural diversity are taboo. (5) One should never admit that he or she has prejudices (Tatum, 1993; Kohls, 1984).

Chapter 2

Substance Abuse and Dependence
Definition, Causation, Epidemiology, and Sequelae

DEFINING ADDICTION

The term "addiction" has been used synonymously with the term "substance dependence." As such, addiction has been defined as "a chronically relapsing [disorder] characterized by compulsive drug taking, an inability to limit the intake of drugs, and the emergence of a withdrawal syndrome during cessation of drug taking (dependence)" (Koob, Sanna, and Bloom, 1998: 1). The World Health Organization, which abandoned its use of the term "addiction," has defined dependence as

a state, a psychic and sometimes also physical [state], resulting from the interaction between a living organism and a drug, characterized by behavioral and other responses that always include a compulsion to take the drug on a continuous or periodic basis in order to experience its psychic effects, and sometimes to avoid the discomfort of its absence (Grinspoon and Balakar, 1976).

"Substance dependence" has been defined with greater precision in the American Psychiatric Association's *Diagnostic and Statistical Manual of Mental Disorders* (DSM) as "a maladaptive pattern of substance use, leading to clinically significant impairment or distress," and characterized by the occurrence within the previous 12 months of three or more of seven elements: (1) tolerance, (2) withdrawal, (3) the use of the substance in increasingly larger amounts or over a longer period of time than was intended,

19

(4) a persistent desire or unsuccessful attempts to reduce the amount or frequency of the substance use, (5) the dedication of a large portion of time to obtaining, using, or recovering from the use of the substance, (6) the elimination or reduction of important social, recreational, or occupational activities due to the use of the substance, and/or (7) the continuing use of the substance, despite knowledge of a persistent or recurrent physical or psychological problem that was initiated or exacerbated by the use of the substance (American Psychiatric Association, 2000).

Tolerance is characterized by a need for increased amounts of the substance to achieve either intoxication or desired effect or by a diminished effect of the substance with the use of the same amount. Withdrawal is manifested by a set of symptoms resulting from the cessation of or reduction in use of a particular substance or by the use of the same or a closely related substance in order to avoid these symptoms. An individual who experiences either tolerance or withdrawal is said to be physiologically dependent (American Psychiatric Association, 2000). It is important to recognize that tolerance, dependence, and withdrawal are normal physiological responses to the repeated use of a drug (Snyder, 1996).

Substance dependence must be distinguished from substance abuse, which is characterized by recurrent substance use (1) that results in a failure to fulfill major role obligations at work, school, or home; (2) that occurs in situations in which it is physically dangerous to use the substance, such as when driving; (3) that results in legal problems, such as arrests for disorderly conduct or driving under the influence; and (4) that results in recurring social or interpersonal difficulties that were initiated by or are exacerbated by the substance use, such as arguments with a domestic partner. The diagnoses of substance abuse and substance dependence are mutually exclusive in that an individual cannot be diagnosed with substance abuse if he or she has once had a diagnosis of substance dependence for the same substance. Depending upon the substance being used and the extent of that use, individuals may experience substance-induced disorders that are independent of abuse or dependence, such as intoxication, delirium associated with intoxication, delirium associated with withdrawal, dementia, amnesia, psychosis, anxiety disorders, sexual dysfunction, sleep disorders, or mood disorders. The use of even substances that may not be associated by the general public with dependence or abuse, such as caffeine, may lead to intoxication, an anxiety disorder, or a sleep disorder.

Substance dependence must also be distinguished from compulsion, which refers to repetitive behaviors, such as hand washing, or mental acts, such as flicking the lights on and off five times, that the person feels he or she must perform in response to an obsession or pursuant to rigidly enforced rules (Snyder, 1996). The distinction between a compulsive behavior and an addiction or dependence is often difficult and may, perhaps, depend upon our understanding of a particular behavior at a given point in time. Pathological gambling, for instance, shares many characteristics with substance dependence, including an aroused euphoric state in association with the behavior, the development of tolerance, and the experience of withdrawal-like symptoms in the absence of betting or gambling (Comings, Rosenthal and Lesieur, 1996). Research relating to pathological gambling has implicated a biochemical dysfunction affecting the reward and reinforcement systems of the brain, similar to that for impulse control and addictive behaviors (Comings, 1998). It remains unclear, however, how substance abuse and gambling behavior are specifically linked. Moreover, these behaviors or mental acts are aimed at preventing or reducing the individual's distress or preventing a dreaded event or situation, but they are not connected in any apparently realistic way with the situation or event that they are designed to neutralize or to avoid or they are clearly in excess of what would be required to do so. Further, this condition cannot be attributable to the abuse of a substance (American Psychiatric Association, 2000).

THE EPIDEMIOLOGY OF ADDICTION

The prevalence of illicit drug use across age and demographic groups varied in a 1994 population survey from 2.7 percent of 12- to 17-year olds who self-identified as being of "other" ethnicity to 14.6 percent of 18- to 25-year old self-identified white respondents (Substance Abuse and Mental Health Services Administration, 1995). Contrary to the impressions of many Americans, African-American respondents under the age of 25 reported rates of illicit drug use that were similar to or lower than the rates reported by individuals of the same age of other ethnicities (Anthony, Warner, and Kesler, 1994; Bachman, Wallace Jr., O'Malley, Johnston, Kurth, and Neighbors, 1991).

It is critical to note, however, that illicit drug use is not synonymous with substance dependence. The National Institute of Mental Health—sponsored National Comorbidity Survey, conducted from 1990 to 1992, utilized a psychiatric diagnostic perspective to obtain population-based rates of diagnoses of abuse and dependence. The study found that among 8,000 Americans ages 15 to 24 years old, the following percentages had developed dependence on various drugs: 7.5 percent, illicit drugs or inhalants; 4.2 percent, cannabis; 2.7 percent cocaine; 24.1 percent, tobacco; and 14.1 percent, alcohol. Approximately 9 percent of men and almost

6 percent of women had a diagnosis of dependence on illicit drugs at some point during their lives (Anthony, Warner, and Kessler, 1994).

THEORIES OF CAUSATION

Numerous theories have been propounded to explain the initiation of addiction. Foremost among these explanations are those related to neurobiology, to genetic factors, and to the role of psychosocial and contextual factors. Although these perspectives are discussed briefly below, it is beyond the scope of this chapter to examine these and other theories in detail, and the reader is referred to additional source material relating to this debate (Elster, 1999; Institute of Medicine, 1996; Edwards and Lader, 1994).

The Neurobiology of Addiction

Addiction is thought to be a disease that, in vulnerable individuals, results from the interaction of the drugs or substances with genetic, environmental, psychosocial, and behavioral factors, resulting in long-term alterations in the biochemical and functional properties of certain groups of neurons in the brain (Institute of Medicine, 2001b).

The biological component of addiction depends, in part, on the functioning of neurons and the release of neurotransmitters. Neurons, one of the major cell types in brain matter, have a nucleus and surrounding cytoplasm but, unlike other cells, they possess axons, which are cellular extensions that project information to other cells. The nerve endings at the end of each axon may divide into tens of thousands of branches, each having contact with yet another neuron, either directly, or through another nerve-cell extension known as a dendrite. Tens of thousands of dendrites may extend from a neuronal cell; each dendrite receives input from a number of neurons (Snyder, 1996). Neurons are able to transmit information to distant locations and to communicate with other neurons through the use of diverse chemical substances known as neurotransmitters (Institute of Medicine, 2001b). Dopamine is one such neurotransmitter.

The transmitting neuron stores the neurotransmitter until the neuron is stimulated, at which time the neurotransmitter is released (Cooper, Bloom, and Roth, 1996). The transmitter is then transfused across a divide known as a synapse and subsequently binds to a receptor, which is a special recognition site. These postsynaptic neurons may be excited, inhibited, or subject to more complex biochemical alterations, depending upon the transmitter.

Drugs that are highly addictive, such as heroin or cocaine, mimic or enhance the action of one or more of the brain's neurotransmitters that are involved in the control of the brain reward circuit (Cooper, Bloom, and Roth, 1996). For instance, alcohol facilitates the activation of a receptor for gamma-aminobutyric acid (GABA), which is one of the most prevalent neurotransmitters throughout the brain. Nicotine mimics the effects of the neurotransmitter acetylcholine at its nicotinic receptors, and heroin mimics endogenous opioid-like compounds known as endorphins. Each of these substances—alcohol, nicotine, and heroin—regulates the activity of the brain reward pathway that extends from the ventral tegmental area within the midbrain to the nucleus accumbens, situated between the limbic system involved in the control of emotion and the stratium, which is involved in the initiation and control of movement (Di Chiara and Imperato, 1988). All addictive drugs act on this pathway, but because they also have unshared sites of action, their subjective and objective behavioral properties differ. This explains, for instance, why both opioids and cocaine are reinforcing but why opioids act as sedatives while cocaine serves as a stimulant (O'Brien, 1996).

The effects of a particular drug depend on the neural locations of the receptors or transporters through which they act, the rapidity with which they reach the brain, and the purity of the drug. The route of administration may determine the rate at which the drug reaches the brain, which explains why smoked cocaine free base (crack cocaine) is more addictive than powdered cocaine that is absorbed more slowly through the nasal mucosa.

Long-term changes in the brain may result from the use of a drug at a sufficient dose with sufficient frequency and chronicity. These long-term changes, such as those seen with opioids and ethyl alcohol, may consist of compensatory adaptations within the brain in areas that control somatic functions; this produces physical dependence. Attempts to withdraw from the drug may result in a physical withdrawal syndrome (O'Brien, 1996). The second type of long-term change that may result relates to adaptations within the brain reward circuitry. Although not well understood, these adaptations appear to relate to the development of tolerance, resulting in attempts to increase the dosage to obtain the same effect; to the development of dependence, so that withdrawal from the drug may result in depressed mood, drug craving, and an inability to experience pleasure; and to the development of sensitization, meaning that the effects of some drugs may become stronger with repeated use (Institute of Medicine, 2001b). Third, some addictive drugs may produce emotional memories of drug use as a function of the activation of dopaminergic circuitry with the use of a particular drug. Consequently, the recall of memories of places, people, and bodily feelings associated with drug use may elicit cravings for the drug (O'Brien, 1996).

The Genetic Contribution to Addiction

Various studies indicate that there may well be a genetic component to vulnerability to addiction. Studies of twins and adopted children indicate that early onset alcoholism is influenced by genetic factors, while alcoholism that commences at a later age is more likely to be associated with environmental and emotional factors (Kendler, Heath, Neale, Kessler and Eaves, 1992; Heath, Meyer, Jardine and Martin, 1991a, 1991b). Genetic studies of alcohol use across various populations have revealed an "alcohol flush reaction," characterized by facial flushing, a rapid heartbeat, headaches and, on occasion, unconsciousness (Thomasson, Edenberg, Crabb, Mai, Jerome, Li, Wang, Lin, Lu and Yin, 1991). This reaction appears to occur among many individuals of Chinese, Japanese, and Korean ancestry. Numerous animal studies also provide support for a genetic basis of vulnerability to addiction (Koob, Sanna, and Bloom, 1998).

Psychosocial Factors Associated with Substance Use

Alcohol use has been associated with various pre-existing characteristics, including aggressivity in childhood (Robins, 1966), lower valuation of education (Brook, Whiteman, Gordon, and Cohen, 1986), lower expectations relating to academic achievement (Jessor and Jessor, 1977), lower levels of religiosity (Webb, Baer, McLaughlin, McKelvey and Caid, 1991), greater rebelliousness (Brook, Whiteman, Gordon, and Cohen, 1986), a rejection of parental authority (Webb, Baer, McLaughlin, McKelvey and Caid, 1991), fewer negative beliefs about the harmfulness of drinking (Margulies, Kessler, and Kandel, 1977), and greater expectations relating to the positive social benefits of drinking. Predictors of frequent drug use among adolescents include rebelliousness and low school achievement. Adolescents who use marijuana also appear to be more inclined to rebelliousness, lower educational expectations, greater opposition to authority, more favorable beliefs about marijuana, and lower levels of religiosity (Brown, Schulenberg, Bachman, O'Malley, and Johnston, 2001). Conduct disorders, depression, and anxiety disorders have been found to be associated with alcoholism and drug abuse (Kessler, Nelson, McGonagle, Edlund, Frank and Leaf, 1996; Riggs, Baker, Mikulich, Young and Crowley, 1995) and a high incidence of substance abuse has been reported among psychiatric patients (Drake and Wallach, 1989; Miller, Busch and Tanebaum, 1989).

Contextual Factors and Substance Use

Parental substance abuse has been found to be associated with an increased risk of substance abuse, including injection drug use, among the children (Moore, 1994; Perez-Arce, 1994; Merikangas, Rounsaville and Prusoff, 1992). Positive parental attitudes regarding substance use and beliefs about the harmlessness of substance use, parental tolerance for adolescent substance use, a lack of close attachment between parents and their children, and a lack of parental involvement in their children's lives have also been found to increase the likelihood that offspring will later engage in substance abuse (Dodgen and Shea, 2000; Hawkins, Catalano and Miller, 1992).

Peers' use of drugs has also been found to play a role in individuals' initiation of substance use. This may be related to the tendency among drug-using adolescents to select similar peers, thereby establishing a mutually reinforcing pattern of substance use (Kaplan and Johnson, 1992). However, the role of peers in the transition from drug use to drug abuse remains unclear (Kaplan, 1986).

Environmental factors, including high rates of crime, the easy availability of drugs, association with drug-using or delinquent peers, and an acceptance of drug use and abuse have been found to be associated with the initiation of drug use (Cohen, Brook, Cohen, Velez and Garcia, 1990; Robins and McEvoy, 1990). The extent to which youth learn about the use of drugs from their social interactions remains unclear. One researcher explained the potential implications of such interactions:

> To see the importance of such endogenous interactions at a deeper level, consider the cocaine epidemic of the 1980s, which appears to have subsided during the 1990s. A plausible explanation of the course of the epidemic begins with positive expectations interactions as youth of the '80s may have observed some of their peers initiate crack usage and apparently enjoy it. There also may have been positive preference interactions of the stigma reducing type. Eventually, however, youth of the '90s may have observed the devastating long-term outcomes experienced by addicts of the '80s and subsequently may have chosen not to initiate crack use themselves. If this story of observational learning is correct, then an information campaign warning of the devastating effects of crack addiction might have been effective in the early stages of the epidemic, but superfluous later on (Manski, 2000: 130).

An inability to access broader educational and employment opportunities may be related to the initiation of drug use and/or its continuation. Among Mexican Americans, lower socioeconomic status, higher school dropout rates, and residence in barrios in large cities have been shown to exacerbate drug use (Carter and Wilson, 1991). African-American women have been found more likely to continue their marijuana use into adulthood, as compared with self-identified white women (Yamaguchi and Kandel, 1985) while Native American youth face high unemployment and school dropout rates (Oetting, Swaim, Edwards, and Beauvais, 1989).

DRUGS: USAGE AND OUTCOMES

The Impact of Alcohol

Use, Abuse, and Effects

Approximately 86.6 percent of men and 77.5 percent of women in the United States have ever consumed alcohol. Lifetime use is highest among those between the ages of 26 and 34 (Substance Use and Mental Health Services Administration, 1998). National research has indicated that 68.7 percent of men and 59.8 percent of women had consumed alcohol during the one year period preceding the investigation, with the highest rates of use again occurring between the ages of 26 and 34. The frequency of alcohol use has been found to vary across subgroups, with whites reporting higher frequency of use in comparison with both African-Americans and Hispanics (Grant, 1997).

A much smaller number of individuals may suffer from alcoholism. Approximately 13.7 percent of people in the United States were believed to fulfill the criteria for alcoholism during the 1980s (Helzer and Burnam, 1991). The lifetime prevalence rate of alcoholism among men has been estimated at 12.5 percent, while for women it is much lower, at 6.4 percent (Kessler, Crum, Warner, Nelson, Schulenberg, and Anthony, 1997). Alcohol abuse has been associated with higher availability of alcohol, peer influences, poverty, lower levels of education, high levels of job-related stress, and lower levels of family interaction (Shuckit, 2000). The prevalence of binge drinking appears to increase substantially during downturns of the economy, implicating economic stress as a significant factor (Dee, 2001).

Alcohol is absorbed primarily in the small intestine and is metabolized in the liver. Depression of the central nervous system constitutes one of the principal effects of alcohol ingestion. Intoxication, which has often been defined in a legal context as having a blood alcohol content of 100 milligrams per deciliter of blood (McGowan, 1997), is characterized by the recent ingestion of alcohol; clinically significant maladaptive behavioral or psychological changes, such as aggressive behavior, that develops during or shortly after the consumption of alcohol; the presence, during or after the use of alcohol, of slurred speech, lack of coordination, unsteady gait, or various other symptoms; and the absence of a general medical condition or other mental disorder that would account for these changes (American Psychiatric Association, 2000).

The potential effects of alcohol ingestion are many. Alcohol consumption during evening hours may increase airway resistance during sleep, resulting in increased inspiratory effort, airway collapse, and obstructive apneas (Aldrich, 1998). Obstructive sleep apnea is often characterized by excessive daytime sleepiness, loud snoring during sleep, and sleep disruption resulting from the closure of the airway. Approximately 2 percent of adult women and 4 percent of adult men suffer from the disorder (Young, Palta, Dempsey, Skatrud, Weber, and Badr, 1993).

Individuals who drink large amounts of alcohol on a repetitive basis may become tolerant of the effects of alcohol, so that intoxication does not occur with the ingestion of the same amounts. Withdrawal, when it is mild, may include symptoms such as tremor, weakness, and sweating. Severe chronic alcoholism may result in subtle disorders of higher intellectual functioning that are detectable with neuropsychological examination: deficits in attentional skills; difficulty in problem-solving; disorders of perceptual-spatial skills; and abnormalities in tactile performance, concept formation, and rule-learning (Grant, Reed and Adams, 1987; Ron, 1983). Additional potential medical and neurological effects include severe malnutrition, cirrhosis, peripheral neuropathy, cerebellar degeneration, and Wernicke-Korsakoff syndrome (Lieber, 1995; Charness, Simon, and Greenberg, 1989; Victor, Adams, and Collins, 1989). The Wernicke-Korsakoff syndrome occurs in two stages. The first stage, Wernicke's encephalopathy, is characterized by ataxia, ophthalmoplegia, and memory deficit. Other symptoms of this stage may include apathy, confusion, and polyneuropathy of the arms and legs. The second phase, Korsakoff syndrome, reflects the residual symptoms of Wernicke's encephalopathy, such as an inability to learn new information (Hartman, 1995).

Alcohol abuse during pregnancy has been associated with spontaneous abortion and with fetal alcohol abuse syndrome (Sokol, Miller, and Martier, 1981). The syndrome is characterized by confirmed maternal consumption of alcohol during pregnancy, characteristic facial features of the child, growth retardation, and abnormalities of the central nervous system (Abel, 1998). Children born to alcohol-abusing mothers may experience neonatal withdrawal symptoms, even in the absence of fetal alcohol abuse syndrome; these symptoms may include jitteriness, increased muscle tone, an increased rate of respiration, exaggerated reflexes, and sleep disturbances. However, the potential effects of the alcohol may vary with the stage of the pregnancy, as well as the amount and frequency of use (Abel, 1998).

Alcohol and Driving

According to statistics of the National Highway Traffic Safety Administration, 17,126 persons were killed in alcohol-related accidents in 1996. This constitutes 40.9 percent of all people killed in traffic accidents that year. If one counts only those deaths in which one or more persons had a blood alcohol content above the legal limit of 0.1 percent at the time of the accident, the figure of alcohol-related deaths is reduced to 13,395, or approximately 32 percent of all fatal crashes (Barr, 1999). In comparison, approximately 15 percent of total road deaths in Great Britain involve accidents in which one or more people have a blood alcohol content (BAC) over the legal limit of .08.

Discussions focusing on the reduction of alcohol-related traffic deaths have generally emphasized a reduction in the allowable BAC to 0.8 and the uniform adoption of a minimum drinking age of 21. However, the adoption of 21 as the minimum age has met with some opposition due, in part, to the existence of "blood borders," which allow individuals under the age of 21 to drive into parts of Canada and Mexico, where the drinking age is 18 (Barr, 1999).

Although the majority of individuals believe that most traffic injuries and fatalities are attributable to drunken driving (Barr, 1999), the National Highway and Traffic Safety Administration has estimated that approximately two-thirds of traffic deaths are associated with aggressive driving and the use of cell phones (Cellar, Nelson, and Yorke, 2000; Irwin, Fitzgerald, and Berg, 2000). However, alcohol-involved pedestrian collisions appear to occur more frequently in areas with greater bar densities, with greater populations, and in which the local population reports drinking greater amounts of alcohol per drinking occasion (LaScala, Johnson, and Greunewald, 2001).

The initiation and publicization of the anti-drunk driving movement has largely been attributed to Mothers Against Drunk Drivers (MADD). The development of this movement, and the role of MADD in the formulation of alcohol-related policy, are discussed in chapter 3.

The Impact of Tobacco

Use, Abuse, and Effects

In 1998, the smoking prevalence among men was 26.4 percent, compared to 22.0 percent among women (United States Surgeon General, 2001). Findings from the National Youth Tobacco Survey in 2000 indicate that tobacco is used by 15.1 percent of middle school students and 34.5 percent of high school students (Anon., 2001b). Approximately 80 percent of tobacco users begin smoking while under the age of 18.

Results of the National Health and Nutrition Examination III from 1989 to 1994 indicate that African-American and non-Hispanic white men have the highest rates (33.3 percent) of regular use of chewing tobacco, followed by rural, higher-income men (14.9 percent). Southern men who began using smokeless tobacco during childhood are least likely to cease their use of the product (Howard-Pitney and Winkleby, 2002).

A study of nicotine use and dependence among 4,414 persons ages 15 to 54 found that 24 percent, or almost half of those who smoked daily for one month or more, were dependent during their lifetimes based on DSM-III-R criteria. The highest risk for dependence occurred during the first 16 years after having initiated smoking (Breslau, Johnson, Hiripi, and Kessler, 2001).

The nicotine contained in tobacco is responsible for the compulsive use of tobacco-containing products (Zevin and Benowitz, 2000). Cigarette smoke itself is composed of volatile and particulate phases. The gaseous phase, which accounts for approximately 95 percent of the weight of cigarette smoke, contains more than 500 gaseous compounds, including carbon monoxide, carbon dioxide, ammonia, and benzene. The particulate phase, which accounts for the remaining 5 percent of the weight of the smoke, consists of 3,500 different compounds, including alkaloid nicotine. The particulate matter minus its alkaloid and water content is known as tar (Zevin and Benowitz, 2000). Increased daily total tar consumption has been linked to an increased risk of myocardial infarction (Sauer et al., 2001).

Nicotine is distilled from burning tobacco. When an individual smokes, he or she inhales small droplets of tar that contain nicotine; these are deposited in the small airways and the alveoli of the lungs. The absorption of nicotine across cell membranes depends on its pH. The pH of most American cigarettes is acidic, so that the nicotine is generally ionized and will not easily cross the membranes. However, the pH of tobacco smoke in pipes and cigars is alkaline, so that the nicotine is not ionized and is easily absorbed from the mouth (Zevin and Benowitz, 2000).

After the nicotine reaches the small airways and alveoli, it is buffered to the physiological pH and is rapidly absorbed. The nicotine then enters the circulation and is distributed to various tissues; it will reach the brain in 10 to 19 seconds. The smoker can manipulate the nicotine intake from each cigarette by varying the puff volume, the number of puffs per cigarette, the intensity of puffing, and the level of inhalation (Herning, Jones, Benowitz, et al., 1983). The absorption of nicotine from gum, chewing tobacco, and snuff occurs slowly through the oral mucosa and results in plasma nicotine levels that are lower than those associated with smoking (McNabb, 1984).

Smoking has been credited with the ability to reduce negative feelings, relieve anxiety, and produce pleasurable effects (Henningfield, 1984). These effects are attributable to the pharmacological effects of nicotine on the brain (Karan and Rosecrans, 2000).

Tobacco use has been linked to excess rate of cardiovascular disease, lung disease, and fatal neoplasms. In the United States, it is the primary cause of illness and premature death (DeLucia, 2001). Cigarette smoking is also the leading risk factor for periodontal disease (Arbes, Agustsdottir, and Slade, 2001).

Secondhand smoke is also associated with adverse health consequences. It has been estimated that, on an annual basis, 3,000 lung cancer deaths and 62,000 deaths from coronary heart disease in adult nonsmokers are attributable to environmental smoke. In addition, secondhand smoke has been shown to be associated with an increased risk in children of asthma (von Maffei et al., 2001), bronchitis, pneumonia, sudden infant death syndrome, low birth weight, and middle ear infections (Anon, 2001a).

Although nicotine is clearly associated with numerous adverse outcomes, research suggests that cigarette smoking is negatively associated with the incidence of Parkinson's disease (Shytle, Baker, Silver, Reid, and Sanberg, 2000). Research with transdermal nicotine seems to suggest that it may also be of use as an adjunct to neuroleptic treatment of Tourette's syndrome, a hyperkinetic movement disorder.

The Impact of Marijuana

Use, Abuse, and Effects

It has been estimated that approximately 32 to 46 percent of the U.S. population over the age of 12 has used marijuana at least once; approximately 5 percent are regular users and an estimated 9 percent have ever developed dependence (Substance Abuse and Mental Health Services Administration, 1998; Anthony, Warner, and Kessler, 1994). Its use is most prevalent among individuals aged 18 to 25 years and, during adolescence, its use is more common among whites than among African-Americans (Kandel, Chem, Warner, Kessler, and Grant, 1992). Recent research has found that higher fines for the possession of marijuana and an increased probability of arrest decrease the likelihood that a young adult will use marijuana (Farrelly, Bray, Zarkin and Wendling, 2001). Research has yielded similar findings with respect to the effect of enforcement of anti-smoking laws on cigarette consumption (Hu, Bai, Keeler, Garnett and Sung, 1994).

Although marijuana usage has been perceived as being the cause of adolescents' problems, research indicates that conduct disorders may exist prior to the commencement of marijuana use (Crowley, McDonald, Whitmore, and Mikulich, 1998). It has been suggested that marijuana acts as a "stepping stone" to the use of other drugs due to its pharmacological effects. However, there is actually no scientific evidence to support this assertion. Rather, marijuana may be used prior to the use of other mood-altering drugs because its effects are milder in comparison with those of other substances. Similarly, marijuana has been labeled a "gateway" to the world of illicit drug use, thereby creating additional otherwise nonexistent opportunities to engage in the use of additional illicit substances (Kandel, Yamaguchi, and Chem, 1992). Research does not support this characterization; marijuana does not appear to be a significant predictor of serious drug use. Rather, the intensity of marijuana use, the co-existence of a psychiatric disorder, and a history of family psychopathology, including alcoholism, are more consistent predictors of serious drug use (Kaplan, Martin, Johnson, and Robbins, 1996; Kandel and Davies, 1992).

Reported effects of marijuana usage include a sense of euphoria, increased talkativeness, periods of lethargy and sleepiness, a sense of enhanced physical and emotional sensitivity, and deficits in short-term memory and learning (Institute of Medicine, 1999). More rarely, users may experience panic, depression, delusions, illusions, or hallucinations (Tart, 1971). Tolerance to most of the effects of marijuana develops relatively quickly, but also disappears relatively quickly. Dependence on marijuana is less likely to occur than dependence on other substances, including alcohol and nicotine, and dependence, when it does occur, appears to be less severe than dependence on other substances (Institute of Medicine, 1999). Although individuals may experience effects of withdrawal, they are relatively minor in comparison with the symptoms associated with withdrawal from alcohol or heroin. For example, marijuana withdrawal is characterized by restlessness, irritability, mild agitation, insomnia, nausea and cramping, while symptoms of alcohol withdrawal include irritability, sleep disturbance, nausea, tachycardia, sweating, seizures, alcohol craving, delirium tremens, tremor, and perceptual distortions (O'Brien, 1996).

The Impact of Cocaine and Crack

Use and Effects

Estimates of the prevalence of cocaine and crack use vary widely, depending upon the context and the source of data. Regional and household surveys have suggested that the prevalence of cocaine use in New York City ranges from 3 to 5 percent (Marzuk, Tardiff, Leon, Stajic, Morgan, and Mann, 1992). An examination of motor fatalities occurring between 1984 and 1987 in New York City indicated that one-fifth of the drivers involved had cocaine in their system at the time of the accident (Marzuk, Tardiff, Leon, Stajic, Morgan, and Mann, 1990). Yet another study that relied exclusively on pregnant women found a prevalence rate of 10 percent (Matera, Warren, Moomjy, Fink, and Fox, 1990).

Cocaine is both short-acting and quick-acting. Injected cocaine reaches the brain quickly, via the bloodstream, and its effects are felt within minutes. The time to the onset of the drug's effect and the peak concentration of its effect are similar when it is inhaled (Jones, 1984). However, the time required to feel cocaine's effects is greater, and the effect is less intense, when the drug is sniffed because it must first pass through the nasal mucosa prior to entering the bloodstream. Similarly, the effect from oral ingestion is both less intense and slower because most of the drug passes through the gastrointestinal tract prior to crossing through cell membranes into the bloodstream. Regardless of the route of administration, the drug's effects are generally felt within 30 to 60 minutes (Morgan and Zimmer, 1997).

Cocaine produces its effect by stimulating both the release of various neurochemical transmitters, especially dopamine, from the nerve cells that produce them and their subsequent binding to receptor sites. Cocaine's stimulant effect is actually an intensification, then, of the body's normal stimulatory mechanism. The effects of the drug, however, are reduced through homeostatic mechanisms that reduce neurotransmitter activity at the receptor sites; this diminution of effect is known as acute tolerance. As a result of acute tolerance, users must employ increasingly larger doses to maintain a stable effect over time. Acute tolerance may develop during even a single period of use.

The intensity of cocaine's impact upon the nervous system depends to a large degree upon the dose administered. At lower doses, cocaine relieves fatigue, increases energy levels, and enhances mental acuity. Even low doses may produce changes in heart rate and blood pressure and, in individuals with pre-existing cardiac or nervous system abnormalities, may prove dangerous (Isner, 1986). Coronary artery or myocardial disease have been found to be common even among chronic cocaine users who are asymptomatic (Roldan, Aliabadi, and Crawford, 2001). Larger doses may produce unwanted affects, such as sleeplessness, agitation, hypervigilance, and paranoia. Large doses have been associated with an increased risk of arrhythmia, coronary artery constriction, seizures, convulsions, and stroke

(Cregler and Mark, 1986). Extremely high doses may produce a psychotic response.

A study of 14,074 births in Greenville County, South Carolina revealed a prevalence of cocaine of 1 percent among the mothers (Weathers, Crane, Sauvain, and Blackhurst, 1993). Prenatal cocaine use has been found to be associated with multiparity, multigravidity, late-onset prenatal care, public assistance, and low academic achievement. Significantly, a nursing professional's opinion regarding a patient's use of cocaine has been found to be a poor predictor of actual use (Rosengreen, Longobucco, Bernstein, Fishman, Cooke, Boctor, and Lewis, 1993). Cocaine use during pregnancy has been linked to fetal hypoxia, intracerebral hemorrhage (Brown, Prager, Lee, and Ramsey, 1992), preterm delivery, premature rupture of the membranes, and longer hospitalizations (Joyce, Racine, McCalla, and Wehbeh, 1995; Neerhof, MacGregor, Retzky, and Sullivan, 1989). These lengthier hospitalizations may account for as much as $500 million in additional health care expenditures (Rizk, Atterbury, and Groome, 1996). Although prematurity may be the major reason for the lengthier hospital stays, adverse social factors have been found to contribute most to inadequate preventive health care and increased stays in the hospital (Forsyth, Leventhal, Qi, Johnson, Schroeder, and Votto, 1998). And, because cocaine use is often correlated with many other potential risk factors, it is difficult to determine whether the use of cocaine poses an independent risk for adverse neonatal outcomes (Frank et al., 1988).

Among adolescents, cocaine use has been found to be associated with being male, living with one or no parent (Wallace, Jr., Forman, Guthrie, Bachman, O'Malley, and Johnston, 1999), being white, having peers who use cocaine, and having ready access to the drug (Yarnold, 1999).

Correlates of cocaine use among adults include employment and recent drug treatment participation. Among women, living with children is negatively related to crack use (Weatherby, McCoy, Metsch, Bletzer, McCoy, and de la Rosa, 1999; Murdoch, 1999). Women are more likely than men to begin, to use, and/or to maintain crack use in the context of intimate opposite sex relationships (Henderson, Boyd, and Mieczkowski, 1994).

Cocaine use has been associated with more unprotected sex, a greater number of sexual partners, and less condom use, thereby increasing the risk of transmission of HIV (Kalichman et al., 1998; Logan, Leukefeld, and Farabee, 1998) and other sexually transmitted diseases (Hibbs and Gunn, 1991). Use of cocaine and crack have also been linked to increased partner violence victimization (Brewer, Fleming, Haggerty, and Catalano, 1998). Those who inject cocaine are more likely to test positive for hepatitis and to report an increased number of emergency department visits to address complications of cocaine use, as compared to users who do not inject (Lexau, Nelson, and Hatsukami, 1998).

The Impact of Hallucinogens

Use, Abuse, and Effects

The term "hallucinogens" encompasses various drugs, such as lysergic acid diethylamide ("acid" or LSD), mescaline, and psilocybin, among others. Researchers have found that many botanical hallucinogens are structurally related to biologically active compounds that occur in the brain. For instance, psilocybine and the psychoactive alkaloids found in morning glory seeds are derivatives of indole-tryptamine and are similar in structure to serotonine. Mescaline is related to noradrenaline, while caffeic acid, derived from chemical found in coffee beans and potatoes, is related structurally to norepinephrine (Furst, 1976). Because of such similarities, it was once thought that LSD, in particular, would offer a potential cure for alcoholism and provide insight into the pathogenesis of schizophrenia (Ulrich and Patten, 1991).

Mescaline, psilocybin, and LSD are administered by swallowing the drug; mescaline can also be smoked. Hallucinogen use results in an altered state of perception and feeling. LSD and mescaline may result in an increase in body temperature, heart rate, and blood pressure; a loss of appetite; sleeplessness; numbness; weakness; and tremors. Psilocybin has been known to produce nervousness and paranoia (National Institute on Drug Abuse, 2000).

Data from the National Household Survey on Drug Abuse for the years 1979 to 1994 indicate that an estimated 5 percent of individuals in the United States have used hallucinogens (Van Etten and Anthony, 1999). Despite this low prevalence rate relative to the use of other substances, hallucinogens, particularly LSD, now represent the drug of choice in many white, middle-class suburbs and their use is now higher than during any other time period since 1975 (Golub and Johnson, 1999).

Hallucinogen use appears to be most common between the ages of 15 and 19, regardless of birth cohort. Use of hallucinogens among adolescents has been associated with being white, having peers who use psychedelics, and involvement in music-related activities (Chilcoat and Schutz, 1996). A survey of 1507 students at several universities in California revealed that 17 percent had used hallucinogenic drugs (Thompson, Anglin, Douglas, Emboden, and Fisher, 1985). Of these, more than 85 percent had use hallucinogenic mushrooms (psilocybin).

The Impact of Heroin

Use, Abuse, and Effects

It has been estimated that 1.3 percent of the U.S. population aged 12 or older, or approximately 2.5 million individuals, have used heroin at some time (National Institute on Drug Abuse, 1992b). Heroin ranks third in drug-caused deaths, after cocaine and alcohol-in-combination (National Institute on Drug Abuse, 1992a).

Unlike alcohol, which is ingested orally, and marijuana, which can be smoked, eaten, or taken in pill form as the prescribed drug Marinol, heroin can be injected as well as smoked or sniffed (Fernandez, 1998). The method by which the drug is administered plays a significant role in its effects; while drugs taken orally may require as much as an hour or more to take effect, the injected drug will act much more quickly since the chemical is delivered directly into the bloodstream (intravenous injection), into a muscle mass (intramuscular injection), or under the upper layers of skin (subcutaneous injection). Injection of the drug is, consequently, more economical because less of the drug is required to achieve the desired effect (Stryker, 1989). For instance, a drug injected into a vein of the arm will reach the brain in 10 to 20 seconds. Many heroin users begin their use by inhaling the drug through smoking or sniffing and only later progress to injection as a result of increased tolerance to the drug (Fernandez, 1998).

Because blood walls are relatively insensitive, irritating substances can be injected. However, the vein may lose its strength and elasticity in the area surrounding the injection site (Ray and Ksir, 1990). If injections are administered into the same area of the vein on a frequent basis, the vein wall may eventually collapse so that blood no longer moves through the vessel. Repeated subcutaneous injections may cause the skin around the injection site to die and shed. The practice of subcutaneous injection is known as "skin popping" (Ray and Ksir, 1990).

The physiological effects of heroin injection occur within 30 to 60 seconds after the drug enters the bloodstream. Following an initial warm rush, the user may experience an instant euphoria accompanied by sleepiness. The pupils of the eyes become constricted, the rate and depth of respiration are decreased, the tone of the anal sphincter is increased, urination becomes difficult, and nausea and vomiting may occur (Milorn, Jr., 1990).

Heroin dependence may occur relatively rapidly, depending upon the purity of the drug, the frequency of its use, and the individual's metabolism. Symptoms of the initial phase of withdrawal from heroin include sleeplessness, muscle aches and spasms, hyperventilation, hypothermia, joint pain, vomiting, and diarrhea. The pain associated with withdrawal is a function of the quantity and frequency of the individual's use (Milorn, Jr., 1990). A secondary withdrawal phase often spans several months.

The use of unsterile needles and injection equipment has been attributed to the limited availability of clean needles due to paraphernalia and prescription laws (Feldman and Biernacki, 1988) and is associated with HIV infection. The probability of infection as the result of each injection with a shared, contaminated needle has been estimated at .0067, based on data from the New Haven, Connecticut legal needle/syringe exchange program (Kaplan and Heimer, 1992a, 1992b). Additionally, the use of unsterile needles and injection equipment may lead to septicemia, hepatitis, bacterial endocarditis, skin abscesses, and tetanus (Fernandez, 1998).

Chapter 3

The Development of Drug Policy

ALCOHOL: USE, ABUSE, AND POLICY

Practice, Perception, and Politics: The Interplay

Alcohol was brought to the English colonies with the very first settlers. Brewing in the colonies similarly occurred early in colonial history. For instance, the first brewery in North America was established in 1612 in New York (Smith, 1998). At the time, alcohol was used as a medicinal remedy for such ailments as headaches and infections (Murdock, 1998) and as a commercial asset in trading with the Indians (Mancall, 1995). Colonial indulgence of alcohol was heavy by current standards, averaging approximately seven shots a day. Alcohol was regarded as an essential part of one's diet in terms of its nutritional and caloric contributions (Heather and Robertson, 2000).

There is some evidence to suggest that numerous circumstances, in addition to dietary needs, contributed to colonists' willingness to drink: rapid population growth, particularly in the cities, which led to feelings of frustration and alienation; the rise of the factory system, which adversely affected skilled craftsmen; economic adversity and, conversely, sudden wealth and prosperity; a decline in the social hierarchy, resulting in perceived threats to professionals' (doctors, clerics, etc.) stature; a developing tradition of celebrating each and every personal and communal event with alcohol; and the use of alcohol as an inducement in trade (Rorabaugh, 1979). Moralists, including Puritan clerics, relied on Biblical passages to warn the colonists of the horrors that would befall them as the result of excessive indulgence: Noah's embarrassment at being found naked and inebriated by his children, and tables covered in vomit after too much wine

(Mancall, 1995). Other clerics, though, celebrated the virtues of alcohol (Heather and Robertson, 2000). Despite the admonitions, however, no serious efforts made to control the use or sale of alcohol until after the Revolution.

Additional evidence suggests that by the 1820s, the custom of men drinking small amounts of liquor communally throughout the day had evolved into a cyclical pattern of communal and/or solo binges, followed by periods of abstinence. It was during this time, in the 1820s, that instances of delirium tremens seemed to have been first noted (Heather and Robertson, 2000). The Temperance Movement of the late 1820s may have been a response to such excesses and to a belief that abstinence provided a form of salvation for women from circumstances thought to be fostered by the use of alcohol, such as poverty, domestic violence, and abandonment (Murdock, 1998). Abstinence may have also signified for some a rejection of working-class norms and the espousal of moral qualities deemed to be consonant with middle-class life: self-control, industriousness, and thrift. In short, a proclamation of abstinence demonstrated both religious adherence and the requisite character to achieve success and status (Gusfield, 1963). As early as 1835, one and one-half million inhabitants of the U.S., of a total of 13 million, had pledged never to indulge in alcohol again (Heather and Robertson, 2000).

During the mid- to late-1800s, an increasing number of states adopted dry laws, which prohibited the commercial manufacture, sale, and public consumption of alcohol. These legal reforms were often in response to the efforts of temperance reformers, many of whom had evolved into prohibitionists (Fahey, 1996). Concurrent with these efforts to reduce and, subsequently, eliminate, the use of alcohol, the American physician Benjamin Rush and the Edinburgh physician Thomas Trotter characterized drunkenness as problematic and the excessive use of alcohol as an addiction (Heather and Robertson, 2000). Addiction was labeled "a disease of the will" that could be cured only by complete abstinence from spirits, so strong was the craving for the substance and so powerless was the individual to reduce its use. Abstinence could be achieved through the infliction of beatings, whippings, threats, and cold showers. In addition, Rush advocated increasingly harsh punishments for intoxication, heavier taxes on alcohol, fewer taverns, and an educational campaign.

The work of Rush and Trotter provided both a framework and a vocabulary for advocates of temperance. Just as Rush and Trotter described the inability of an habitual drunkard to control his disease, so did those in the Temperance Movement portray the unsatisfied craving of alcohol's victim for yet more alcohol. The emphasis on abstinence as the only cure for this dependence foreshadowed the approach that was to be embraced at a later date by Alcoholics Anonymous. For instance, one temperance author wrote in 1833:

> In their sober intervals they reason justly, of their own situation and its danger; they know that for them, there can be no temperate drinking: They resolve to abstain altogether, and thus avoid temptation they are too weak to resist. By degrees they grow confident, and secure in their own strength, and ... they taste a little wine. From that moment the nicely adjusted balance of self control is deranged, the demon returns in power, reason is cast out, and the man is destroyed (Quoted in Heather and Robertson, 2000: 22).

Many temperance advocates subscribed to the then-current scientific theory that alcohol addiction was an inherited trait that would worsen with succeeding generations (Heather and Robertson, 2000; Murdock, 1998). Accordingly, women's use of alcohol, even in moderation, could result in race suicide. The descent of women into the horrors of drunkenness was variously attributed to male selfishness, insensitivity, and cruelty; to physicians' thoughtless prescription of alcohol as a remedy for a wide range of female ailments, such as the pain of menstruation, pregnancy, and childbirth; to sedentary habits, improper diet, and other forms of hygienic neglect; and to the cultural oppression of women. Women suffering from drunkenness were portrayed as physical and mental degenerates, whose only hope for salvation lay in sterilization (Murdock, 1998).

Inebriate homes or asylums, some designated specifically for women, were established in order to provide a setting in which drunkards could receive medical attention and abstinence could be enforced (Heather and Robertson, 2000). The first such asylum was established in 1841 and, by the end of the 19th century, more than 50 others had been opened. However, women were often denied admission to the private facilities and, even among drinkers, remained marginalized. In fact, women's public use of alcohol was associated with sexual depravity, with prostitution, and with intrusion into what was considered to be male space (Murdock, 1998). Other treatments, such as Keeley's cure of "double chloride of gold," were heralded as the ultimate answer to alcohol addiction, despite the lack of scientific evidence to support such claims (Heather and Robertson, 2000).

Gradually, from the 1830s through the beginning of the 20th century, academic psychiatry integrated the concept of inebriety as a disease necessitating treatment (Paredes, 1976). The recognition of alcohol as a disease was not embraced, however, by the Temperance Movement, whose mission of temperance through education had metamorphosized into one of prohibition and regulation of the liquor industry and the saloon (Heather and Robertson, 2000). As a result of this new-found vigor for prohibition, the disease theory of alcoholism remained essentially dormant until the mid-1930s, following the repeal of Prohibition in 1933.

Although some women's groups had initially championed Prohibition as a mechanism for their protection, many later campaigned actively in favor of its repeal. Popular magazines shifted from their moralistic view of alcoholism in the early part of the 20th century to a more "naturalistic" approach in the 1960s (Linsky, 1971). Accordingly, alcoholism, which was once attributed to internal biological and/or psychological causes, was explained by reference to external causes. Public attention to the causes and consequences of alcohol use similarly experienced a shift, moving from an emphasis in the 1950s on alcohol's impact on private life to issues related to drunken driving in the 1960s, with a later focus in the 1970s on the economic impact of drinking (McKenzie and Giesbrecht, 1981). Concurrently, the number of articles related to driving while under the influence of alcohol rose from fewer than 20 in 1980 to greater than 150 in 1983 and 1984 (Hingson, Howland, Morelock, and Heeren, 1988). Alcohol-related articles in 5 national newspapers during the period from 1985 to 1991 increasingly emphasized public health issues, de-emphasized clinical aspects of alcoholism, and have shifted towards an emphasis on external environmental factors to define or explain alcohol-related behavior (Lemmens, Vaeth, and Greenfield, 1999). As an example, cultural norms have been found to be associated with patterns of alcohol consumption (Thaller, Buljan, Breitenfeld, Marusic, Breitenfeld, De-Syo, and Zoricic, 1998; Engs, Hanson, Gliksman, and Smythe, 1990). Greater levels of acculturation among immigrants have been found to be associated with current drinking, while educational level and occupational status have been found to correlate with alcohol-related problems (Li and Rosenblood, 1994; Nawakami, Harataniu, Hemi, and Araki, 1992).

Most recently, public health policy has focused on driving while under the influence of alcohol. This emphasis is not surprising in view of recent research findings indicating an increasing unwillingness on the part of the public to tolerate or escuse alcohol-related misbehaviors and aggression (Paglia and Room, 1998). As indicated previously (see chapter 2), the initiation and publicization of the anti-drunk driving movement has been attributed in large degree to the efforts of MADD, Mothers Against Drunk Driving.

MADD came into being as a nonprofit organization in August 1980, largely through the single-minded efforts of Candy Lightner, who had lost her 13-year old daughter as the result of a car accident caused by a drunk driver. At the time of the accident, the driver was on probation for previous DUI (driving under the influence) convictions and had been released on bail, posted by his wife, for another hit-and-run DUI offense that had occurred several days prior to the accident involving Cari Lightner (Reinarman, 1988). The organization was funded with the proceeds from Cari's insurance settlement, Candy Lightner's own savings, and various small grants from the American Council on Alcohol Problems, the National Highway Traffic Safety Administration, and the Levy Foundation (Reinarman, 1988).

From its inception, MADD portrayed itself as the voice of the victim. Weed has identified three categories of victim status reflective of MADD membership, with each type of victimhood giving rise to a different status: the individually harmed victim who survived an accident caused by a drunken driver; the bereaved victim, who has lost a loved one as the result of a drunk driving incident; and the general community activist, who often views the drunken driver as an individual whose lack of responsibility poses a danger to the entire community (Weed, 1990). One self-identified harmed victim explained:

> I am not on crutches. I am not in a wheelchair. I do not have brain damage.
> I see, hear, feel and think as well as ever. In fact, I have no remaining visible
> injuries. But I do bear the scars inside as the victim of a drunk driving crash.
>   Because I am President of MADD, most people assume that one of my
> children was killed in a drunk driving crash. I can never pretend to know
> the pain of having a child killed. But I do know the pain of being an injured
> victim (Sadoff, 1989: 4).

The moral authority of the bereaved victim is heightened if the deceased was "an innocent victim:" weak, in the process of doing something respectable, blameless, with no connection to the "bad" offender (Christie, 1986).

MADD's almost unprecedented success has been attributed to its legislative and media advocacy efforts, rather than to the actual incidence or prevalence of alcohol-related injuries or deaths (Reinarman, 1988). As an example, MADD designed a "Rating the States" (RTS) Program to publicize the efforts of each of the states to combat alcohol-impaired driving. As part of this 1993 program, MADD rated each state in the following areas: gubernatorial leadership, statistics and records, enforcement, administrative and criminal sanctions, regulatory control and availability, legislative efforts, prevention and public awareness efforts, youth issues, self-sufficiency programs, innovative programs, and victim issues. Each state was assigned a grade, ranging from F (the lowest) to A (the highest). Publication of the report often led to renewed efforts by the states to address alcohol-impaired driving (Russell, Voas, DeJong, and Chaloupka, 1995). Several factors have been identified that were critical to the success of this program: (1) the high degree of credibility already associated with MADD as an organization;

(2) the high degree of interest that the public generally has in knowing how their own state compares with others; (3) the use of a rating system from A to F that is familiar to almost everyone; (4) a focus on specific political leaders, resulting in political controversy and increased attention and action; and (5) reliance on outside consultants with expertise in marketing and extensive media contacts (Reinarman, 1988).

MADD'S orientation, with its emphasis on individual responsibility and refusal to address systemic aspects of drunken driving, was in harmony with the policies and rhetoric of the agenda of both Reagan and the New Right. Consequently, the timing of the movement contributed to its success (Marshall and Oleson, 1994; Reinarman, 1988). MADD used its political credibility to achieve major successes: the elimination of plea bargaining for drunken driving offenses, the institution of mandatory jail sentences, the reclassification of alcohol related injuries and death accidents to felonies, the development and implementation of "dram shop" (server) liability laws, the institution of random sobriety checkpoints, and the adoption of mandatory treatment laws and of 21 as the minimum drinking age (Reinarman, 1988). Research findings indicate that regulations related to alcohol accessibility, the licensure of alcohol outlets, the disciplinary procedures of alcohol outlets, and the enforcement of blood alcohol concentration laws are associated with lower rates of traffic fatalities (Cohen, Mason, and Scribner, 2001).

The Economics of Alcohol Use, Abuse, and Dependence

Our approach to the use of alcohol, particularly in light of its potential adverse effects, may be difficult to understand absent at least a brief examination of the economic aspects of alcohol use, dependence, and our current state of regulation.

Four phases of government regulatory response to alcohol that coincide with distinct historical periods and social influences have been identified. Colonial times to the 1850s was characterized by a focus on the availability of a safe form of alcohol and the imposition of excise taxes. The period of Prohibition, from the 1859s through 1933, reflected increasing government involvement, while from 1933 to 1985, there was increased social tolerance of alcohol use, together with the adoption of age and site restrictions. Currently, there is an emphasis on drunk driving, with the corresponding passage of anti-drunk driving laws (McGowan, 1997).

Additionally, since Prohibition, the federal government has essentially yielded regulation of the alcohol industry to the state and local governments, which currently maintain, in general, a three-pronged approach that includes: (1) the supervision of the sale and distribution of alcoholic products, (2) the determination of what constitutes the "reasonable" use of alcoholic beverages, and (3) the accumulation of revenue. The attainment of these goals has generally been effectuated through reliance on one or more of three strategies: (1) the imposition of restriction on sites for the sale of alcohol and on the age at which alcohol may be consumed; (2) the establishment of a definition of "drunk driving" and of penalties for driving while intoxicated; and (3) the imposition of excise taxes on the sale of alcoholic products.

The revenue raised through the sale of alcoholic beverages is far from inconsequential. In 1995 alone, a total of $95,335,000 was spent on alcoholic beverages in the United States; this constitutes approximately 2.8 percent of all disposable income in the U.S. during that year. Almost one-third of this amount, constituting 1 percent of the nation's 1995 disposable income, was for distilled spirits. Only soft drinks and beer grossed higher revenues from larger sales that year. Accordingly, excise tax revenues have risen consistently from approximately $7.7 billion in 1970 for the beer, wine, and distilled spirits industries combined, to approximately $16 billion in 1995 (McGowan, 1997).

Industry response to government concerns has varied by industry segment. The wine industry has portrayed its product as "the alcoholic beverage of moderation," in sharp contrast to the "party" image of beer (Cohen, Mason, and Scribner, 2001). Accordingly, unlike the beer and distilled spirit industries, the wine industry has been able to avoid the drunk driving issue and, instead, has focused on the numerous medical reports that have documented the beneficial health effects of wine consumption in moderation (McGowan, 1997). In contrast, the beer industry has aligned itself with advocates for stricter anti-drunk driving laws, in an effort to avoid potential increases in excise sales tax (McGowan, 1997).

The cost of alcohol abuse, however, is far from inconsequential. It has been estimated that in 1980, the cost of alcohol abuse in the United States was $152.51 billion (Harwood, Napolitano, Kristiansen, and Collins, 1984). Morbidity and premature mortality resulted in reduced productivity estimated at $121.93 billion. More recent estimates place the total cost of alcohol abuse in the U.S. at $91.71 billion, with estimated productivity losses resulting from alcohol-related morbidity and mortality at $71.10 billion (Rice, Sander, Kelman, Miller, and Dunmeyer, 1991).

TOBACCO: USE, ABUSE, AND POLICY

The Beginnings

Records of tobacco use date back at least several centuries. Tobacco was used in various forms by shamans in South America at least as early as the 17th century, according to records of various missionaries and chroniclers of events (Wilbert, 1987). Columbus and other explorers noted the use of this substance following their arrival in the New World. One commentator of the time described the practice of smoking:

> the Indians have one [habit] that is especially harmful, the inhaling of a certain kind of smoke which they call tobacco, in order to produce a state of stupor. . . . The caciques employed a tube, shaped like a Y, inserting the forked extremities in their nostrils and the tube itself in the lighted weed; in this way they would inhale the smoke until they became unconscious and lay sprawling on the earth like men in a drunken slumber. Those who could not procure the right sort of wood took their smoke through a hollow reed (cañuela); it is this the Indians call *tobacco*, and not the weed nor its effects, as some have supposed. They prize this herb very highly, and plant it in their orchards or on their farms for the purpose mentioned above.
>   I cannot imagine what pleasure they derive from this practice (Oviedo, *Historia general y natural de las Indias* [General and Natural History of the Indias], quoted in Corti, 1931).

Despite the apparent rejection of smoking, tobacco use soon flourished in the Old World. Spanish sailors recounted the glories of the practice. Tobacco was frequently used in the Old World as a remedy for numerous ailments, including coughs, asthma, headache, stomach cramps, and gout. By the end of the 16th century, smoking had become widespread among all economic classes in Europe (Corti, 1931).

Tobacco soon flourished as a crop in the colonies of Maryland, Virginia, and South Carolina (Prince, Jr., 2000). In South Carolina, for instance, exports of tobacco leaf had risen to half a million pounds per year by 1773. Following the War for Independence, tobacco exports increased even further.

Three centuries later, by the 1940s, "cigarette smoking rivaled baseball as America's national pastime," (Kagan and Nelson, 2001: 11), encouraged in part by the appearance of glamorous movie stars dangling their exotic-appearing cigarettes on screen. In addition, the tobacco industry consistently engaged in aggressive marketing campaigns to promote their product. Strategies included claims of health benefits attributable to smoking (1933: "Give your throat a Kool vacation! Like a week by the sea, this mild menthol is a tonic to hot, tired throats"); appeals to youth through the use of cartoon characters, such as Joe Camel; and an emphasis on the alleged (and nonexistent) benefits of smoking cigarette with a lighter tar content (1954: "L&M Filters are Just What the Doctor Ordered!" [Philip Morris] (Institute of Medicine, 2001a: 62–65; Slade, 2001). By 1965, over one-half of the adult men in the United States were smokers (Kagan and Nelson, 2001).

Regulatory Efforts

Tobacco was originally listed as a drug in the 1890 edition of the United States Pharmacopoeia, but was subsequently removed from the 1905 edition and has not been included in the official listing of drugs since that time. Consequently, tobacco was not among the drugs that the Food and Drug Administration (FDA) was to regulate at the time that the Food and Drug Act of 1906 was passed (Neuberger, 1963). In general, the FDA did not attempt to regulate tobacco prior to the 1980s. In fact, the FDA specifically stated that it would attempt to regulate cigarettes as drugs only if they were promoted as having beneficial effects on the body (Public Health Cigarette Amendments of 1971, 1972). This had occurred previously in the 1950s, in response to the claims of several cigarette manufacturers that cigarettes could be used to reduce body weight and reduce the frequency of respiratory disease (*United States v. 354 Bulk Cartons*, 1959; *United States v. 46 Cartons*, 1953). The Federal Trade Commission (FTC), which had been regulating cigarette advertising since the 1930s, issued guidelines in 1955 that prohibited false claims in cigarette advertising (*In re Philip Morris and Co.*, 1955).

The British researcher Sir Richard Doll published a study in 1952 that reported a link between smoking and cancer (Doll and Hill, 1952). The tobacco industry responded to the public concern generated by this report by introducing filtered cigarettes and by lowering the tar content (Federal Register, 1995). However, even though the tar levels dropped, the nicotine levels consistently increased.

Efforts to control tobacco can be traced back to the first report of the Surgeon General, issued in 1964. Although the tobacco industry had known for years of the dangers and the addictive nature of smoking, the information had not been made known to the public; this report represented the first major public disclosure of such risks.

In 1964, following this publication of the Surgeon General's Report on Smoking and Health, the FTC began proceedings to require that cigarette manufacturers place warning labels on all cigarette packages and in all cigarette advertisements, to advise potential consumers that smoking could affect their health. The FTC claimed that the failure to warn consumers of the smoking-related dangers constituted "an unfair and deceptive trade practice" within the meaning of the Federal Trade Commission Act. Packages were to state: "Cigarette smoking is dangerous to health and may cause death from cancer and other diseases" (29 Federal Register 8325, 1964). Later, in 1969, the Federal Communications Commission (FCC) issued a notice of proposed rulemaking that would have prohibited cigarette advertising on radio and television (34 Fed. Reg. 1959, 1969). Both of these attempts to regulate smoking advertisements were ultimately impeded and obstructed by Congress (see Kelder and Daynard, 1997). Subsequent efforts to further regulate the advertisement and sale of tobacco under the Consumer Product Safety Act similarly failed (Kelder and Daynard, 1997).

The FDA rejected an attempt by the anti-smoking group Action on Smoking and Health in the late 1970s to have the FDA regulate tobacco as a drug. The FDA concluded at that time that there was insufficient evidence to indicate that cigarettes were intended to affect the structure or the function of the body (*Action on Smoking and Health v. Harris*, 1980).

The American Heart Association later petitioned the FDA in 1988 to regulate low tar cigarettes as drugs; the FDA concurred with this position in 1996 (Food and Drug Administration, 1996). In making this determination, the FDA relied on the findings of numerous epidemiological studies that suggested that smoking was responsible for hundreds of thousands of premature deaths each year, as well as a multitude of adverse physical effects. By the time that the FDA rendered this decision, the American Psychiatric Association, the American Psychological Association, and the United States Surgeon General, among others, had concluded that nicotine is an addictive substance. The FDA further noted that tobacco companies had seemed to be aware of the adverse effects of tobacco for some time and, in fact, had intended that nicotine have the stimulating and sedating effects that were associated with tobacco use (FDA, 1996). For instance, as early as 1963, the General Counsel of Brown and Williamson Tobacco Company had written in an internal document that remained undiscovered publicly until a much later date: "We are, then, in the business of selling nicotine, an addictive drug . . . (Federal Register, 1995: 41,611).

In addition to finding that tobacco is a drug, the FDA concluded that tobacco was also subject to FDA regulation as a drug delivery device because "the primary purpose of parts of the cigarette . . . is to effectuate the delivery of a carefully controlled amount of the nicotine to a site in the human body where it can be absorbed" (Food and Drug Administration, 1995a). The controlling statute defines a device as

> an instrument, apparatus, implement, machine, contrivance, implant, in vitro reagent, or other similar or related article, including any component, part, or accessory, which is- . . .
> (3) intended to affect the structure or any function of the body of man or other animals, and which does not achieve its primary intended purposes through chemical action within or on the body of man or other animals and which is not dependent upon being metabolized for the achievement of its primary intended purposes (21 U.S.C. §321(h), 1994).

This position was not unreasonable, in view of tobacco manufacturers' efforts to manipulate the nicotine levels in the cigarettes. The FDA found, for instance, in its examination of patents filed by various tobacco companies, that the level of nicotine was increased by adding nicotine to the cigarettes' filters and wrappers (Kessler, 1995). Manufacturers increased the nicotine levels in cigarettes with low tar because consumers were known to smoke fewer of these cigarettes. Certain tobacco plants were bred specifically to increase the nicotine levels. The R.J. Reynolds executive Claude E. Teague, Jr. had even written:

> In a sense, the tobacco industry may be thought of as being a specialized, highly ritualized, and stylized segment of the pharmaceutical industry. Tobacco products contain and deliver nicotine, a potent drug with a variety of physiological effects (Federal Register, 1995: 41,617–41,618).

Despite these findings, the FDA decided not to ban the use of tobacco, believing that such a ban would be circumvented through smuggling and black market sales. Additionally, adverse health consequences could befall the individuals who were already addicted to the use of nicotine. Accordingly, it adopted a strategy to prevent the initiation of smoking behavior in children and adolescents by restricting the sale of tobacco products to individuals under the age of 18, requiring that vendors verify purchasers' age with identification, prohibiting the distribution of free samples and the sale of cigarettes through vending machines, and implementing restrictions on the advertising and promotion of cigarettes (21 C.F.R. §§897.14, 897.30, 897.32, 897.34, 1996).

Whether smoking regulations should be implemented at all has stimulated significant ethical debate. There is general consensus with the premise that the government has the power to regulate smoking in order to protect the health of the public; what remains unsettled is the scope and implementation of that power (Jacobson and Wasserman, 1997) and how to balance that power with individuals' right to "make life-style choices" (Leichter, 1991: 3). The regulation of the use of tobacco has been justified based upon the harm it causes to others, such as from secondhand smoke; the harm that it may do to smokers who are uninformed of the health-associated risks; the need to protect children; and the need to protect those who are coerced, that is, those who are addicted to nicotine (Pope, 2000). Such regulations are analogous to laws that mandate the use of helmets for motorcycle riders and seat belts for drivers and passengers of automobiles. Nevertheless, the tobacco industry has mocked the need for regulations, maintaining that the regulation of smoking behavior is just the beginning of a slide down the slippery slope, eventually leading to the regulation of alcohol use, butter, and bungee jumping, using exactly the same rationale

(Ezra, 1993). An advertisement in Philip Morris Magazine quipped:

> Smoking is a civil right,
> Those who don't should join the fight.
> For if one right does disappear,
> The loss of others may be near....
> Too many calories can cause you to die,
> So let's have a ban on apple pie.
> Once a government restricts a right,
> The end will never be near in sight.
> There's a lesson here...this is no joke,
> I once had a right to smoke! (Mroz, 1987: 29).

Despite these activities, federal regulatory agencies have been characterized as "weakly involved" in the formulation of tobacco policy in the United States (Kagan and Nelson, 2001: 30). Instead, tobacco policy in recent years has been shaped by the interplay of numerous groups with conflicting agendas and interests. These groups include environmentalists, antitobacco activists, health researchers, governmental public health officials, nonprofit organizations such as the American Cancer Society and, of course, the tobacco industry and its allies, particularly those in Congress.

As an example, numerous state and local jurisdictions have enhanced their efforts to control cigarette sales and smoking. Voters in various jurisdictions, including California, Massachusetts, and Michigan, approved an increase in cigarette taxes. In 1998, California became the first state in the country to ban smoking in all bars (Kagan and Nelson, 2001).

In addition, numerous states filed lawsuits against the tobacco industry to recover the costs of Medicaid payments for the treatment of smoking-related illness of their citizens. By June 1, 1998, the tobacco industry was facing 897 legal actions, which included numerous state cases, 55 class actions lawsuits, 62 lawsuits brought by union health plans, 613 individual claims, and various other actions (Mather, 1998). Ultimately the majority of the states reached a settlement with the industry that year. And, although the tobacco industry had almost always prevailed in lawsuits against it by smokers seeking damages for injuries alleged to have resulted from cigarettes, by the year 2000, the tobacco industry was facing large jury verdicts against it in several states (Kagan and Nelson, 2001).

MARIJUANA: USE, ABUSE, AND POLICY

Practice, Perceptions, and Politics

Marijuana has been used as a medicinal drug in various cultures for thousands of years for the treatment of a variety of ailments, including cramps, lack of appetite, and rheumatism (Bloomquist, 1971). Its active ingredient, delta-9-tetrahydrocannibol (THC) has been isolated for use in Marinol, which has been available to AIDS and cancer patients to combat nausea and to glaucoma patients to help reduce intraocular pressure (Timpone, Wright, Li, Egorin, Enama, Mayers, Galetto, and DATRI 004 Study Group, 1997; Jones, Benowitz, and Herning, 1981). Marijuana use does not appear to lead to dependence in most individuals (Perkonigg, Lieb, Hofler, Schuster, Sonntag, and Wittchen, 1999). Additionally, as compared with Marinol, smoked marijuana or marijuana ingested with food is cheaper, acts more quickly and is easier to regulate or adjust in terms of the dosage (Bergstrom, 1997; Satel, 1997).

United States physicians first recognized the potential therapeutic value of marijuana as early as 1840 (Grinspoon and Bakalar, 1997; Grinspoon and Bakalar, 1995). It was identified in the 1851 edition of the *United States Dispensatory* as a remedy for numerous disorders, including neuralgia, gout, rheumatism, tetanus, hydrophobia, epidemic cholera, convulsions, chorea, hysteria, mental depression, delirium tremens, insanity, and uterine hemorrhage. Until 1942, it was included in the United States Pharmacopoeia as a remedy for poor appetite (Grinspoon and Bakalar, 1997; Grinspoon and Bakalar, 1995).

The eventual adoption of provisions prohibiting and criminalizing marijuana must be understood in the context of the social and political climate prevailing at the time of their inception. Opiates, and especially morphine, were widely used during the Civil War period to alleviate the suffering that accompanied battle-related injuries. The indiscriminate use of these drugs, even for relatively common gastrointestinal complaints, may have led to addiction in many Civil War veterans, resulting in what came to be called "morphinomania" (Bonnie and Whitebread II, 1999).

This situation was aggravated by the lack of restrictions placed on druggists who refilled morphine-containing prescriptions. It is believed that the numbers of individuals addicted to opiates was further increased through the indiscriminate sale of medicinal remedies to consumers who were often unaware of their opiate content, resulting in an increasing number of addicts among whites, women, and members of the middle class. Concurrently, the use of alcohol and tobacco became increasingly widespread and accepted.

The Initiation of Drug Regulations

The first drug regulations were effectuated by the states and essentially represented a reaction to the individuals perceived to be the primary users of the drugs, rather than the effects of the drugs themselves. Opium use among the Chinese became the focus of state legislation in the late

1800s in Nevada, the Dakotas, California, Montana, Wyoming, Arizona, New Mexico, and Washington. Cocaine use among African Americans in the South was identified as the source of criminal conduct. Ultimately, morphine and cocaine came to be associated with the immoral underworld of pimps, gamblers, and prostitutes. States responded with the enactment of legislation designed to restrict pharmacies' ability to dispense morphine-containing drugs. Federal legislation was adopted in 1909 to prohibit the importation of opium other than at designated ports and for any use that was not medicinal in nature.

The use of marijuana, though, was unregulated by either the federal government or by any state government until the early 1900s, when the state of California first prohibited its possession or sale and various other states adopted restrictions on the dispensing of cannabis without a prescription or on the refilling of prescriptions containing the substance (Bonnie and Whitebread II, 1999). The American Medical Association opposed a federal prohibition against the use of marijuana, which was vigorously supported by members of law enforcement, who argued that the use of the drug would result in higher levels of crime due to its courage-enhancing properties. For instance, a district attorney in New Orleans alleged in 1931 that

> the underworld [had realized] the value of [marijuana] in subjugating the will of human derelicts to that of a master mind. Its use sweeps away all restraint, and its influence may be attributed to many of our present-day crimes. It has been the experience of the Police and Prosecuting Officials in the South that immediately before the commission of many crimes the use of marihuana cigarettes had been indulged in by criminals so as to relieve themselves from the natural restraint which might deter them from the commission of criminal acts, and to give them the false courage necessary to commit the contemplated crime.

This same district attorney further urged that federal aid be provided to the states to aid them in their "effort to suppress a traffic as deadly and as destructive to society . . ." (Stanley, 1931: 257). Similar, but more cautious, assumptions about the effects of the drug are reflected in a report of the same era by the then Surgeon General of the United States:

> While the effects of the drug are definitely narcotic in nature, it is habitually taken for the stimulating effects obtained and the individual satisfaction experienced through the temporary inflation of the personality. No evidence exists that the drug is accumulative in its effect or that a tolerance may be developed through its continued use. . . . The sudden discontinuance of its use . . . does not give rise to any "withdrawal" symptoms . . . (Cummings, 1929, quoted in Bonnie and Whitebread II, 1999: 129).

The initial restrictions on the use of marijuana, even for medicinal purposes, stemmed from its classification as a narcotic. That classification rested, in turn, on the association of the drug with "ethnic minorities" and those who were "immoral." This association between the foreign-born and the use and evils of marihuana reflected an already-existing American preoccupation with lawlessness among foreigners (Bonnie and Whitebread II, 1999). The association of marijuana with Mexicans and with crime, in an era of fervent xenophobia, provided ample incentive for the promulgation of restrictive legislation. Eventually, however, law enforcement personnel urged the adoption of restrictions due to the effects of the drug itself, not merely the characteristics of those who were perceived to be users. Marijuana was to become labeled "the most dangerous of all drugs," with the ability to "excite a state of frenzy leading to actions of uncontrollable violence or even murder (Hayes and Bowery, cited in Bonnie and Whitebread II, 1999).

Prohibitions against the use of marijuana were eventually implemented by the federal government through the enactment of the Marijuana Tax Act of 1937, which attempted to reduce the use of marijuana through the imposition of a tax. The passage of the Act reflected the triumph of those who had campaigned for regulation on the basis of an alleged association between marijuana use, alienage, crime, and moral depravity, over those who presented a more reasoned and studied response. For instance, a 1931 medical journal stated:

> The debasing and baneful influence of hashish and opium is not restricted to individuals but has manifested itself in nations and races as well. The dominant race and most enlightened countries are alcoholic, whilst the races and nations addicted to hemp and opium, some of which once attained to heights of culture and civilization have deteriorated both mentally and physically (Fossier, 1931, quoted in Bonnie and Whitebread II, 1999: 152).

In contrast, a report of the League of Nations Advisory Committee stated:

> Cannabis indica does not produce a dependence such as in opium addiction. In opium addiction there is a complete dependence and when it is withdrawn there is actual physical pain which is not the case with cannabis. Alcohol more nearly produces the same effect as cannabis in that there is an excitement or general feeling of lifting of personality, followed by a delirious stage, and a subsequent narcosis. There is no dependence or increased tolerance such as in opium addiction. As to the social or moral degradation associated with cannabis it probably belongs in the same category as alcohol. As with alcohol, it may be taken a relatively long time without social or emotional breakdown. Marihuana is habit-forming, although not addicting, in the same sense as alcohol might be with some people, or sugar or coffee. Marihuana produces

a delirium with a frenzy which might result in violence; but this is also true of alcohol (League of Nations, June 1937, quoted in Bonnie and Whitebread II, 1999: 152).

Following the passage of the Tax Act, the Federal Bureau of Narcotics sought to reduce the level of marijuana-associated sensationalism in the press and to control the cultivation of marijuana for legitimate purposes. This shift in position would render it more difficult for defense attorneys who, prior to the Act's passage, had been able to rely on the government's science-clothed rhetoric to support the insanity defenses offered by their criminal clients (Bonnie and Whitebread II, 1999). Additionally, judges were to be educated to the dangers of marijuana use and the need to impose long-term sentences on would-be violators. The Boggs Act of 1951 sought to discourage further the use of marijuana through the establishment of mandatory prison sentences and monetary fines. These consequences were rendered even more severe with the passage of the 1956 Narcotics Control Act. The subsequent 1970 Controlled Substances Act (CSA) effectively prohibited even the medicinal use of marijuana.

The National Organization for the Reform of Marijuana Laws sought in 1972 to have marijuana reclassified as a Schedule II drug, which would permit its use by prescription (Grinspoon and Bakalar, 1995). Public hearings on the issue were commenced in 1986 by the Drug Enforcement Agency (DEA), which had been previously known as the Bureau of Narcotics and Dangerous Drugs. The DEA's administrative law judge, after hearing extensive testimony from patients and physicians, found in 1988 that the natural form of marijuana was generally therapeutically safe and ordered that the drug be reclassified as a Schedule II substance. However, this decision was overridden by the DEA in 1992 (Grinspoon and Bakalar, 1995). The DEA Administrator relied on the following criteria in rendering his decision: (1) a drug's chemistry must be known and reproducible; (2) there must be adequate safety studies; (3) there must be adequate and well-controlled studies proving efficacy; (4) the drug must be accepted by qualified experts; and (5) the scientific evidence that the drug has a currently accepted medical use must be widely available (Grinspoon and Bakalar, 1997).

The decision of the DEA was appealed by the Alliance for Cannabis Therapeutics (ACT). ACT argued that marijuana was beneficial in alleviating various side effects of chemotherapy for cancer patients, muscle spasticity in multiple sclerosis patients, and the effects of glaucoma. The court upheld the DEA standards and found that the medicinal use of marijuana failed to comply with these standards. First, there was a dearth of safety studies in humans. Second, well-controlled evaluations of the therapeutic value of marijuana were lacking. Third, the drug's chemistry was unlikely to be known and reproducible due to variations in the plant composition as a function of differences by geographic region in the soil, the light, the water, and harvesting and storage conditions (Margolis, 1994).

Changing Times

A number of states have recently adopted legislation that has decriminalized the use of marijuana (Institute of Medicine, 1999). And, despite the ongoing existence of federal prohibitions against the use of marijuana in any form other than the prescribed pill Marinol, several states have enacted legislation permitting the use of smoked marijuana in the context of medical treatment (Institute of Medicine, 1999). In other states, courts have refused to sanction physicians who recommend the medical use of marijuana to their patients (*Conant v. McCaffrey*, 2000). For instance, California voters passed on November 5, 1996 the Compassionate Use Act of 1996, also known as Proposition 215 (California Health and Safety Code, 2000). The statute permits patients suffering from serious illnesses to possess small quantities of marijuana for their medical use, provides that the primary caregivers of these patients will not be subject to sanctions or criminal prosecution for recommending the use of marijuana, and further protects physicians in California from punishment or loss of rights or privileges for recommending marijuana to a patient for medical use. It is critical to note that the law does not permit physicians to prescribe marijuana to their patients, but permits only a discussion with the patient of the possible benefits and risks, including arrest, of using marijuana for medical purposes. The Clinton administration responded with a threat to prosecute any physician who recommended the use of marijuana, as well as any patients who were found to be using marijuana medicinally (Savage and Warren, 1996). The U.S. Supreme Court ultimately concluded that federal law that regulates controlled substances may not be nullified by legislative actions of states (*United States v. Oakland Cannabis Buyers' Coop*, 2001).

HIV/AIDS and Marijuana. Much of the impetus for the legalization of marijuana in the medical context has come from the suffering of individuals with HIV infection and AIDS disease. The human immunodeficiency virus, or HIV, is believed to be the causative agent of the disease known as acquired immune deficiency syndrome, or AIDS. The first clinical cases of AIDS were recognized in the United States in 1981, when physicians began to see young gay men infected with *Pneumocystis carinii* pneumonia (PCP) and Kaposi's sarcoma (KS), both of which were highly unusual in young men. These individuals, as well as later-identified hemophiliacs and injecting drug users, shared a critical symptom: immunodeficiency. It was not until 1983, however, that the virus was itself identified. And, although the syndrome AIDS was not recognized as such until the early 1980s, it appears that the disease was present in individuals as early as the 1950s.

The definition of the syndrome that has come to be known as AIDS has been revised several times since the initial recognition of the disease, in order to accommodate increasing knowledge regarding the effects of the virus. For instance, the initial definition of AIDS did not include HIV wasting and HIV encephalopathy, which were added to the definition of AIDS in 1987; invasive cervical cancer was not included as an AIDS-defining disease until the 1993 revision.

Initially, the vast majority of identified AIDS cases were attributed to men who had had unprotected sexual intercourse with men, individuals who had shared injection equipment with others, and hemophiliacs and others who had received contaminated blood or blood products. Most recently, an increasing proportion of AIDS cases are occurring among women, among heterosexuals, and among members of communities of color. The greatest proportionate increases since the beginning of the epidemic have occurred in the south and in the Midwest. By 1993, AIDS had become the eighth leading cause of death overall and the leading cause of death among persons aged 25 to 44 (Osmond, 1999b).

A survey of 100 members of the San Francisco Cannabis Cultivator Club, each of whom used marijuana at least once a week, found that 60 of the 100 used the marijuana for the relief of symptoms associated with HIV and the medications used to treat HIV; these symptoms included wasting, nausea, weight loss, chronic diarrhea, alterations in taste perceptions, and painful oral ulcers. Wasting involves a weight loss of at least 10 percent or more in the presence of diarrhea or chronic weakness, together with documented fever for at least 30 days that is not attributable to a concurrent condition other than infection with HIV (Mulligan and Schambelan, 1999). Prior to the development and adoption of antiretrovirals, the prevalence of wasting was estimated to be as high as 37%. Weight loss also results from nausea from the medication regimen, from candidiasis and other oral manifestations of AIDS that may make eating physically painful, from chronic diarrhea resulting from the illness, from social isolation, and from altered taste perception. Numerous drugs have been utilized in an attempt to stimulate individuals' appetites and/or to reduce the nausea including growth hormone, anabolic steroids, thalidomide, fish oil, and Marinol (Koch, Kim, and Scott, 1999). Similar use was reported among the members of the Los Angeles buyers club (Institute of Medicine, 1999). Some, but not all, of the individuals using marijuana for the relief of symptoms had previously used the drug recreationally.

The use of marijuana to alleviate both the symptoms of AIDS and the side effects of their medications was also reported to the Institute of Medicine during testimony related to the medical use of marijuana. One man recounted his many symptoms, which included skin rashes, a metallic aftertaste, dizziness, anemia, headaches, spiking fevers, depression, and neuropathy, as well as uncontrollable nausea, vomiting, and diarrhea. In discussing marijuana, this gentleman stated:

> The pot calmed my stomach against a handful of pills. The pot made me hungry so I could eat without a tube. The pot eased the pain of crippling neural side effects so I could dial the phone by myself. The pot calmed my soul and allowed me to accept that I would probably die soon. Because I smoked pot I have lived long enough to see the development of the first truly effective HIV therapies. I lived to gain 50 lb., regain my vigor, and celebrate my 35th birthday (Testimony of G.S., Institute of Medicine, 1999: 27).

Use of Marijuana for Other Disorders. In a study of San Francisco Cannabis Cultivator Club members, it was found that approximately 40 percent of the medicinal marijuana users relied on smoked marijuana to alleviate symptoms of disorders other than HIV/AIDS, including musculoskeletal disorders and arthritis, depression, neurological disorders, gastrointestinal disorders, glaucoma, cancer, and skin manifestations of Reiter's syndrome (Institute of Medicine, 1999). Members of the Los Angeles Cannabis Resource Center reported usage of medicinal marijuana for these and additional disorders, including epilepsy, Tourette syndrome, and multiple sclerosis.

Speakers at public workshops conducted by the Institute of Medicine also reported the use of marijuana to treat anorexia, nausea, and vomiting associated with cancer, migraines, Wilson's disease, and multiple sclerosis; to treat mood disorders such as depression, anxiety, bipolar disorder, and posttraumatic stress disorder; for the management of pain associated with migraine, injury, postpolio syndrome, degenerative disk disease, rheumatoid arthritis, nail-patella syndrome, the effects of Gulf War chemical exposure, multiple congenital cartilaginous exostosis; to reduce muscle spasticity associated with multiple sclerosis, paralysis, spinal cord injuries, and spasmodic torticollis; to relieve intraocular pressure associated with glaucoma; and to relieve diarrhea associated with Crohn's disease (Institute of Medicine, 1999). Other research has indicated that marijuana is used by individuals to alleviate chronic pain, depression, and menstrual cramps (Osborne, Smart, Weber, and Birchmore-Timney, 2000).

The Politics of Marijuana as Medicine. Following an exhaustive review of scientific research and testimony at its own hearings, the Institute of

Medicine recommended in 1999 that research be conducted relating to the physiological effects of marijuana, the risks of smoking marijuana, and the effectiveness of marijuana in the reduction or alleviation of various disease symptoms (Institute of Medicine, 1999). Although this report had been commissioned by the federal Office of Drug Control Policy (Hamilton, 1999), then-"Drug Czar" Barry McCaffrey flatly refuted the possibility that marijuana could have any legitimate medicinal use (Rivera Live, 1999). Even more recently, lawmakers have rejected the potential usefulness of marijuana, characterizing it as significantly dissimilar to alcohol because of its inherent "mind-altering" properties. For instance, Congressman Bob Barr has asserted that the "difference between mind-altering drugs [such as marijuana] and alcohol is any use of mind-altering drugs alters your mind and poses the danger that is the essence of society's need to protect itself and to protect its citizens" (Barr, Sterling, and Williams, 2001).

The Economics of Marijuana Use, Abuse, and Dependence

The economic impact of marijuana use, as well as other specific illegal drugs, is difficult to estimate due to the nonexistence of data critical to such an analysis. Data are lacking, for instance, on such basic issues as the frequency, amount, and intensity of use and the numbers of heavy users (National Research Council, 2001). Data relating to the risks that attend drug use are also necessary but, again, are noticeably absent. These risks include the acute risks associated with a given incident of drug use; the chronic risks of a career of drug use; the delayed effects of drug use; and variations of risk associated with differences in the demographic character-istics of users, in geographical areas, by manner of drug administration, by purity of the drug, and by temporal context (National Research Council, 2001). The calculation of cost is rendered still more difficult due to the multi-faceted nature of such an analysis which, depending upon the drug at issue, may include costs associated with mental and physical illness, the transmission of disease to others, accident victimization, reduced produc-tivity, child abuse, and crime or violence that is economically motivated or associated with the psychopharmacological properties of the drug, and criminal justice costs. Too, the value of a number of harms, such as in-fringements on liberty and privacy and the corruption of legal authorities, is difficult to quantify (MacCoun, Reuter, and Schelling, 1996). An estimate of marijuana's impact is rendered yet more difficult due to users' frequent reliance on multiple drugs and the aggregation of economic data across multiple drug categories.

As a result, estimates of the annual economic cost of drug abuse vary widely. A report of the American Medical Association (1993) estimated that more than $171 billion is expended each year on problems related to alcohol, tobacco, and drug abuse. Other researchers estimated that, in 1988, the cost of health care, law enforcement, and lost productivity due to drug abuse reached $58.3 billion, as compared to 1985 expenditures of $85.8 billion for similar costs associated with alcohol abuse alone (Rice, Kelman, and Miller, 1991). The National Institute of Drug Abuse estimated in 1999 that the 1992 cost of drug abuse was $98 billion and, by 1995, the annual cost had risen to $110 billion after adjusting for inflation and population change (Cartwright, 1999). The cost of crime associated with illicit drug abuse has been estimated at $57.1 billion, of which $39.1 billion represents lost wages due to incarceration, criminal careers, and crime-related victimization (Cartwright, 1999).

COCAINE AND CRACK: USE, ABUSE, AND POLICY

The Medical Era of Cocaine Use

Cocaine is a psychoactive alkaloid that is found in the leaves of Erythroxylon coca, a plant that is indigenous to Peru, Bolivia, and Colombia (Quinones-Jenab, 2001). Evidence suggests that the use of cocaine as a psychostimulant dates back as far as 5,000 years. During the sixteenth century, travelers to South America from Europe observed the use of coca leaves to reduce fatigue and to increase stamina (Spillane, 2000). In fact, the "world's first antidrug campaign" was directed against coca by the Catholic church in 1552, in an attempt to ban its use in Latin America (Streatfield, 2001).

In the United States, following the Civil War, a group of physicians investigated the therapeutic value of coca. Experimentation was impeded, however, due to difficulties encountered in obtaining coca and the inability to control the quality of the product. Because of the variation in the quality of the coca leaves obtained, researchers were often unable to duplicate in the laboratory the effects of coca that were being reported by its users. Dowdeswell, an English physician, finally concluded that coca had no therapeutic or popular value and a "more decided effect" could be had by ingesting "tea, milk-and-water, and even plain water, hot, tepid, and cold" (Dowdeswell, 1876: 664). Edward R. Squibb, a member of both the American Medical Association and the American Pharmaceutical Association and the head of a pharmaceutical house, denounced the quality of the United States' drug supply as "low grade" and demanded increased regulation and inspection.

Later, in 1884, the Austrian physician Carl Koller reported the results of an experiment during which he had anesthetized the surface of an eye with cocaine. Prior to this discovery that cocaine could be used as a local anesthetic, physicians performing surgery had few choices: no anesthetic or a general anesthetic, such as ether or chloroform. The use of cocaine as a local anesthetic permitted physicians to perform more delicate operations, without the dangers associated with the use of general anesthesia, such as vomiting, which would cause uncontrollable movement in the patient. Cocaine also allowed patients to remain awake during the procedures (Streatfield, 2001; Spillane, 2000). Ultimately, the use of cocaine was extended to many types of surgical procedures and to nonsurgical procedures that required assessment in sensitive areas.

In the late 1800s, prior to the development of modern psychotherapy, neurologists shared responsibility for the treatment of "nervous" diseases. The condition of neurasthenia represented both a cause and an effect of nervousness. Conditions believed to be linked to neurasthenia included hay fever, hypochondria, headache, hysteria, epilepsy, and insanity, among others. This "nervousness," thought to be prevalent among "brain workers," was attributed to overstimulation and exhausting work habits. As such, it was a disorder that affected men and women in the middle and upper classes. As nervousness was believed to have some physical basis, after 1884 drug therapy for the condition included the use of cocaine (Spillane, 2000).

Two significant events occurred during this time that would ultimately change cocaine use. First, von Anrep described the analgesic properties of cocaine (Quinones-Jenab, 2001). Second, Freud described the psychomotor and euphoric effects of the drug and recommended its use in the treatment of hypochondria, hysteria, and melancholy (Freud, 1884). Cocaine use became widespread as an antidepressant, as a tonic, and as a mental stimulant. Coca was also used as a tonic and a stimulant to treat debility, exhaustion, neurasthenia, and overwork.

Cocaine was also introduced as a treatment for opiate addiction; it was believed to confer both stimulation and support during withdrawal and to be directly antagonistic to the physiological effects of morphine (Freud, 1884). Although the initial response of addicts to this use of cocaine was favorable, medical opinion remained divided on the benefits of coca or cocaine in the treatment of opiate addiction. (Streatfield, 2001; Spillane, 2000). Even more dangerous, opiate addicts introduced to cocaine had invented "speedballs," a cocktail of cocaine and heroin or morphine (Streatfield, 2001).

The "medical era" of cocaine extended for almost a decade. However, indications that cocaine could be addictive appeared even in the late 1880s (Mattison, 1886–87). Despite the identification of the dangers associated with cocaine use, many physicians continued to utilize the drug as a remedy for a wide range of ailments, from sinus problems to nervousness. However, physicians began to advocate for strict medical control and conservative usage in order to avoid "cocaine poisoning" and the creation of a "cocaine habit." Physicians were particularly concerned about the rapidity with which a cocaine habit seemed to appear, the euphoric properties of the drug that encouraged its use, the dramatic physical deterioration associated with cocaine overuse, the startling behavioral changes that often accompanied its use, and the difficulty of effectuating a cure from cocaine use (Spillane, 2000).

During this medical era, the United States relied heavily on the coca crops of Peru and Bolivia, resulting in an expansion of its cultivation in those countries. British manufacturers obtained their coca supplies from Ceylon and India, while growers in Java supplied their product to the Netherlands. In fact, the United States was one of the leading consumers, producers, and promoters of cocaine for both medical and popular usage (Gootenberg, 1999). Coca imports to the United States peaked at 1,277,604 pounds in 1905. Prior to World War I, Germany, the United States, and the Netherlands represented the world's three largest cocaine manufacturers (Spillane, 2000). It is critical to remember that, at this point in time, the importation of coca and the manufacture of cocaine were both legal.

Manufacturers often touted the drug's benefits and not infrequently downplayed reports detailing cocaine's negative effects. Parke, Davis, a pharmaceutical company that was heavily invested in the marketing of cocaine, developed coca leaf cigars and cigarettes and distributed free cocaine to physicians in exchange for reports of the drug's effectiveness (Streatfield, 2001). In its early advertising, Coca-Cola stressed the appeal of its product as a vehicle for the stimulant and therapeutic properties of coca. The success of Coca-Cola led to the development of imitation products that also utilized fluid extract of coca (Streatfield, 2001). Coca wines and patents medical preparations also gained marketplace prominence (Spillane, 2000).

The Popular Era of Cocaine Use

New patterns of cocaine use soon appeared, such as cocaine sniffing in New Orleans. The typical cocaine abuser had been a white male professional, aged 30 or older, the profile of the medical era cocaine user. By 1903, however, the level of cocaine consumption had increased five-fold compared to what it had been in 1890, and the vast majority of the increase was attributable to nonmedical usage. The image of cocaine users metamorphosized from that of overtaxed "brain workers" needing relief from stress to that of blacks, criminals, and common laborers using cocaine for their own pleasure. The "popular era" of cocaine use (1895–1920) had begun (Spillane, 2000).

As in Latin America, cocaine was adopted for use as a stimulant by laborers. Many of these waterfront laborers, or roustabouts as they were called, were black; their use of cocaine reinforced perceptions of them as better able to endure physical labor and environmental conditions that would be physically unbearable to whites. Employers in the textile, mining, and road construction industries soon made cocaine available for sale to their employees in their company commissaries.

By 1900, cocaine had become the hard drug of choice among prostitutes in New Orleans, in an area of town frequented by the roustabouts. The city passed an ordinance prohibiting the sale of cocaine, following the police chief's farfetched claim that 15,000 to 25,000 "cocaine fiends," representing 4.5 to 7 percent of the city's population, resided there.

A hostile response soon emerged to blacks' use of cocaine, which was perceived as the manifestation of a more assertive attitude among younger blacks, an attitude that seemed to threaten existing social restraints. One pharmaceutical journal reported:

> The use of cocaine by Negroes in certain parts of the country is simply appalling. . . . The police officers of questionable districts tell us that habitués are made wild by cocaine, which they have no difficulty at all in obtaining (Streatfield, 2001: 140, quoting *American Pharmaceutical Journal*, 1901).

The original introduction of cocaine into black communities through its provision by employers to black laborers was forgotten or overlooked.

Concern was also raised both about the use of cocaine by children and the danger that cocaine posed to young women, who might unwittingly be forced into prostitution after having been offered the drug. Prostitutes soon became the central figure of the "moral contagion model." Then-New York City Police Commissioner Bingham asserted that

> the classes of the community most addicted to the habitual use of cocaine are parasites who live on the earnings of prostitutes, prostitutes of the lowest order, and young degenerates who acquire the habit through their connection with prostitutes and parasites (Quoted in Spillane, 2000: 98).

Increasing pressure from law enforcement during this time both served to reduce opium smoking (see heroin, below) and to encourage cocaine sniffing, which was more convenient and less likely to be detected. Users of morphine found the injection of cocaine and morphine and, later, heroin irresistible. Heroin, which was readily available for a decade following its initial introduction, (see below), could be sniffed or injected before, after, or concurrent with cocaine use.

Unlike opium and morphine use, which public health and law enforcement authorities viewed as an addiction, cocaine use was perceived as a vice within the control of the individual. Distinctions were made between opiate addicts who had become such through use associated with chronic ailments; those who relied on the drug to address acute and relapsing illness; and those who utilized the drug as a means of escaping depression or experiencing a new sensation (Powers, 1915). Cocaine use increasingly became associated with individuals seeking both pleasure and a deviant identity, a characterization that served to absolve the medical profession of any responsibility for the users' predicament (Burnham, 1993). Concurrently, police efforts to control cocaine use and users were intensified, as users of cocaine were likened to carriers of an infectious disease, necessitating their quarantine to protect the general public.

The passage of the Harrison Act in 1914 essentially rendered all cocaine use illegal. Users were often arrested on vagrancy charges, since the sale, but not the possession, of cocaine was prohibited and sales were difficult to detect. Although even the police complained that users should be cared for in institutions, cocaine users were far less likely than either opiate users or addicts to be committed to public asylums or long-term care facilities due, in part, to the perception of cocaine use as a chosen vice rather than a physical addiction.

Law enforcement, in assessing the relationship between cocaine use and crime, concluded that most criminal activity was conducted in order to gain funds to purchase more drugs. Cocaine also came to be associated with violent, unpredictable, and antisocial behavior. This association was particularly strong in the South, where police departments attempted to hold in check those blacks who came under the influence of cocaine, "sexual desires are increased and perverted, peaceful negroes become quarrelsome, and timid negroes develop a degree of "Dutch courage" that is sometimes almost incredible" (Williams, 1914: 247).

J.L. Lynch, a federal food and drug inspector, observing the growing habitual use of cocaine- and coca-containing products, such as Coca-Cola, joined a coalition that had as its aim the restriction of access to cocaine. This goal became part of a larger movement to institute regulations for the development and distribution of new drug products. The movement reflected two goals: the minimization of harms resulting from the widespread availability of cocaine and the creation of a system for the regulation of drugs. Other voices joined the demand for drug regulation: journalists, the federal government, and reform-minded physicians and their professional organizations.

The passage of the Pure Food and Drug Act of 1906, under which Lynch had been permitted to conduct his investigation, provided the basis for the prosecutions of soft drink and patent medicine manufacturers who had used coca or cocaine in their products and had neglected to disclose the ingredient in the package labeling. By the time the Harrison Act went into effect, most manufacturers had eliminated cocaine as an ingredient in their products or ceased their production. Fear of adverse publicity and prosecution, as well as declining sales, provided sufficient motivation.

Concurrently, local jurisdictions promulgated ordinance prohibiting the sale of cocaine (New Orleans), restricting the quantity that druggists could dispense at any one time (New York State), limiting the amount of the drug that could be held in stock (New York), or prohibiting the sale of the drug to habitual users (Chicago). Druggists, clearly, had become the target of the anticocaine forces. Ultimately, druggists joined the anticocaine movement, not only as a response to this hostility, but also as a means of reinforcing their professional status and exerting influence over the content of any new legislation that might be considered (Spillane, 2000).

Because restrictions were imposed on the sale, but not on the possession, of cocaine, and sales were difficult to observe, an underground system of distribution soon developed. Sellers operated from parks, drugstores, hotels, restaurants, bars, theaters, public buildings, newsstands, pool halls, and streets. The cocaine sold underground varied on cost, depending on location, and was often of lesser purity in an attempt to stretch the supply and to increase the profit.

Current policy prohibits the sale and possession of cocaine in any amount. As was seen in the discussion of alcohol and marijuana, above, and as indicated in the discussion of heroin, below, alcohol, marijuana, cocaine, and heroin

> were all advanced partly on the idea that their users were deviant, dangerous "others" whom no society could safely tolerate. Each substance was once a significant part of the therapeutic arsenal of "legitimate" medicine, and each was subsequently identified as "illegitimate" because of concerns that were at least as influenced by fear and prejudice as by objective evaluations of the harms they caused (Spillane, 2000: 158).

The Age of Crack

The mid-1970s heralded a return to increased cocaine consumption, followed by the "Age of Crack" and the associated domestic and foreign drug wars (Gootenberg, 1999: 5). By the mid-1980s, drugs and drug use were perceived as threats to national security (Walker, 1996). Commissioner

Anslinger had asserted, in fact, that drug control was critical to security, and charged that Communist China and Cuba both sought to weaken the United States by using drugs as a weapon of war (Kinder, 1981).

Crack, a smokeable form of cocaine, first appeared in inner-city neighborhoods in New York, Los Angeles, and Miami in late 1984 (Reinarman and Levine, 1997b). It is produced by cooking down in a pot a mixture of powder cocaine, water, and baking soda, making a crackling sound when it is heated, giving the drug its name. Crack itself represented neither a new form of cocaine, which had previously been used in smoke form, nor a new drug, as it was entirely cocaine. Rather, the innovation lay in its marketing and marketability: $5 to $20 for a small vial or envelope that could produce a very brief, but extremely intense, high. Too, the crack business offered people in lower income neighborhoods greater pay than they might otherwise earn (Bourgois, 1997).

The news media and politicians, including former Presidents Ronald Reagan and George Bush, decried America's use of drugs and called for an "all-out war on drugs." Although the media reported that crack was "flooding America" and had become the "drug of choice" (NBC Nightly News, May 23, 1986), a 1986 survey of high school students found that only 4.1 percent had even tried crack during the previous year (Johnston, O'Malley, and Bachman, 1988). Reagan and his administration characterized drug use as an individual moral choice and the result of individual deviance and weakness. Unemployment, poverty, violence, and depression did not beget drug usage; rather, they were the consequences of individuals gone morally astray (Reinarman and Levine, 1997a).

HALLUCINOGENS: USE, ABUSE, AND POLICY

Hallucinogens have been in use for thousands of years. Peyote, for example, has been represented in an archaeological tomb dating back to the period from 100 B.C. to 100 A.D. (Furst, 1976). Use of the Sophora secundiflora, which produces a red, bean-like seed known as the "mescal bean," dates back to the end of the Late Pleistocene period, approximately 10,000 years ago (Adovasio and Fry, 1975). These seeds contain a quinolizidine alkaloid known as cystisine which, in high doses, can produce hallucinations, convulsions, and respiratory failure (Schultes, 1972).

The Spaniards arriving in the New World perceived the continued use of hallucinogens by the native peoples as a validation of their traditional religion and a repudiation of Christianity. The missionaries attributed the "supernatural" effects of the substances to the work of the Devil. The preaching and the torture that were inflicted on the natives in an effort to abolish hallucinogen use served, instead, to encourage the practice in secrecy (Furst, 1976).

LSD was discovered in 1938 by Albert Hofmann and colleagues. The drug has been called "the most potent psychoactive or 'psychedelic' compound known up to that time" (Furst, 1976: 59).

HEROIN: USE ABUSE, AND POLICY

Practice, Perception, and Politics

A discussion of heroin use in the United States must necessarily begin with an examination of the use of opiates. As early as the mid-1500s, men and women in the United States used a liquid form of opium, known as Laudanum, or "black drop," to experience a high (Fernandez, 1998). Later, both men and women used liquid opium as their drug of choice; women could avoid the stigmatization associated with frequenting a saloon and men could similarly avoid the social consequences of appearing to be drunkards. By the mid-1800s, many patent medicines, including those marketed to remedy children's coughs and diarrhea, contained liquid opium.

Although intended to alleviate pain and discomfort, the use of these preparations led to widespread addiction (Fernandez, 1998). It has been estimated that by 1885, approximately 71 percent of those addicted to opiates in the United States were middle- and upper-class white women who had purchased the drug legally. The rate of addiction was 4.59 persons per 1,000 Americans, compared with a rate of 2.04 per 1,000 persons today (Attias, cited in Fernandez, 1998). The number of individuals addicted to opiates increased even more with the inadvertent addiction of Civil War soldiers who became addicted to the morphine used to soothe the pain from their war wounds (Fernandez, 1998).

Opium dens, although frequented by those born in the United States, came to be associated with Chinese immigrants, who often established the dens in their Chinatowns in major cities, such as San Francisco and New York. Chinese immigrants became the target of propaganda that arose in response to the United States' depressed economy and the fear that Chinese immigrants were usurping employment opportunities from American workers. The propaganda extended to the opium dens, said to have been organized by "yellow fiends" to force "unsuspecting white women to become enslaved" to the drug (Attias, cited in Fernandez, 1998).

Heroin itself was discovered in 1874 (Durlacher, 2000). Heroin powder proved to be even more potent and addictive than the liquid opium that had been an ingredient of patent medicines. In 1898, it was introduced by Bayer and Company as a nonprescription remedy for a wide range of maladies, including chest pain, pneumonia, and tuberculosis. These medicines were available in powder and liquid forms and, owing to the invention of the hypodermic syringe in 1853, in injectable form (Durlacher, 2000; Fernandez, 1998).

During the late 19th and early 20th centuries, a growing reform and prohibitionist movement campaigned against the manufacturers of products containing such drugs. Prior to this time, the medical community had not yet understood the extent of addiction and its potential consequences. It was not until 1906, with the passage of the Pure Food and Drug Act, that the sale of medicine containing opium, morphine, or heroin became regulated (Musto, 1987). The later passage of the Harrison Act in 1914 rendered the use of opium and related products criminal by providing for the licensure and taxation of all individuals who "produce, import, manufacture, compound, deal in, dispense, sell, distribute, or give away opium or coca leaves, their salts, derivatives, or preparations...." Although the Act excluded "the dispensing or distribution of any of the aforesaid drugs to a patient by a physician, dentist, or veterinary surgeon registered under [the] Act in the course of his professional practice...," addiction was not perceived as a disease and, therefore, the maintenance of addiction was not encompassed within this exclusion. An editorial in *American Medicine* was harsh in its condemnation of this new law:

> Narcotic drug addiction is one of the gravest and most important questions confronting the medical profession today. Instead of improving conditions, the laws recently passed have made the problem more complex. Honest medical men have found such handicaps and dangers to themselves and their reputations in these laws...that they have simply decided to have as little to do as possible with drug addicts or their needs...The druggists are in the same position and for similar reasons many of them have discontinued entirely the sale of narcotic drugs. [The addict] is denied the medical care he urgently needs.... (Durlacher, 2000: 16).

It has been estimated that, as a result of the passage of such laws and the associated domestic law enforcement effort, that the number of "addicts" was reduced from 200,000 in 1924 to 20,000 in 1945 (McCoy, 1991). The post-World War II resurgence of heroin use in the United States has been attributed to the CIA's three decade-long anti-communist collaboration with foreign armed forces sympathetic to opium growers and heroin traffickers; the use of heroin by American soldiers in Vietnam during the 1960s and 1970s (Fernandez, 1998); and the emulation of heroin-addicted jazz musicians during the 1940s and 1950s, of rock musicians during the

1960s and 1970s, and of grunge musicians during the late 1980s (Durlacher, 2000). Increased law enforcement and treatment efforts reduced the estimated number of heroin addicts in the United States from 500,000 in the late 1960s to 200,000 by the mid-1970s. However, the CIA's subsequent support of Afghan rebels against the Soviet occupation in Afghanistan and its corresponding willingness to ignore the Afghan heroin trade contributed to yet another upsurge in heroin use (McCoy, 1991). By 1980, the number of heroin addicts in the United States had once again grown to 500,000 (Fernandez, 1998). Most recently, heroin has developed a following among middle-class users, many of whom believe that they will not become addicted to the drug if they do not inject it (Fernandez, 1998).

The Economic Impact of Heroin

As with marijuana, it is difficult to estimate the economic impact of heroin alone. The economic cost of substance use discussed in the context of marijuana encompass the costs associated with heroin due to the aggregation of all illicit substances in the published analyses. Nonetheless, a number of identifiable costs are associated with the use of heroin itself, while still others are associated with the use of injected drugs, which includes heroin.

It has been estimated that, for fiscal year 1993, a total of $480 million from all sources was expended for methadone treatment for heroin (Stoller and Bigelow, 1999). Methadone treatment, which is highly regulated by the federal government (Institute of Medicine, 1995), mimics to a degree the effects of heroin, such as euphoria, but may also result in significant adverse effects, such as respiratory failure and death (Walsh and Strain, 1999). Treatment with methadone does not address co-existing non-heroin substance disorders, such as cocaine abuse or the use of sedatives or alcohol (Stitzer and Chutuape, 1999).

The average annual cost of continuous methadone maintenance treatment per client, adjusted to 1994 dollars, is approximately $4,722; the average cost per treatment episode per client for methadone maintenance treatment is approximately $6,742 (French and Martin, 1996). In 1992, 3,600 injection drug users died from hepatitis B and C, while an additional 10,737 deaths were attributable to AIDS among injection drug users (Cartwright, 1999). The morbidity costs associated with drug-related diseases range from $31 for a mild infection with a sexually transmitted disease other than HIV/AIDS, to $220,038 for the treatment of severe tuberculosis. Significant costs may also be incurred in conjunction with the provision of prenatal care to low birthweight infants of substance-using mothers (French and Martin, 1996). Criminal activity, consisting of both drug dealing/possession and "victimless" offenses, as well as personal and property offenses, has also been associated with heroin use (Department of Health and Human Services, 1991).

CURRENT POLICIES AND POLICY OPTIONS: PUNISH OR TREAT?

Numerous strategies are currently in use to address addiction within both the criminal and treatment contexts. Additional approaches focus on substance use-associated crime, such as trafficking in illicit drugs and violent crime, and on the imposition of collateral sanctions for drug use, such as the withholding of public benefits. A discussion of these additional approaches is beyond the scope of this article and the reader is referred elsewhere for this analysis (Demleitner, 2002; Rah, 2002). Instead, this section focuses on various strategies currently utilized to address addiction to legal and illegal substances within the criminal context: prison and prison-based treatment, involuntary civil commitment, drug courts, and therapeutic communities and, in addition, discusses the need to integrate research findings relating to behavior change into the penal-based treatment framework.

Prison and Prison-Based Treatment

Imprisonment has been our traditional response to the purchase, possession for personal use, and use of illegal drugs or of legal drugs without the requisite prescription. In 1996 alone, 1.5 million individuals entered the criminal justice system following their arrests for drug-related offenses. It is unclear, however, what proportion of these individuals were imprisoned for possession for personal use alone. It has been estimated that 60 percent of federal inmates are serving sentences for drug-related offenses (Office of National Drug Control Policy, 1999), resulting in the annual expenditure of $2 billion by the United States Bureau of Prisons (Massing, 1998), and that almost one-half million of the nation's inmates are addicted to drugs (Lewis, 2000; Wren, 1999). The National Center on Addiction and Substance Abuse has estimated "that if rates of incarceration continue to rise at their current pace, 1 out of every 20 Americans born in 1997 will serve time in prison . . . " (National Center on Addiction and Substance Abuse, 1998).

It has been argued that our predilection to imprison substance abusers constitutes cruel and unusual punishment within the meaning of the Eighth Amendment because imprisonment under such circumstances constitutes, in essence, punishment for offenses that are related to the status of being a drug addict, rather than offenses related to conduct (Brennan, 1998). Although several judicial decisions lend credence to this view (*Powell v. Texas*, 1968; *Robinson v. California*, 1962), more recent opinions have emphasized the individual's free will in the initial decision to use an illegal substance (*United States v. Moore*, 1973).

Treatment is potentially available to substance abusers housed in federal prisons and in jails. In 1998, approximately 34,0000 prisoners were enrolled in the residential treatment programs available at 40 federal prisons (Office of National Drug Control Policy, 1999). Participants in these programs have been found to be less likely to use drugs and less likely to be arrested, compared to nonparticipants (Office of National Drug Control Policy, 1999). The situation is much bleaker, however, in the jails. Although more than 50 percent of the largest jail systems in the U.S. offer alcohol or drug treatment, less than 10 percent of those eligible actually participate and the success of the treatment, as measured by rates of rearrest, appears negligible (National Institute of Justice, 1996).

Numerous barriers attend the provision of effective drug treatment in the prison setting. Limited resources impede institutions' ability to address the specific needs of the many inmates who are polydrug users and to identify those who may be suffering from undiagnosed mental illness, in addition to their substance abuse. Violent or difficult prisoners may be prohibited from participating in the treatment programs, which are voluntary. The separation of participating inmates from the general prison population may not be possible, rendering the recovery process more difficult. Despite the recent proclivity towards the arrest and imprisonment of substance-using pregnant women, few prisons are equipped to provide substance abuse treatment that considers the special needs of pregnant women (Platt, 1995). Too, the sentence to be served may require less time than the treatment program demands, resulting in a decreased probability of recovery due to the premature termination of treatment (National Institute of Justice, 1996).

Civil Commitment

Compulsory civil commitment for substance abusers is premised on the belief that "some heroin and other substance abusers are motivated for treatment, but most are not. As such, there must be some lever for diverting into treatment those who ordinarily would not seek assistance on a voluntary basis" (Inciardi, 1988: 549).

Compulsory civil commitment, in lieu of criminal sentencing, was utilized during the 1930s and again during the 1960s. The Public Health Service-established "narcotics farms" of the 1930s, located in rural areas, provided treatment to substance abusers who had entered voluntarily or who were committed involuntarily following a federal conviction (Platt et al., 1998). Individuals were provided with up to one year of residential substance abuse treatment and long-term community-based aftercare, with parole supervision, as appropriate. Many of the voluntary patients left prior to the completion of the treatment protocol and relapse among all of the patients was common (Platt, 1986).

Several formal commitment schemes were later implemented in California and in New York. The California Civil Addict Program was based on a seven-year commitment program that was initiated during incarceration in a medium security prison; three-fourths of the 7 years was often spent on parole under community supervision (Anglin, 1988). An evaluation of the program revealed that individuals in the commitment program utilized narcotics at a slower rate than did the comparison nonparticipants and this difference in the rate of narcotics use was maintained during the 5-year supervision period. However, increased daily use of narcotics occurred in both the commitment group and the comparison group after the 5-year supervision period (Inciardi, 1988).

Neither the New York Parole Project (NYPP) nor the New York Addiction Control Commission (NACC) could claim the same level of success. The NYPP, which was the precursor of the NACC, was compromised by a lack of adequate officer training, biased case selection for the program, and the use of rearrest for a new crime, rather than drug use, as the basis for parole failure. The NACC was similarly unsuccessful, due to the maintenance of a correctional, rather than a therapeutic, atmosphere; the inexperience of the facility administration; the modeling of the aftercare program on the parole system, rather than on a therapeutic framework; and the loss of public support due to efforts to camouflage the program's difficulties (Inciardi, 1988).

Involuntary commitment may be possible even apart from such defunct programs. A number of states permit the postprison indefinite civil commitment of sexually violent predators, who are deemed to be suffering from a "mental abnormality" that renders it likely that they will again engage in predatory sexual violence (Arizona Revised Statutes Annotated §§36–3701 to 36–3716, 1999; California Welfare and Institutions Code §§6600–6609.3, 2000). Such crimes include rape, indecent liberties with a child, indecent solicitation of a child, and sexual exploitation of a child.238. These laws, founded upon the police power of the state rather than on the concept of *parens patriae* (La Fond, 1999), have been upheld against numerous constitutional challenges (*Kansas v. Hendricks*, 1997).

The parameters of these statutes are sufficiently expansive so as to permit the involuntary commitment of substance users. First, "mental

abnormality" is legislatively defined and may bear no relation to clinical classifications of mental illness (La Fond, 1999). Accordingly, the term
"mental abnormality" essentially serves to collapse "all badness into mad-
ness" (Morse, 1998), thereby permitting the term to be applied to any
behavior and ensuring "that the class of individuals potentially subject to
involuntary civil commitment can be defined by the political process rather
than through a system based on demonstrable medical expertise and limited by effective judicial review (La Fond, 1999). For instance, the legitima-
tion of the legislative determination that pedophiles are unable to control
their sexual urges, despite the nonexistence of any empirical or theoretical
support for this thesis, permits the legislature to similarly classify others
with undesirable behaviors as suffering from a mental abnormality and au-
thorize their indefinite postprison civil commitment (Winick, 1998). These
statutes essentially permit reliance on incapacitation as a nonpunitive objective, without a corollary right to treatment, thereby "transforming therapeutic civil commitment into a broad, inexpensive quarantine scheme"
(La Fond, 1999: 4). Involuntary commitment becomes premised merely
upon a finding of dangerousness, without a concomitant finding of mental illness (Dorsett, 1998), potentially authorizing the similar disposition of
any and all individuals deemed by society to be dangerous in some manner.

Various judicial determinations lend credence to this possibility. The
Supreme Court of Virginia, for instance, has held that an individual who
has engaged in aggressive behavior and is likely to do so again and to harm
others may be involuntarily confined as an inpatient, despite disagreement
as to whether her polydrug use constitutes mental illness within the meaning of the relevant statute (*Mercer v. Commonwealth of Virginia*, 2000). The
possibility of involuntary civil commitment is rendered more likely in view
of the inclusion of various substance-related disorders as categories of mental illness in the *Diagnostic and Statistical Manual of Mental Disorders, Fourth
Edition, Text Revision* (DSM-IV-R-T) (American Psychiatric Association,
2000), thereby ensuring in the context of such a proceeding that substance
abuse is subsumed under one or both the classifications of mental illness
or mental abnormality.

The wisdom of such an approach is, however, questionable. Civil
commitment does not necessarily mandate treatment during the period
of commitment (*In re Mental Health of K.K.B.*, 1980). Even though sufficient
treatment would be provided to support an individual's medical needs, it
is unclear whether, in this context, the substance-using individual would
be provided with additional treatment components, such as counseling
and vocational training (*Youngberg v. Romeo*, 1982). Further, research seems
to indicate that the effectiveness of mandated treatment may be less than
desired because coercion may compel an individual's presence, but does

not assure the active participation necessary to complete treatment successfully (Maddux, 1988).

Drug Courts

As of June 1, 1998, a total of 430 drug courts were in various stages of planning or operation in 48 states, the District of Columbia, Puerto Rico, Guam and several Native American tribal courts (Drug Court Clearinghouse and Technical Assistance Project, 1998). The concept of the drug court derives from the theory of therapeutic jurisprudence. Therapeutic jurisprudence, defined as "the study of the role of law as a therapeutic agent" (Winick, 1997), relies on the social sciences to provide information that is critical to the attainment of specified goals and the examination and prioritization of competing values (Wexler and Schopp, 1992). The drug court is predicated on two underlying assumptions: that drug usage has become epidemic, requiring that "something" be done, and that drug addiction is a treatable disease (Hoffman, 2000). Further, the establishment of the drug court as a mechanism for the disposition of drug-related cases constitutes an acknowledgement of the failure of the usual adjudication process to address substance use, the failure of the probation system to identify and provide necessary services in the context of community supervision, and the failure of the private and public drug treatment provider systems to address in a meaningful way the substance abuse treatment needs of the criminal justice population (Goldkamp, 2000).

Initially, drug treatment courts adhered to one of two paradigms. The differentiated case management (DCM) model, reflected in New York City's approach to drug cases, requires that specialized case management courts handle a high volume of cases in a rather traditional manner, without a treatment component. In contrast, the treatment-based approach, as implemented in Dade County, Florida, targets nonviolent felony drug offenders for a one-year diversion and treatment program that includes counseling, fellowship meetings, education, acupuncture, vocational services, intense judicial review, and frequent review of urinalysis results. Currently, most drug courts are hybrids of these two models (Hoffman, 2000).

Eligibility criteria for participation in drug court programs differ in many respects, including the qualifying offenses, the stage of the criminal process at which a defendant may be accepted into the program, the extent of system-wide support, the structure and content of treatment, the sanctions and incentives utilized to encourage substance users to complete the program, and the court's level of productivity (Goldkamp, 2000). Generally, however, drug treatment courts share 5 core elements: (1) immediate intervention, (2) a nonadversarial adjudication process, (3) judicial involvement in the defendant's treatment program, (4) clearly defined rules and structured goals for treatment program participants, and (5) a collaborative team approach that includes the judge, prosecutor defense counsel, treatment provider, and corrections personnel (Hora, Schma and Rosenthal, 1999).

Evaluations of the effectiveness of drug courts have included informal surveys of a single drug court conducted by its own personnel, court-commissioned studies of a single court conducted by non-court personnel, and formal studies of several drug courts by non-court professionals that were not commissioned by the courts themselves (Hoffman, 2000). The majority of the studies suffer from one or more methodological weaknesses, such as the failure to select an appropriate comparison court and/or court population, the choice of the measure or measures to be utilized to judge success, and a relatively short follow-up period (Hoffman, 2000).

Nonetheless, several of the more rigorous evaluations have noted the relative lack of success of drug treatment courts. A 1991 study by the American Bar Association examined the DCM-based drug courts in Cook County, Illinois, Milwaukee, and Philadelphia, as well as the treatment-based court in Dade County, Florida. Although the drug courts had successfully reduced the amount of time required for the processing of cases, there was no reduction in the rate of recidivism (Smith, 1991). A later study of the Dade County system found lower rates of recidivism associated with the drug court but, alarmingly, higher rates of defendant failure to report. A study of the Baltimore drug court indicated decreases in recidivism rates in both the traditional and the drug courts (Hoffman, 2000). A later study conducted by the United States General Accounting Office concluded that insufficient data exist to determine whether drug courts aid in reducing recidivism and preventing relapse (United States General Accounting Office, 1997).

Critics of the drug court have emphasized the system's shortcomings, including daunting caseloads, the failure of the program to reduce the prison population, the failure of judges to individualize sentences due to the burgeoning caseloads, the inconsistent handling of cases resulting from frequent changes in judges, and the imposition of sentences on individuals illegally in the United States that are designed to meet the goals of the Immigration and Naturalization Service, rather than to fulfill the philosophy of the drug court (Hoffman, 2000). Supporters, however, have noted that drug treatment courts provide an incentive to substance abusers to remain in treatment, because a failure to do so will result in a conviction (Hora, Schma, and Rosenthal, 1999). While acknowledging the less than stellar performance of the drug courts in reducing recidivism, supporters have stressed the impact of drug courts in reducing time in probation and the lower proportion of offenders who are sentenced to prison as a result of a new arrest. Additionally, reliance on drug courts reduced the costs associated with incarceration, with health care, and with drug-related criminal activity (Hora, Schma, and Rosenthal, 1999).

Unfortunately, it appears that we have failed to utilize our experience with behavior change to inform our disposition of addiction-related cases within the criminal context. Research has indicated that behavior change is often viewed as a process that consists of sequential, incremental small changes, rather than as a discrete overt behavioral outcome (Fisher and Fisher, 2000). Additionally, change is not linear but involves, instead, recycling through various stages of change. Accordingly, relapse is seen as a component part of the effort to modify behavior and, in particular, to modify addictive behavior (Taylor, 1994).

The transtheoretical model is one such model of behavior change. This theory posits that an individual moves through the following stages of change in an attempt to change behavior: (1) precontemplation, during which there is no intent to change behavior; (2) contemplation, during which an individual intends to change behavior during the upcoming 6 months; (3) preparation, involving an intent to take effective action to change; (4) action, during which time an individual will make modifications in his or her behavior; and (5) maintenance, which commences 6 months after the initiation of consistent behavior change (Prochaska and Velicer, 1997).

A number of drug courts have expanded into the juvenile and family court contexts (Danziger and Kuhn, 1999). Many of these specialized courts are premised on the belief that continuous intervention is necessary; that intervention may include the requirements of child and family participation in treatment, frequent drug testing, and frequent court status hearings (Office of Justice Programs, 1998). This approach recognizes the critical role of the family and the context in which substance use is occurring (Cohen, Brook, Cohen, Velez, and Garcia, 1990). The demanding nature of this integrated approach requires that judges and judicial personnel receive appropriate training in multiple areas, including child development, substance abuse treatment and prevention modalities, and interviewing techniques (Danziger and Kuhn, 1999).

Harm Reduction

The theory of harm reduction is premised on the concept of addiction as a continuum, with abstinence at one end. For some individuals, the management of their addiction and their health may constitute movement in the direction of abstinence (Sorge, 1991). The concept of harm reduction necessarily demands varying manifestations according to location, client demographics, the drugs being used, and the local legal and political milieus. It conceives of the major problem as one of the effects of drug use on lifestyle, rather than of drug use per se. Accordingly, no single approach can be adopted and the implementation of a program must be tailored to the specific context.

Within this framework, intermediate steps towards an ultimate goal of abstinence are seen as having value. Accordingly, relapse is not perceived as a failure but, instead, is recognized as a common feature of the progression towards abstinence. Additionally, along the continuum from abstinence to abuse exists a range of behaviors that can be ranked in terms of safety. Harm reduction focuses on the social and environmental aspects of drug taking, helping substance users to make use of their social contexts and communities to enhance their survival. This approach recognizes that the drug user has the ability to act responsibly and to make choices to stop or modify risky behaviors. Harm reduction further posits that such changes can occur at the individual, network, and cultural levels. Although harm reduction can assume any number of forms, much of the United States has been unwilling to examine or to adopt this approach in any of its possible manifestations.

Needle Exchange Programs and Syringe Prescriptions

Harm reduction can be operationalized through the establishment of needle exchange programs (NEPs). While not treating addiction directly, such programs often distribute information about substance abuse treatment and provide appropriate treatment referrals in the course of providing sterile needles and syringes to injection drug users in exchange for their used equipment (School of Public health, University of California, Berkeley, 1993). As of 2000, 112 NEPs were operating in 29 states and the District of Columbia, involving at least 71 cities in the U.S. (Ferrini, 2000). The organization of these programs varies widely, ranging from formal, government-sponsored endeavors to illegal, underground programs (Burris, Finucane, Gallagher, and Grace, 1996). Exchanges may occur in pharmacies or other fixed sites or in mobile vans or via vending machines. More than 5.4 million syringes have been exchanged since 1989, despite the federal government's ban against the use of its funds for this purpose (Ferrini, 2000).

Numerous objections have been raised against the establishment of such programs, including fears that the programs will increase the frequency of injections among users, provoke violent behavior at the exchange sites, increase the numbers of injection drug users, and result in the disposal of an increased number of needles on the streets (Ferrini, 2000). However, research has indicated that, in addition to providing referrals for substance abuse, NEPs have been effective in reducing the numbers of improperly discarded needles by injection drug users (Doherty, Junge, Rathouz, Garfein, Riley, and Vlahov, 2000), in reducing the median frequency of injections (Guydish et al., 1993), in reducing the frequency of sharing injection equipment (Schwartz, 1993), and in reducing the rate of transmission of HIV/AIDS and hepatitis (Hagan, Des Jarlais, Friedman et al., 1995).

Harm reduction may also take the form of syringe prescription by physicians (Rich, Macalino, McKenzie, Taylor, and Burris, 2001). This approach facilitates the use of sterile equipment in order to reduce the transmission of HIV and other blood-born diseases among injection drug users, their sexual partners, and their offspring. In addition, the physician-patient interaction relating to the prescription provides the health care professional with an opportunity to discuss substance abuse treatment and, potentially, to make an appropriate referral (Rich, Macalino, McKenzie, Taylor, and Burris, 2001).

The Treatment Approach

In sharp contrast to the U.S. approach criminalizing the use of illicit substances, various European countries have provided for the availability of specified substances by prescription to individuals diagnosed as substance abusers. Switzerland, for instance, has initiated an experimental program whereby a predetermined number of substance abusers may receive prescriptions for specified drugs (Durlacher, 2000). It is hypothesized that, if successful, the program will result in the commission of fewer drug-associated crimes, decreased transmission of HIV/AIDS, and improved health among injection drug users. In addition, the experiment will assess the likelihood that a black market in diverted heroin may develop as an unintended result of the program (Durlacher, 2000).

Great Britain has established a somewhat similar approach. Individuals who are addicted to drugs may obtain a sufficient quantity of the drug to enable them to remain comfortable, but only through a clinic licensed to provide this service (Goode, 1999). One clinic in Liverpool dispenses heroin to addicted individuals, believing that the dispensation of the drug, together with clean needles in exchange for used ones, will help the addicted individuals maintain healthy lives until they are able to give up heroin.

The Normalization Approach

The Netherlands has adopted yet a third approach, that of normalization (Platt, 1995). This approach entails the decriminalization of the use and retail trade in cannabis products such as marijuana and hashish; the separation of drug markets, thereby avoiding the marginalization of cannabis users and the consequent potential for their introduction to harder drugs; and the normalization of drug problems. This latter element essentially acknowledges the widespread use of various drugs in addition to alcohol and tobacco, and attempts to minimize the harm associated with their use (van Vliet, 1990).

The U.S. Controversy

Needle Exchange and Syringe Prescriptions. Despite several federally commissioned investigations that have recommended the implementation of needle exchange programs, the federal government continues to prohibit the use of federal funds for this purpose. Consequently, state and local governments have relied on their own public funds or on privately donated sums to support these efforts (School of Public Health, University of California, Berkeley, 1993). Opponents believe that the establishment of such programs implies a social acceptance of illegal substance use and requires the decriminalization of needle possession (Ferrini, 2000). The dire outcomes once predicted to occur as a result of such programs have been demonstrated to be essentially nonexistent, while the cost savings is significant. One model, for example, estimated a 5-year cost savings of $1.3 million to one community, with a cost saving to cost ratio of 4 to 1; this model was based only on a consideration of medical costs associated with HIV infection and did not encompass potential cost savings associated with lost productivity or the prevention of hepatitis (Gold, Gafni, Nelligan, and Millson, 1997). Needle exchange programs have received the endorsement of numerous professional medical groups, including the American Medical Association, the American Public Health Association, the American Society of Addiction Medicine, the Centers for Disease Control and Prevention, and the American Academy of Pediatrics. The American Medical Association, the National Research Council, and the Institute of Medicine support the repeal of the ban in the use of federal funds for these programs (Ferrini, 2000).

Normalization/Legalization, Decriminalization, or Treatment? Significant controversy has also attended discussion relating to the use of now-illicit drugs, such as marijuana and the legalization or normalization of that use

(Evans and Berent, 1992). These often acerbic debates not infrequently reflect a lack of understanding of both the dynamics of drug use and the chemistry of specific drugs at issue (Barr, Sterling, and Williams, 2001), a failure to distinguish between the decriminalization and the legalization of a drug (Goode, 1999), and a failure to draw distinctions between various drugs, such as heroin and marijuana (Goode, 1999). Arguments are often premised on moral grounds (Bennett, 1998), and doubts are frequently voiced with respect to claims that such (relatively undefined) drug reform measures will eliminate drug-associated crime and promote the betterment of the community's health (Courtwright, 1998).

Consider, for instance, the various responses to the content of the Ohio Drug Treatment Initiative, a proposed amendment to Ohio's constitution that was placed on the ballot in November 2002. The proposed amendment had as its purpose (1) the intervention in the cycle of drug use, addiction, and crime through the provision of treatment in lieu of prison for nonviolent drug users; (2) the cessation of wasteful spending associated with the incarceration of nonviolent drug users; (3) the provision of qualified treatment to nonviolent defendants charged with possession or use, while understanding that these individuals may relapse during their recovery process; (4) the enhancement of the public safety through the preservation of jail space for violent offenders; and (5) the assurance of adequate funding levels for substance abuse treatment in the state of Ohio. Briefly, with regard to the disposition of charges related to possession or use, the proposed amendment provided for a judicial determination of eligibility for treatment; a stay of all criminal proceedings pending that determination; the provision of an appropriate assessment of the defendant; the recommendation of an appropriate treatment plan by a qualified treatment professional; the appointment of a qualified treatment professional to monitor the defendant's progress; the imposition of sanctions, including up to 90 days' incarceration, for failure to comply with the treatment plan; and the dismissal of the stayed proceedings following successful completion of the treatment plan.

The proposed scheme sought to decriminalize possession or use for first or second-time nonviolent offenders, that is, remove existing criminal penalties for specified behaviors. In contrast to decriminalization, legalization entails the control by the state or other governmental entity over specific aspects of the behavior at issue (Goode, 1999). Such is the case, for instance, with alcohol and tobacco, which have been legalized but are highly regulated in terms of who may purchase the products, the locations at which they may be purchased, the manner in which they may be advertised, and so on. Decriminalization is also to be distinguished from Britain's treatment approach, whereby narcotics are dispensed under specified conditions at authorized clinics to individuals deemed to be addicted, and California's approach to the medical use of marijuana, which permits the use of marijuana under specified conditions. Despite these critical distinctions, the governor of Ohio has labeled the amendment a "de-facto legalization, not just of marijuana but a whole range of other drugs..." (Taft, 2002).

Chapter 4

Considering the Historical and Cultural Context
Race and Ethnicity

O ne might wonder about the relevance to substance abuse treatment and research today of events that took place a century ago, or why "culture" has or should have anything to do with one's willingness to participate in research or the ability of a treatment plan to succeed. Two examples, discussed in significantly greater detail below, are illustrative.

First, consider the history of alcohol use among Native Americans. It was brought to them by white settlers, sometimes for legitimate trade purposes, but often to assist in gaining an unfair advantage in negotiations. Concomitantly, Native Americans saw the loss of their homelands, the breach of numerous agreements, and the violation of their culture. Although each individual bears responsibility for his or her own behavior, it may be critical for some individuals that treatment include a recognition and acknowledgement of this betrayal. Some individuals, as a consequence of this historical legacy and the resulting community wound, may be reluctant or even unwilling to accept treatment from a non-Native American provider or participate in research that is not being conducted by a Native American.

In the research context some individuals may be reluctant to volunteer their participation in research due to the past complicity of various entities within the United States government in misrepresentations that resulted in significant harm to the research participants. In some cases, the "participants" were never informed that they were participating in research. The Public Health Service-led Tuskegee syphilis study with African-American men, the radiation experiments on civilians by the Department of Defense, together with private universities, and the LSD experiments on members of the United States military, all come to mind. How, one might ask, could anyone possibly trust a researcher and research with this legacy in the United States?

As indicated previously, one cannot—or should not—ascribe particular sensitivities or practices to all individuals of a particular group. It is critical, however, that one be sensitive to issues that may arise so that, when and if they do, they can be acknowledged and addressed respectfully.

AFRICAN-AMERICANS: HISTORICAL AND CULTURAL CONTEXT

The Historical Context

African-American Health during Slavery

Many Southern physicians believed that significant medical differences existed between blacks and whites. Some physicians argued that blacks were immune from certain diseases that affected whites, such as malaria, but were especially susceptible to other conditions, such as frostbite (Savitt, 1985). For instance, one northern physician observed of blacks that:

> God has adapted him, both in his physical and mental structure, to the tropics.... His head is protected from the rays of a vertical sun by a dense mat of woolly hair, wholly impervious to its fiercest heats, while his entire surface, studded with innumerable sebaceous glands, forming a complete excretory system, relieves him from all those climatic influences so fatal, under the same circumstances, to the sensitive and highly organized white man. Instead of seeking to shelter himself from the burning sun of the tropics, he courts it, enjoys it, delights in its fiercest heats (Van Evrie, 1861: 251, 256).

African-Americans suffered from several causes of mortality, including pulmonary tuberculosis and neonatal tetanus, more so than whites. One particular form of tuberculosis, characterized by difficulty in breathing, abdominal pain, progressive debility and emaciation, and ultimately death, was so common among blacks that it became known as Negro Consumption or *Struma Africana*. Various explanations have been offered in attempts to explain the impact of this form of tuberculosis on blacks, including lack of an immune response to the disease due to lack of exposure and an increased susceptibility to serious first attacks of tuberculosis due to various factors, including malnutrition and pre-existing illness (Savitt, 1985).

Epidemics of cholera, yellow fever, and typhoid were of special concern among slaves. Slaves were often particularly vulnerable to cholera as a result of the increased consumption of water required by their strenuous work. The water, however, was often contaminated and the slaves frequently suffered from nutritional deficiencies that adversely affected their ability to recover from cholera (Lee and Lee, 1977).

The especial vulnerability to a number of diseases was used by some as an illustration of blacks' inferiority (Savitt, 1985). The harsh conditions to which black slaves were subjected were rarely mentioned as contributing to their susceptibility to specific diseases or to their poor health.

Male slaves were valued for their work, while the value of female slaves was determined not only by their capacity for work, but their capacity to reproduce and to increase the human property that formed the basis for the slave economy. Because female slaves were property, without any degree of autonomy, they were subject to their masters' sexual desires (Jacobs, 1988; Smith, 1988). Slaves were physically mutilated for real and imagined offenses (Hurmence, 1984; Jacobs, 1988). Lavinia Bell's treatment as a slave was all too common:

> After that time she was sent into the cotton field with the other field hands, where the treatment was cruelly severe. No clothes whatever were allowed them, their hair was cut off close to their head, and thus were exposed to the glare of a southern sun from early morn until late at night. Scarcely a day passed without their receiving fifty lashes, whether they worked or whether they did not. They were also compelled to go down on their knees, and harnessed to a plough, to plough up the land, with boys for riders, to whip them when they flagged in their work. At other times, they were compelled to walk on hackles, used for hackling flax. Her feet are now dotted over with scars, caused by their brutality.... Still later, for some disobedience on her part, they hoisted her into a tree, locked a chain round her neck, and handcuffed her wrists, the marks being yet visible. There she was left for two days and nights, without a morsel to eat, being taunted with such questions as to whether she was hungry and would like something to eat.... (Blassingame, 1977: 342–343).

This failure to provide food for a slave was regarded as "the most aggravated development of meanness even among slaveholders" (Douglass, 1968: 34).

Disagreement exists with respect to the medical treatment that slaves received. Accounts from slaves seem to indicate that, even as judged by the standards of the time, medical care was often poor. Midwives or doctors were rarely in attendance at the birth of a slave's child. At least one author, however, has argued that medical care of slaves was often superior to that received by their owners, if only because the slave represented a financial investment which could be threatened by ill health (Kolchin, 1993). Slaves not infrequently resorted to remedies at home rather than report their illness to the person in charge and be required to submit to the medical care provided at the behest of the owner. Consequently, a dual system of health care developed (Savitt, 1985).

Poor living conditions exacerbated existing health problems. Although slaves were provided with housing, they were rarely provided with toilets (Blassingame, 1977). The housing itself was often characterized by poor ventilation, lack of light, and damp, earthen floors (Semmes, 1996). There was little opportunity to bathe or to wash clothes, resulting in the promotion of bedbugs and body lice. The soil and water were often infested with worms and larvae, to which the slaves were particularly vulnerable due to the lack of shoes and the poor sanitation (Blassingame, 1979; Savitt, 1978). Roundworm, threadworm, tapeworm, and hookworm infestations plagued many slaves. The practice of eating soil (geophagy), which was continued from West Africa, further promoted infestation with worms (Savitt, 1978).

Poor diets and food shortages further contributed to the development of poor health. Slaveowners frequently provided the slaves with pork, which was the preferred source of protein for the owners. However, the slaveowners retained the leanest cuts for themselves, and passed on the fatty portions, together with cornmeal, to the slaves. On some plantations, slaves rarely had dairy products, fruits, or vegetables (Stampp, 1956). Not surprisingly, the slaves' poor diet often resulted in deficiencies in vitamins, including vitamins A, B, C, and D. These deficiencies, in turn, led to disease such as scurvy, beriberi, and pellagra (Savitt, 1978).

Slaves were the unwilling subjects of scientific experimentation. When compensation was offered, it was provided to the master owning the slave, rather than to the slave participating in the experiment. As an example, the physician J. Marion Sims reached an agreement with one slaveowner to maintain several of his female slaves at his expense in exchange for their use in experiments intended to design strategies for the repair of vesicovaginal fistulas (Sims, 1894).

African-American Health during Reconstruction

Poor housing and poor sanitation continued into the period of Reconstruction (Blassingame, 1973; Morais, 1967). African-Americans suffered from pellagra and other nutritional-deficiency diseases (Johnson, 1966), for which they were themselves held responsible. One physician opined

His [the Negro] diet is fatty; he revels in fat; every pore of his sleek, contented face wreaks with unctuousness. To him the force-producing quality of the fats has the seductive fascination that opium leaves about the Oriental . . . (Tipton, 1886, quoted in Charatz-Litt, 1992: 717).

The high rates of death among African-Americans were attributable primarily to heart disease, tuberculosis, influenza, nephritis, cancer, pellagra, and malaria (Johnson, 1966). In fact, New York Life's and Equitable's actuaries predicted that blacks would be extinct by the year 2000 as the result of the extremely high mortality rate (Haller, 1971). Congress responded to the high death rates among African-Americans with the passage of the Freedmen's legislation, which opened universities, hospitals, soup kitchens, and clinics in the South (Blassingame, 1973; Morais, 1967).

Science and scientists were neither more benevolent nor more astute in their observations concerning African-Americans than they had been during previous eras. Dr. G. Frank Lydston, a professor of genitourinary surgery and syphilology at the Chicago College of Physicians, decried the rape of white women by African-American men and attributed such events to characteristics deemed to be innate to African-Americans:

When all inhibitions of a high order have been removed by sexual excitement, I fail to see any difference from a physical standpoint between the sexual furor of the negro and that which prevails among the lower animals in certain instances and at certain periods . . . namely, that the *furor sexualis* in the negro resembles similar sexual attacks in the bull and elephant, and the running amuck of the Malay race. This *furor sexualis* has been especially frequent among the negroes in States cursed by carpetbag statesmanship, in which frequent changes in the social and commercial status of the Negro race have occurred (McGuire and Lydston, 1893: 111, quoted in Haller, Jr., 1971: 53) (italics in original).

African-American Health during the Twentieth Century

The late 1800s and the beginning of the 1900s were characterized by significant migration of African-Americans from rural to urban areas. The Great Migration to northern urban areas, which began in 1915, was associated with pull factors in the North, such as employment opportunities, and push factors from the South, including a depressed demand for labor, low wages, floods, segregation, discrimination, lynching, and poor educational opportunities (Woodson, 1969).

African-Americans continued to suffer from serious health problems despite migration to urban areas. During the early 1920s, for instance, tuberculosis was responsible for three times as many deaths among blacks as among whites in New York City. Harlem's rate of infant mortality from

1923 to 1927 was 111 per 1,000, compared to a rate of 64.5 per 1,000 for the entire city of New York (Osofsky, 1966). Such disparities, particularly in the South, have been attributed in part to the actions of the white medical community (Charatz-Litt, 1992). White physicians often refused to treat black patients. Black physicians were rendered less effective in treating patients due to their inferior medical training and their exclusion from membership in many medical associations and societies, thereby precluding them from accessing new techniques (Byrd and Clayton, 1992; Charatz-Litt, 1992; Seham, 1964).

The National Hospital Association (NHA) was organized in 1923 as a member of the National Medical Association (NMA). Although the NMA's mission emphasized the education of its black physician members, the NHA focused on equality for blacks in the southern health care system (Charatz-Litt, 1992). It was not until the mid-1960s, however, that the American Medical Association (AMA) reaffirmed its intent to cease racially discriminatory exclusion policies and practices (Anonymous, 1965). The movement toward recognition of black physicians was due in large measure to the passage of federal legislation, such as the Civil Rights Act, requiring cessation of discriminatory and exclusionary policies and practices (Byrd and Clayton, 1992).

Blacks were often solicited as subjects of medical experiments. M. Robert Hines, for instance, obtained spinal fluid from 423 sick and healthy black infants at an Atlanta hospital, apparently without the consent of the children's parents or guardians. A number of children suffered trauma, including blood in the spinal fluid, as the result of the needle puncture (Roberts, 1925).

The Tuskegee syphilis study is perhaps the most notorious scientific experiment conducted with blacks as subjects of research. In 1929, the United States Public Health Service (USPHS) conducted a study to examine the prevalence of syphilis among blacks and possible mechanisms for treatment. The town of Tuskegee, located in Macon County in Alabama, was found to have the highest rate of syphilis among the six counties that had been included in the study (Gill, 1932; Jones, 1981). This study, funded by the Julius Rosenwald Fund, concluded that mass treatment of syphilis would be feasible. However, funding became inadequate for the continuation of the project and the implementation of the treatment due to the economic depression that commenced in 1929 and which devastated the Fund's financial resources (Thomas and Quinn, 1991).

The Tuskegee study was initiated in 1932 by the USPHS to follow the natural history of untreated, latent syphilis in black males. The impetus for the study derived in part from conflict between the prevailing scientific view in the United States of the progression of syphilis in blacks and the results of a study by Bruusgard in Norway. The U.S. view held that syphilis affected the neurological functioning in whites, but the cardiovascular system in blacks. Bruusgaard, however, had found from his retrospective study of white men with untreated syphilis that cardiovascular effects were common and neurological complications rare (Clark and Danbolt, 1955). However, even at the time that the Tuskegee study was initiated, there existed general consensus within the medical community that syphilis required treatment even in its latent stages, despite the toxic effects of treatment. Moore (1933: 237), a venereologist, observed:

> Though it imposes a slight though measurable risk of its own, treatment markedly diminishes the risk from syphilis. In latent syphilis . . . the probability of progression, relapse, or death is reduced from a probable 25–30 percent without treatment to about 5 percent with it; and the gravity of the relapse if it occurs, is markedly diminished.

Interest in other racial differences also provided impetus to continue with the study. Blacks were believed to possess an excessive sexual desire, a lack of morality (Hazen, 1914; Quillian, 1906), and an attraction to white women stemming from "racial instincts that are about as amenable to ethical culture as is the inherent odor of the race . . . " (Howard, 1903: 424).

The original Tuskegee study was to include black males between the ages of 25 and 60 who were infected with syphilis. The study required a physical examination, x-rays, and a spinal tap. The original design did not contemplate the provision of treatment to those enrolled in the study, despite existing consensus in the medical community regarding the necessity of treatment (Brandt, 1985). However, those recruited for the study were advised that they were ill with "bad blood," a term referring to syphilis, and would be provided with treatment. The mercurial ointment and neoarsphenamine provided to subjects as treatment were ineffective and intended to be ineffective. Similarly, the spinal tap which was administered for diagnostic purposes only was portrayed as a "special treatment" to encourage participation. A control group of healthy uninfected men was added to the study as controls in 1933, following USPHS' approval to continue with the study (Brandt, 1985).

The researchers themselves noted the conditions that made this extended study possible: follow-up by a nurse who was known to the participants and who came from the community from which they were recruited; the provision to the subjects of the research burial assistance, which they might not have otherwise been able to afford; the provision of transportation to the subjects by the nurse; and government sponsorship of the "care" that the subjects believed, and had been led to believe, was being furnished to them (Rivers, Schuman, Simpson, and Olansky, 1953).

The Tuskegee study continued for 40 years, despite various events that should have signaled its termination. First, the USPHS had begun to administer penicillin to some syphilitic patients in various treatment clinics (Mahoney, Arnold, Sterner, Harris, and Zwally, 1944). By at least 1945, it was clear in the professional literature that syphilis infections would respond to treatment with penicillin, even in cases that had been resistant to treatment with bismuth subsalicylate and mapharsen, a then-standard treatment (Noojin, Callaway, and Flower, 1945). Yet, subjects of the Tuskegee study were not only not offered penicillin treatment, but were also prevented from receiving care when they sought it out (Thomas and Quinn, 1991). Second, a series of articles had been published in professional journals indicating that the subjects were suffering to a much greater degree than the controls with increased morbidity and a reduction in life expectancy (Deibert and Bruyere, 1946; Heler and Bruyere, 1946; Pesare, Buer, and Gleeson, 1950; Vonderlehr, Clark, Wenger, and Heller, 1950). Yet, defenders of the study asserted as late as 1974 that there was inadequate basis for treatment with either penicillin or other regimens during the course of the study and that it was the "*shibboleth* of informed consent...born in court decisions in California (1957) and Kansas (1960)" that provoked the furor over the study (Kampmeier, 1974: 1352). Clearly, the Nuremberg Code of 1949 was ignored.

It was not until 1972 that the then-existing Department of Health, Education, and Welfare convened an advisory panel in response to the criticism triggered by media coverage of the experiment (Brandt, 1985). The report of that committee focused on the failure to provide penicillin treatment and the failure to obtain informed consent. According to Brandt (1985), this emphasis obscured the historical facts regarding the availability of drug treatment for syphilis prior to the advent of penicillin and ignored the fact that the men believed that they were receiving clinical care and did not know that they were part of an experiment (Brandt, 1985).

The Tuskegee study has had a far-reaching impact. The study has, for many blacks, become a "symbol of their mistreatment by the medical establishment, a metaphor for deceit, conspiracy, malpractice, and neglect, if not outright racial genocide" (Jones, 1992: 38). As a consequence, educational programs designed to combat HIV in black communities have been met with distrust and a belief that AIDS and/or AIDS prevention and care represent forms of racial genocide (Jones, 1992; Thomas and Quinn, 1991).

Perhaps not coincidentally, the Tuskegee study had been initiated during a time, the 1920s and 1930s, when the eugenics movement provided a scientific platform from which those deemed to be inferior could be controlled politically. The eugenicists of the time reflected a diversity of professions, including biologists, animal breeders, psychologists, criminologists, social workers, and activists of racist and nativist organizations (Tucker, 1994). Unlike the scientist Galton's plea for the use of "better stocks" to improve the condition of the human race, American eugenicists focused on those groups and individuals believed to be "unfit." State legislation permitting the involuntary sterilization of "degenerates," promulgated largely in response to the efforts of eugenicists, ultimately resulted in the sterilization of over 45,000 individuals in 30 states (Gurch and Pendell, 1947). The eugenicists assured the American public that such laws would disproportionately affect blacks and immigrants, allowing those Americans of "good stock" to continue propagating (Tucker, 1994: 61).

But African-Americans were impacted by more than the Tuskegee study, and still yet in the name of science. As late as the 1960s, a number of scientists claimed that African-Americans suffered as a result of biology, not political oppression and racism: "It is what he is that makes the Negro a second class citizen, not segregation" (Putnam, 1961). Dwight Ingle, a physiologist with the University of Chicago, proposed in 1964 that because "the very high birth rate among indolent incompetent Negroes" posed "a threat to the future success of this race," that "conception control [be imposed] for all who, either because of genetic limitations or because of poor cultural heritage, are unable to endow children with a reasonable chance to achieve happiness, self-sufficiency and good citizenship" (Ingle, 1964: 378).

William Shockley, a professor of engineering at Stanford University and one of the recipients of the Nobel Prize for the development of the transistor, argued vociferously that "the major deficit in Negro intellectual performance must be primarily of hereditary origin and thus relatively irremediable by practical improvements in environment "(Schockley, 1968: 87–88). As late as 1988, scientists continued to argue that evolution was responsible for the supposed intellectual inferiority of African-Americans (Rushotn, 1988). These scientific assertions were not without political consequence, as they were ultimately utilized to support segregationist policies; the platforms of extremeist organizations, such as the Ku Klux Klan and the American Nazi Party; and the ideology of politicians such as Lousiana's David Duke (Tucker, 1994).

Substance Use and Health

Infectious Disease

HIV/AIDS. Although African-Americans represent only 12 percent of the total United States population, they account for almost 38 percent of all

AIDS cases reported in this country (Centers for Disease Control and Prevention, 2002b). For the year 2000, African-American women represented almost two-thirds of all women reported with AIDS. The rate of reported AIDS cases among African-Americans in the year 2000 was 58.1 per 100,000, more than two times the rate among Hispanics and eight times the rate for whites (Centers for Disease Control and Prevention, 2002b). The sharing of needles and the trading of sex for drugs have been implicated as factors in these high rates; these behaviors place not only the substance user, but his or her sexual partner and children at risk of infection as well. In the year 2000, AIDS cases associated with injection drug use accounted for 26 percent of all AIDS cases among African-Americans (Centers for Disease Control and Prevention, 2002a). A study of mortality resulting from AIDS in South Carolina found that African-Americans with AIDS were at increased risk of death at one year as compared to whites (Scott, Sy, Jackson, Macera, and Harris, 1997).

Syphilis. The incidence rate of syphilis, which can be transmitted through needlesharing as well as through sexual contact, is high among African-Americans. In the year 2000, 70.8 percent of all cases of primary and secondary syphilis reported to the Centers for Disease Control and Prevention occurred among African-Americans. The rate of syphilis in the year 2000 among African-Americans was 12.8 cases per 100,000 persons, which is 21 times greater than the rate among non-Hispanic whites (Centers for Disease Control and Prevention, 2002f).

Hepatitis B and C. African-Americans experience a higher incidence rate of hepatitis C than do non-Hispanic whites (Kinzie et al., 2001), but have been found to be less likely to report injection drug use as a risk factor (Bonacini, Groshen, Yu, Govindarajan, and Lindsay, 2001).

Tuberculosis. In the year 2001, a total of 2.3 percent of all persons reported to have tuberculosis were known to have injected drugs, and 7.2 percent had used noninjecting drugs (Centers for Disease Control and Prevention, 2002g). In the same year, slightly more than 15 percent of individuals reported to have tuberculosis had an excess of alcohol use. A breakdown of these categories by ethnic group is unavailable. However, for the year 2001, the largest proportion of tuberculosis cases were reported among African-Americans (4,796 of a total of 15,989 cases).

Substance Use

Alcohol advertising targeting the African-American communities in the United States has emphasized the sale of malt liquor to young adults through the use of "power" and gang-related images (Alaniz and Wilkes, 1998). Nevertheless, African-American teens have been found less likely than those of other ethnic groups to misuse alcohol (Ellickson, McGuigan, Adams, Bell, and Hays, 1996).

Among young African-Americans, those who drop out of high school have been found to be at elevated risk for alcohol disorders, as compared to those who have an associate's degree or greater. In comparison, among non-Hispanic whites, individuals who enter college but do not graduate with a degree appear to be at increased risk of alcohol disorders (Crum and Anthony, 2000). Research further suggests that, among African-Americans, those who do not complete high school are twice as likely to engage in injecting drug use. The award of a graduate equivalency certificate (GED) in lieu of high school completion does not appear to reduce this increased risk (Obot, Hubbard, and Anthony, 1999). However, a study involving a diverse sample of high school students found that African-American youth are less likely than others to engage in simultaneous polydrug use (Collins, Ellickson, and Bell, 1998).

Various factors have been found to be protective against alcohol misuse. Data from a 1984 national survey of subsamples of 1,224 African American women and 1,034 non-Hispanic women indicate that African Americans tend to have more conservative drinking norms for women (Herd, 1997). Adolescent religious involvement appears to reduce the likelihood of alcohol use (Heath, Madden, Grant, McLaughlin, Todorov, and Bucholz, 1999).

A study of 708 patients admitted to treatment at a health maintenance organization's chemical dependency program found that, compared to non-Hispanic whites, African-Americans were more likely to be dependent on both alcohol and drugs, rather than either alcohol or drugs (Tam, Weisner, and Mertens, 2000). However, it was demonstrated in a study of primary care patients enrolled in a trial of brief interventions for problem drinking that, when alcohol problems do occur, African-Americans may be better able than non-Hispanic whites to address the drinking problems due to increased familiarity with coping mechanisms (Conigliaro, Maisto, McNeil, Kraemer, Kelley, Conigliaro, and O'Connor, 2000).

A study of tobacco advertising through the use of billboards in St. Louis noted that tobacco billboards are most likely to be found in low income areas and areas with a higher percentage of African-Americans. Approximately 74 percent of the billboards in St. Louis were found to be located within 2000 feet of public school property (Luke, Esmundo, and Bloom, 2000). Despite such advertising efforts, it appears that receptivity to protobacco media is lower among African-American youth ages 12 to 17, as compared with non-Hispanic whites of the same age group (Chen, Cruz, Schuster, Unger, and Johnson, 2002).

Research findings regarding the rates of cigarette use among African-American youth have been inconsistent. Research has demonstrated that the use of cigarettes and smokeless tobacco appears to be less common among African-American youth than among adolescents from other ethnic groups (Griesler, Kandel, and Davies, 2002; Hu, Hedeker, Flay, Sussman, Day, and Siddiqui, 1996; Khoury, Warheit, Zimmerman, Vega, and Gil, 1996) and, when smoking is initiated, it occurs at a later age among African-American youth as compared with youth of other ethnic groups (Lando, Haddock, Robinson, Klesges, and Talcott, 2000). Other studies, however, appear to indicate that there is a higher prevalence of smoking among African-Americans as compared with other groups (Richardson, 1997; Emont, Dorrell, Bishop, and McClain, 1995). Being African-American has been associated with an increased likelihood of using mentholated cigarettes (Hyland, Garten, Giovino, and Cummings, 2002).

Compared to women in other ethnic groups, African-American women are more likely to view not smoking as a positive identity marker (Mermelstein, 1999). This may also hold true for adolescents, as research indicates that the perception of looking different from other ethnic groups has been associated among African-American teens with the avoidance of peer tobacco use (Parker, Sussman, Crippens, Elder, and Scholl, 1998). Lower rates of current smoking have been found among pregnant African-American women as compared with non-Hispanic white women (Arnold, Davis, Berkel, Jackson, Nandy, and London, 2001).

Research suggests that individuals who use crack may be particularly vulnerable to drug-associated difficulties. A study of 203 African-American women who used crack cocaine found that, although they may have entered prostitution in order to obtain funds for their drugs, their increase in drug usage was often linked to efforts to deal with the distress caused by activities associated with the prostitution (Young, Boyd, and Hubbell, 2000). Another study of 602 African-American individuals who used and/or sold powder cocaine, crack cocaine, and/or heroin found that frequent crack and multiple hard drug users were equally likely to be involved in drug distribution activities. However, those using crack were less likely to be employed either on a part-time or a full-time basis and were also less likely to be recipients of any form of public assistance (Cross, Johnson, Davis, and Liberty, 2001).

ASIANS AND PACIFIC ISLANDERS: HISTORICAL AND CULTURAL CONTEXT

Although Asians and Pacific Islanders, as defined by the U.S. census, constitute only 3 percent of the U.S. population, they are the fastest growing minority group in the United States (1990 Census in Lum, 1995; Takaki, 1989). This increase is attributable to several factors, including the passage and implementation of the Immigration Act of 1965, which removed provisions excluding Asians from entry into the United States, and the influx of refugees from Southeast Asia beginning in 1975 (Burr and Mutchler, 1993; Lin-Fu, 1988; McKeney and Bennett, 1994; Takaki, 1989).

The Asian and Pacific Islander population of the United States is extremely diverse, encompassing at last count 29 different Asian groups and 20 different Pacific Islander groups, which together speak over 100 languages (Loue, Lloyd, and Loh, 1996). According to the 1980 census, 6 subgroups accounted for more than 95 percent of the Asian Pacific Islander population: Chinese, Filipino, Japanese, Asian Indian, Korean, and Vietnamese (Lin-Fu, 1988).

The Asian and Pacific Islander population is equally diverse with respect to socioeconomic status, migration patterns, access to health care, and risk for specific diseases; these factors are inter-related. For example, as a group, Japanese Americans tend to be more highly acculturated and of higher socioeconomic status. This is not surprising, in view of their migration to the U.S. since the late nineteenth century. In contrast, recent arrivals from Southeast Asia tend to be poor, less acculturated, and face increased barriers to health care, such as language (Takada, Ford, and Lloyd, 1998). Southeast Asian refugees may have also suffered higher levels of stress and trauma in migration, which may, in turn, affect their health.

As a group, Asians and Pacific Islanders appear to have few health problems and to be well insured for health care (Mayeno and Hirota, 1994; Smith and Ryan, 1987). Unfortunately, these aggregated data mask the large variation within the Asian and Pacific Islander population. The 1980 census, for instance, indicated that 7.5 percent of all Asian Americans have an annual family income over $50,000 (Mayeno and Hirota, 1994). However, Asian Americans also had the highest proportion of unrelated persons (individuals not living in the same household) with yearly incomes below $2,000 (Mayeno and Hirota, 1994). A San Diego survey of Asian Americans found that 75.8 percent lived below the poverty level, while 53 percent of the Vietnamese in a San Francisco Bay area survey reported incomes below the federal poverty level (Mayeno and Hirota, 1994).

Many Asians and Pacific Islanders work in low wage jobs, such as factory and service industry positions, which often do not provide either employer-sponsored health insurance or sufficient resources to permit the employees to purchase health insurance. A recent study in Boston's Chinatown found that 61 percent of the employed uninsured earned less than $10,000 per year (Mayeno and Hirota, 1994). Studies conducted in California and Chicago have similarly found that high proportions of some

Asian American groups lacked health insurance coverage (Mayeno and Hirota, 1994).

The Cultural and Historical Context

Language and Acculturation

Language may constitute a significant barrier to care. Limited reading skills in both one's native language and in English may reduce one's ability to read and understand signs in health care facilities, paperwork and informational materials, as well as provider instructions (Mayeno and Hirota, 1994). A study conducted in San Diego in 1988 found that 60 percent of the individuals surveyed attributed difficulty in obtaining health care to language (Mayeno and Hirota, 1994).

Levels of acculturation differ not only between individuals but across groups as well. Individuals who are more acculturated to U.S. society tend to rely to a greater degree on Western medicine. Less acculturated groups and individuals are more likely to rely on alternative explanatory models of health and illness and, consequently, more traditional methods of care. For instance, many Southeast Asians view health as a state of equilibrium or balance with disease and illness resulting from disequilibrium or an imbalance of specific forces or elements (Jenkins, Le, McPhee, et al., 1996; Miller, 1995; Shimada, Jackson, Goldstein, and Buchwald, 1995; Uba, 1992), often treatable with herbal medicines (Jenkins et al., 1996). The lack of health professionals who understand the cultural context of Asians and Pacific Islanders may interact with the difficulties in communication due to language differences to further compound the problems faced in accessing care (Takada, Ford, and Lloyd, 1998).

Explanatory Models of Health and Illness

An understanding of culture-specific explanatory models for health and illness is critical to understanding how individuals interpret and respond to illness episodes, including those occasioned in connection with substance use. These conceptualizations of health and illness, which differ from the Western medical perspective, may impact individual's willingness to seek care and to adhere to the medical recommendations that they receive.

Numerous studies of health beliefs among Southeast Asians have often failed to distinguish between various Southeast Asian groups, e.g., Thai, Lao, Cambodian, etc., but have dealt instead with health and illness beliefs as if they were alike across all groups. Not infrequently, researchers have failed to specify which Southeast Asian groups are being discussed, making cross-study comparisons difficult.

Mattson (1995) has identified three categories of illness causation common to many Southeast Asians: (1) physical causes, such as accidents or spoiled food; (2) metaphysical causes, such as an imbalance of *yin* and *yang*, of hot and cold energy, of diet, or of emotions; and (3) supernatural causes, such as evil spirits or soul loss. Disease results from imbalance and disharmony and illness is attributed to deficiencies or excesses of physical, spiritual, or natural elements. These beliefs impact upon individuals' health seeking behaviors and utilization of services. For instance, Mattson (1995) notes that many Southeast Asian women will avoid pelvic examinations because they believe that dilation of the vagina with a speculum will expose the woman to wind and result in the loss of heat and the influx of cold. In situations in which an illness is believed to have been brought about by an imbalance of *yin* and *yang*, individuals are more likely to self-medicate with herbs than to seek out a traditional or religious healer or Western health care provider (Uba, 1992).

The Mien, a Southeast Asian hill people, originally migrated from China to various parts of Southeast Asia in the 13th century. Although they have continued to live predominantly in Thailand and in Laos, Mien have immigrated to various countries beginning in the mid-1970s (Moore and Boehnlein, 1991). The Mien believe that illness may result from environmental exposures, such as dampness, inadequate food, or germs. Such illnesses can be cured by using herbal remedies or by modifying the environmental factors. An illness that does not respond to such treatment is thought to be a disorder of the spirit world, such as soul loss, requiring treatment by a shaman. Regardless of the postulated cause of the illness, emotional distress tends to be expressed through the verbalization of somatic symptoms (Moore and Boehnlein, 1991). This manner of expressing emotional distress has been noted among other Asian groups as well.

The Hmong, another hill tribe of Southeast Asia, emigrated from China into Vietnam, Laos, Thailand, and Myanmar (Quincy, 1988). Until recent years, the Hmong's cultivation and use of opium in their traditional residences in the highland areas of these countries was legal (Lintner, 1999). These activities continue today in many of the villages, albeit less openly than once occurred. Opium as a crop offers significant advantages because it requires neither sophisticated mechanisms to prevent spoilage nor specific types of packaging (Lintner, 1999).

The Hmong, and other hill tribes, often ate raw opium after mixing it with other substances, such as garlic. Ingested opium was used as a remedy for pain, cough, dysentery, and to alleviate the symptoms of malaria. The

Hmong began smoking opium recreationally after having seen tobacco smoking (Renard, 2001). Eating, however, permitted greater absorption of the opium compound and was generally seen as more convenient and more pleasurable. Westermeyer (1982: 57) has described the Hmong practice of smoking opium:

> Regular opium smokers usually had a small glass kerosene lamp, although older Hmong said that a lamp of pig fat was decidedly superior. Each ball of opium is placed on a small iron skewer and heated over the flame. As it begins to bubble and fume, it is deftly placed in the small aperture of the pipe. The smoker then places the pipe in his mouth as the flame is applied to the opium wad. With an opium lamp, this process is facilitated by reclining on one's side and holding the pipe so the aperture is horizontal to the ground... At the moment when the opium volatizes from the heat, the smoker inhales deeply. Experienced users then contract their chest, abdominal and diaphragmatic muscles against a closed glottis so to realize an optimal effect. This operation, called the Val Salva maneuver by physiologists, increases the intrapulmonary pressure and facilitates the rapid absorption of the active opiate compounds across the pulmonary membranes directly into the blood stream. These compounds can be absorbed only from the pulmonary alveoli, not across the trachea and the bronchial tree.

Opium in its volatized form was used as a remedy for children for their fever, diarrhea, and cough (Westermeyer, 1982). It has been hypothesized that increasing government pressure beginning in the 1980s on the Hmong and other hill tribes to reduce opium production contributed to the increase in heroin use (Renard, 2001).

The CIA of the U.S. began recruiting Hmong assistance for the "secret army" beginning in 1962. This effort and the subsequent series of events resulted in Hmong resettlement in the U.S. Capps (1994) has examined the impact of migration to the U.S. on the Hmong traditional health and illness beliefs, one of the few studies to concern itself with modifications to health beliefs following migration from a developing to a developed nation.

Capps found that many Hmong converted to Christianity and abandoned animistic practices following relocation to Kansas City. Although Hmong individuals frequently continued to attribute illness to a "traditional" cause, such as sorcery or ancestral spirits' removal of their protection of individuals in response to improper behavior, individuals refused to consult a shaman for healing because of fear that they would be ostracized from the now-converted Hmong community. Interestingly, consultation with a shaman has been replaced by prayer.

Fright illness (*ceeb*) continues to be a common illness among the immigrated Hmong. This syndrome results from immersion in cold water, a car accident, or other unexpected and similarly startling events. *Ceeb* is believed to tighten the veins, resulting in a reduced flow of blood and cold extremities. The Kansas City Hmong no longer treat *ceeb* with soul-calling rituals, but rely instead on massage and prayer (Capps, 1994).

Koucharang, believed by Cambodians to be the result of turbulent emotions or of "thinking too much," is characterized by intrusive thoughts, headaches, and suicidal ideation. It is not, however, perceived to be a kind of mental illness or problem. The syndrome has most often been noted among Cambodians exposed to severe violence in their home countries and has been documented among Cambodian refugees in California and Massachusetts (Frye and D'Avanzo, 1994b). Because it is not perceived as a mental disorder, individuals suffering from *koucharang* are unlikely to seek out either counseling or medical services.

Chinese, including Chinese in the United States, have been found to have five basic explanations for disease causation: wind, which is thought to enter the body when it is in an especially vulnerable state; an imbalance of hot and cold; poison; blockages of *ch'i*, the energy force; and fright. Gould-Martin and Ngin (1981) have found that Chinese Americans are often able to reconcile the popular Chinese explanation for specific illnesses with the popular American explanation, such as wind as a cause of illness (Chinese) and wind-borne dust as a cause of illness (American).

Many East Indians subscribe to the precepts of ayurvedic medicine. A detailed review of Ayurvedic principles is beyond the scope of this chapter. Briefly, Ayurveda enumerates five elements in the universe: water, fire, earth, wind, and ether. Fire, water, and wind constitute the three humors found in the body as bile, phlegm, and wind, respectively. An imbalance in these humors results in illness, whereas homeostasis maintains health. Humoral equilibrium can be lost due to the consumption of foods that are inappropriately "hot" or "cold", *i.e.*, the nature of the food is such that it increases or decreases the heat in the body (Ramakrishna and Weiss, 1992). This emphasis on diet may impact patient expectations of the patient-provider relationship in that patients may expect physicians to conduct not only a complete examination and history, but also a complete dietary history as well (Ramakrishna and Weiss, 1992).

However, expectations and values are not governed by tradition alone, but are also subject to other influences. Many patients may believe, for instance, that capsules are stronger than tablets and that injections are superior to all other forms of treatment (Ramakrishna and Weiss, 1992). Such beliefs impact on patients' willingness to seek out care, the acceptability of the care received, and willingness to adhere to medical recommendations (Shimada et al., 1995).

The Historical Context

The migration experience of Asians and Pacific Islanders clearly differs between individuals and between specific groups; broad generalizations are, therefore, suspect. Too, the large number of subgroups classified as Asian and Pacific Islander renders impossible an examination of the migration experience and historical context of each group. This section presents a brief overview of three Asian and Pacific Islander subgroups. We must ask ourselves whether and how the migration experience of these populations relates to their current health and health care and the potential implications for substance abuse treatment and research.

Chinese Americans

Early Chinese migrants to the United States often came as laborers, intending to work temporarily in the U.S. and to return home with their earnings. During the latter half of the nineteenth century, approximately 46,000 Chinese migrated to Hawaii, while about 380,000 migrated to the U.S. mainland between 1849 and 1930 (Takaki, 1989). Many of these individuals sought refuge from ongoing conflict, including the British Opium Wars (1839–1842, 1856–1864) and peasant rebellions such as the Red Turban Rebellion (1854–1864), and from harsh economic conditions. The typical immigrant of this period was male, married, and generally unaccompanied by his wife and family due to the expense and, in the mainland U.S., to legislation restricting the entry of Chinese women (Osumi, 1982; Peffer, 1986; Wu, 1972).

The Chinese lived predominantly in rural areas for several decades, many of them settling in California and other areas in the West (Takaki, 1989). Gradually, the Chinese became an urban population, representing a wide range of socioeconomic statuses (Cao and Novas, 1996).

Initially, Chinese were welcomed into California as workers in the gold fields, in railroad construction, and in manufacturing (Cao and Novas, 1996). By the late 1860s, Chinese workers in San Francisco constituted almost half of those employed in four major industries: boots and shoes, woolens, tobacco, and sewing (Takaki, 1989). The Chinese population also became increasingly active in agriculture, primarily as laborers (Cao and Novas, 1996). However, the growing "ethnic antagonism" (Takaki, 1989: 92) that confronted the Chinese in mines, fields, and factories ultimately propelled them into self-employment situations, often in laundry, retail, or restaurants.

In the South, Chinese laborers were seen as role models for black workers due to their hard work and sense of economy. In the Northeast, the

Chinese population often worked in factories. Women were frequently employed as housekeepers, servants, cooks, miners, seamstresses, and laundresses. And, in a world dominated by men, many women were employed as prostitutes. Many of these women were treated as slaves and not infrequently became addicted to opium (Takaki, 1989).

As indicated in the preceding chapter, opium dens came to be associated with Chinese immigrants, who established some dens in the Chinatowns of major cities. At the time of their establishment, such enterprises were legally permitted. However, opium dens became the target of anti-Chinese propaganda that characterized Chinese immigrants as "yellow fiends" intending to enslave white women (Attias, cited in Fernandez, 1998).

Despite the growing reliance on the Chinese workforce in the late 1800s and early 1900s, the Chinese remained an "internal colony" (Takaki, 1989: 99), excluded from full participation in what was perceived to be a homogenous white society. This exclusion was premised on the perception of the Chinese as inferior, undesirable, and a threat to the survival of American society as a result of a myriad of potent and incurable diseases that they brought with them to the U.S. ("yellow peril") (Gussow, 1989). Their subordinate position was reinforced through various legal and political mechanisms, including court decisions disregarding the testimony of Chinese witnesses (Heizer and Almquist, 1977), the Chinese Exclusion Act of 1882 (Takaki, 1989), the Geary Act of 1892, which required the registration of all Chinese persons in the United States (Cao and Novas, 1996), the establishment of segregated schools, and political rhetoric (Lyman, 1971).

Although the Chinese were often perceived by others as temporary settlers, many immigrants formed Chinatowns and *fongs*, groupings of village associations. Recreation often took the form of Chinese theater and festivals. Viewed from the outside, Chinatowns were ghettos. In San Francisco's Chinatown in 1934, an average of 20.4 persons shared each bathroom and an average of 12.3 persons shared each kitchen. Over three quarters of Chinatown dwellings were found to be substandard, compared to one fifth of the dwellings in other parts of the city. The rate of tuberculosis was three times higher in Chinatown than in San Francisco's other residential areas (Lee, 1938).

One of the major issues remained the separation of China-born and U.S.-born Chinese from each other. Even as late as 1930, 80 percent of the U.S. Chinese population was male (Takaki, 1989). Under then-existing immigration laws, those Chinese born in the United States could bring in their overseas-born children, but could not bring in their China-born wives. Some such children came as "paper sons," claiming U.S. citizenship based on forged or purchased identity papers.

Education was seen as a bridge for second-generation Chinese Americans to improve their situation. Second generation Chinese were often caught between two worlds, uncomfortable with Chinese despite their Chinese appearance, but denied social and economic opportunities because of their appearance. Second generation Chinese often found themselves confined to a low-skill job market (Takaki, 1989).

The situation changed significantly with the advent of World War II and the development of animosities between the United States and Germany and Japan. Chinese became friends. Employment opportunities became available to Chinese in the armed services and in the defense industries. The exclusion laws that had been in place to prevent the entry of Chinese into the United States were repealed and Chinese immigrants were, for the first time, eligible to apply for naturalization as citizens of the United States (Takaki, 1989).

Japanese Americans

At the time the Chinese Exclusion Act of 1882 came into effect, there were just over 2,000 Japanese on the U.S. mainland. Within 40 years, the population reached an estimated 138,834 (Takaki, 1989). By 1930, approximately half of the Japanese population consisted of first generation immigrants (*Issei*), while the second half comprised second generation Japanese (*Nisei*). Almost half of the Japanese population resided in California. Many of the immigrants were farmers, merchants, and students, and many were quite well-educated (Spickard, 1996). Many, including the farm laborers and cannery workers, worked under harsh conditions characterized by long hours. Their poor diets not infrequently led to malnutrition and night blindness (Takaki, 1989).

The Japanese urban economy expanded greatly during the early 1900s. Enterprises, which included barber shops, poolrooms, laundries, hotels, and stores, provided the Japanese community with employment. Other Japanese entered farming on a large scale, obtaining land to farm through contracts, sharing, leasing, or ownership (Spickard, 1996).

The Japanese were often the target of both verbal and physical discrimination. Japanese were seen as competitors and a menace to American labor, so much so that labor organizations called for the expansion of the Chinese Exclusion Act to include the Japanese. The California legislature in 1913 passed legislation denying land ownership to "aliens ineligible to citizenship," which included the Japanese (California Statutes, 1913). A 1920 law prohibited these individuals from leasing agricultural land or acquiring it under the names of U.S.-born minor children, a strategy that had been used earlier to avoid the impact of the 1913 land ownership law (Takaki,

1989). The 1921 "Ladies' Agreement" barred the immigration of picture brides and sharply curtailed Japanese immigration to the U.S. (Kanzaki, 1921). The 1924 general immigration law specifically excluded from entry aliens ineligible to citizenship, *i.e.*, the Japanese.

Numerous other, more personal, objections were voiced against the *Issei*. The Japanese were seen as incapable of being good Americans, as "unassimilable... with great pride of race, [having] no idea of assimilating in the sense of amalgamation" (McClatchy, quoted in Daniels, 1962: 99). The Japanese were characterized as filthy individuals whose "nests pollute the communities like the running sores of leprosy" (*American Defender*, quoted in Ogawa, 1971: 13). Japanese men were perceived as sexually aggressive, lusting after white women (*Los Angeles Times*, quoted in Ogawa, 1971: 15) and, additionally, represented new, devious attempts by Japan to take over American territory (Spickard, 1996).

As with the Chinese, education was seen as a way out, a bridge to something better. Despite efforts to acquire higher education, however, *Nisei* were often trapped in the ethnic labor market, often due to racism and discrimination (Spickard, 1996). Numerous strategies were developed in an attempt to overcome these barriers, including the promotion of U.S. nationalism within the Japanese-American community, and the cultivation of an "American" lifestyle (Takaki, 1989).

The Japanese attack of Pearl Harbor during World War II fueled fears of the Japanese and ultimately resulted in the mass internment of Japanese Americans on the mainland U.S., but not Hawaii. Japanese, many of them native-born American citizens, were ordered to report to evacuation centers, from which they were transported to one of ten internment camps and housed in barracks and stalls that were often filthy and congested (Commission on Wartime Relocation and Internment of Civilians, 1997; Spickard, 1996; Takaki, 1989). Adults worked as wage earners for the government. It has been estimated that those who were interned suffered approximately $370 million in direct property losses, equivalent to between $1 billion and $3 billion in 1983 dollars, not including lost income and lost opportunities (Taylor, 1986). Despite their treatment by the U.S. government, about 33,000 *Nisei* served in the Armed Forces during the Second World War. It was not until 1988, though, that the U.S. government acknowledged the wrong committed by the internment (Reagan, 1988).

The Filipino Community

Unlike the Chinese and Japanese migrants to the United States, Filipino migrants came to Hawaii and to the mainland U.S. from what was a U.S. territory. Approximately 110,000 Filipinos had migrated to Hawaii by the mid-1930s; approximately 40,000 had arrived on the mainland. Most were poor and uneducated men, who saw themselves as temporary sojourners (Takaki, 1989).

On the mainland, most Filipinos worked in agriculture, with the remainder employed as service workers or in the Alaska salmon fisheries. Work in the fields entailed long hours, low pay, and often unsatisfactory conditions. Workers were often housed in crowded, flimsy bunkhouses that lacked insulation and sewage disposal. Continuing poor conditions ultimately prompted the Filipino workers in some areas to organize, demonstrate, and win concessions from the growers (Takaki, 1989).

Despite their status as "little brown brothers" in the Philippines, Filipinos encountered intense racial discrimination in the United States. They were often segregated or refused service altogether, prohibited from living in certain areas, and were ineligible to apply for citizenship. The passage of the Tydings McDuffie Act of 1934 granted commonwealth status to the protectorate of the Philippines and all Filipinos were subsequently reclassified as aliens, rather than nationals, laying the foundation for efforts to deport and repatriate them to their original home (Cao and Novas, 1996). Fears of Filipino sexuality and the resulting threat to white racial purity sparked and fueled racial violence (Takaki, 1989). Anti-miscegenation laws in many states prohibited intermarriage between Filipinos and whites. Those who intermarried often experienced social ostracism (Takaki, 1989).

World War II appears to have been somewhat of a watershed in Americans' perceptions of Filipinos. Filipino loyalty and patriotism prompted revisions to states' land laws that had prohibited the sale or leasing of land to Filipinos, the expansion of immigration provisions to permit the entry of Filipinos, and the revision of the citizenship laws to allow for the eligibility of Filipinos (Takaki, 1989).

Substance Use and Health

Infectious Disease

HIV/AIDS.   Initially, little attention was focused on HIV/AIDS in the Asian and Pacific Islander populations, due to both the relatively few cases that had been reported in this population and the erroneous belief that Asians and Pacific Islanders might be genetically immune to the infection (Gock, 1994; Lee and Fong, 1990). As of December 2001, a total of 6,157 AIDS cases among Asians and Pacific Islanders had been reported to the Centers for Disease Control and Prevention (Centers for Disease Control and Prevention, 2002f). For 1997, Asians and Pacific Islanders had the lowest rate of AIDS cases among all ethnic groups, 4.5 per 100,000 (Centers for Disease

Control and Prevention, 1997). These data mask, however, an alarming increase in the rate of reported AIDS cases among Asians and Pacific Islanders which, for the years 1987 through 1990, was similar to all other ethnic groups combined (Gock, 1994). Additionally, in large metropolitan areas with large Asian and Pacific Islander populations, the Asian and Pacific Islander communities have experienced the highest rate of increase in reported AIDS cases of any ethnic group (Toleran, 1991).

Numerous factors may contribute to the increase in HIV transmission among Asians and Pacific Islanders, including persistent stereotypes regarding immunity to the infection (Gock, 1994), low levels of knowledge about HIV and its transmission and prevention (Albrecht, Levy, Sugrue, Prohaska, and Ostrow, 1989; DiClemente, Zorn, and Temoshok, 1986; Siegel, Lazarus, Krasnovsky, Dubin, and Chesney, 1991; Strunin, 1991), risky sexual behaviors (Cochran, Mays, and Leung, 1991), and a belief in the inability to prevent infection stemming from a belief in karmic destiny (Loue, Lloyd, and Loh, 1996). Prevention efforts are rendered more challenging due to the cultural and linguistic diversity of the Asian and Pacific Islander communities (Brown, 1992; Gock, 1994; Loue, Lloyd, and Loh, 1996), cultural taboos related to sex communication (Brown, 1992; Loue et al., 1996), and the need to develop specific strategies for those engaging in higher risk behaviors within the broader Asian and Pacific Islander communities (Brown, 1992).

Hepatitis B.   The great majority of the 200 million individuals chronically infected with hepatitis B virus (HBV) worldwide are in Asia (Hann, 1994), so it is not surprising that hepatitis B infection is more common among Asian Americans than among other U.S. ethnic groups. Untreated, HBV may lead to hepatocellular carcinoma, chronic active hepatitis, and chronic liver disease (Hann, 1994; Mayeno and Hirota, 1994). HBV chronic carrier rates ranging from 5 percent to 15 percent have been reported in various Asian and Pacific Islander subpopulations (Franks, Berg, Kane, et al., 1989; London, 1990; McGlynn, London, Hann, and Sharrar, 1986; Szmuness, Stevens, Ikram, Much et al., 1978). Several studies have indicated that the death rate among Chinese American males suffering from hepatocellular carcinoma is significantly higher than the rate among whites (Fraumeni and Mason, 1974; Szmuness et al., 1978).

HBV is often transmitted in the Asian and Pacific population perinatally. Data indicate that the risk of perinatal transmission is 16 times greater among Asians and Pacific Islanders than it is for the entire U.S. population (Mayeno and Hirota, 1994). Barriers to the prevention of transmission include lack of knowledge about HBV and/or the relationship between HBV and liver disease (Jackson, Rhodes, Inui, and Buchwald, 1997; Jenkins, Le,

McPhee, and Stewart, 1996; Sworts and Riccitelli, 1997), and lack of immunization (Jenkins, McPhee, Bird, and Bonilla, 1990).

Tuberculosis. Asian Americans are also disproportionately affected by tuberculosis. The incidence rate among Asians and Pacific Islanders is more than 6 times that of the U.S. population as a whole, due in part to the high prevalence of tuberculosis in the countries of origin (Mayeno and Hirota, 1994). For the year 2001, Asians and Pacific Islanders experienced the highest case rate of any ethnic group: 32.7 cases per 100,000 persons, as compared to a rate of 1.6 per 100,000 among non-Hispanic whites. Of the 15,989 cases of tuberculosis reported that year, 3,552 were attributable to Asians and Pacific Islanders (Centers for Disease Control and Prevention, 2002g).

Mental Health and Illness

As indicated previously, mental illness is often relevant to substance abuse treatment and research due to the relatively high frequency of co-occurring disorders. Diagnosis of mental or emotional disorders among Asians and Pacific Islanders is often complex, due to language differences, difficulties in the application of Western diagnostic criteria to the presenting symptoms, and a lack of understanding by mental health professionals of the cultural context of the presenting symptoms (Ong, 1995). Additionally, many Asians and Pacific Islanders may be reluctant to utilize Western mental health services, often due to differing concepts of mental health and illness and the appropriate treatment for such disorders. For instance, many Asians and Pacific Islanders may express depression and anxiety somatically, perhaps due to the stigma associated with mental illness (Cheung and Dobkin de Rios, 1982; Flaskerud and Soldevilla, 1986; Kim and Rew, 1994). Typical presenting symptoms include anxiety, dizziness, fatigue, irritability, and lack of appetite (Flaskerud and Soldevilla, 1986; Kim and Rew, 1994). These symptoms may be attributed to karma, the actions of ancestral spirits (Ong, 1995), possession by evil spirits (Flaskerud and Soldevilla, 1986), character weakness or misdeeds (Flaskerud and Soldevilla, 1986; Kim and Renfrew, 1994). Treatment may consist of praying to ancestors, avoiding "thinking too much," and reliance on traditional techniques to restore balance in the body and in the environment (Flaskerud and Soldevilla, 1986; Frye and D'Avanzo, 1994a; Kim and Rew, 1994; Ong, 1995).

Mental health problems most commonly reported among Asians and Pacific Islanders are depression, schizophrenia, and problems associated with family discord, loss of status, and loss of self-esteem

(Agbayani-Siewert, 1994; Flaskerud and Soldevilla, 1986; Kim and Rew, 1994; Kuo, 1984; Ying, 1990). The experience of immigration itself, isolation from peers, poverty, and alienation from younger family members have been identified as risk factors for mental illness among Asians and Pacific Islanders (Lum 1995). Southeast Asians, in particular, have been found to have high rates of anxiety, depression, and post-traumatic stress disorder (PTSD), often in response to their escape experiences or the events that occurred during their resettlement in refugee camps (Carlson and Rosser-Hogan, 1993; Clarke et al., 1993; Palinkas and Pickwell, 1995; Lin-Fu, 1988; Sack et al., 1993; Tran, 1993). Racism has also been identified as a potential risk factor for impaired mental health and a barrier to the receipt of appropriate mental health services (Cheung and Dobkin de Rios, 1982).

Health care providers may not associate their patients' varied somatic complaints with a mental health disorder. Chronic headache has been found to be associated with depression among a sample of Cambodians (Handelman and Yeo, 1996). "Extreme sadness" and "thinking too much" are "culture-bound syndromes" among Cambodians that are associated with PTSD (Frye and D'Avanzo, 1994a; Moore and Boehnlein, 1991). "Thinking too much" is characterized by headache, chest pain, palpitations, shortness of breath, excess sleeping, and withdrawal. Alcohol and drugs may be used to cope with "thinking too much," although suicide may also be viewed as an option (Frye and D'Avanzo, 1994a).

Substance Use

Research has indicated that rates of alcohol misuse may be lower among Asians compared with other groups (Ellickson, McGuigan, Adams, Bell, and Hays, 1996; Akutsu, Sue, Zane, and Nakamura, 1989). Lower rates of alcohol use and alcoholism have been found among some Asians with a specific mutation in the aldehyde dehydrogenase (ALDH2) gene. Asian individuals with this gene may experience severe hangovers compared to those without the gene, leading researchers to hypothesize that the ALDH2*2 allele may serve to protect these individuals against problematic drinking (Wall, Horn, Johnson, Smith, and Carr, 2000). Alcohol consumption patterns appear to be heavier among individuals of Japanese ethnicity in comparison with other subgroups. Heavier drinking has been associated with having friends who drink (Chi, Lubben, and Kitano, 1989).

Asians seem to experience difficulty in accessing care for alcohol disorders in comparison with other ethnic groups. This has been attributed to poor case recognition among primary care providers and consequent lack of referral (Commander, Odell, Williams, Sashidharan, and Surtees, 1999). Language and lack of health insurance may also constitute barriers to accessing care. HMO-based research indicates that, compared with other groups, Asian patients are more likely to be dissatisfied with the performance of their primary care physicians (Murray-Garcia, Selby, Schmittdiel, Grumbach, and Quesenberry, 2000). Participation in health research, including clinical trials, has been low, although the reasons for the lack of participation are unclear (Ray-Mazumder, 2001).

Data from the National Youth Tobacco Survey conducted during 2000 indicate that during the last year of high school, approximately one-third of Asian American youth are smokers (Appleyard, Messeri, and Haviland, 2001). Findings from the 1990–1996 California Tobacco Survey and the California Youth Tobacco Survey, which assessed smoking behaviors among California youth in grades 7 through 10, indicate that the lifetime prevalence of smoking among Asian youth is 16.1 percent, compared to 26.1 percent among non-Asians, while the 30-day smoking rate was 6.9 percent, compared to 14.2 percent among non-Asians. The lifetime prevalence of smoking was highest among Filipino youth, compared to other Asian Americans (Chen, Unger, Cruz, and Johnson, 1999). Research in other areas of the country similarly found the lowest prevalence of smoking among Asian youth, compared to others (French and Perry, 1996; Giovino et al., 1994; Foreyt, Jackson, Squires, et al., 1993). Higher levels of acculturation have been found to be associated with higher prevalence rates of smoking and earlier age of smoking onset (Chen, Unger, Cruz, and Johnson, 1999). However, increased length of time in the United States appears to be associated with decreased smoking prevalence among young Vietnamese males (Wiecha, 1996).

A recent study of tobacco use among Chinese Americans in Chicago found that 34 percent of the male respondents and 2 percent of the female respondents reported smoking. Smoking among men was found to be significantly associated with a low level of education, the use of a non-Western physician or clinic for health care, and a lack of knowledge about the early warning signs and symptoms of cancer (Yu, Chen, Kim, and Abdulrahim, 2002).

Relatively little research has focused on the use of specific drugs. Poor grades have been found to be predictive of inhalant use among Asian youth (Mackesy-Amiti and Fendrich, 2000).

Several factors may impact on reported prevalence rates, in addition to the methodological difficulties usually associated with such research. First, foreign-born populations may define substance differently than do U.S.-born groups. Researchers conducting a telephone survey of a Japanese community in southern California found that Japanese-born respondents defined "substance abuse" as referring to hard drugs, such as marijuana and heroin, but did not believe that the term encompassed the abuse of alcohol and tobacco. U.S.-born respondents, however, included tobacco and alcohol in their view of substance abuse (Sasao, 1989). Second, shame and stigma are associated with substance abuse problems. As a result, individuals may not seek care or may be reluctant to self-report abuse in the context of research (Sue and Morishima, 1982; Kim, 1978). Finally, a feeling of fatalism may predominate among some groups, so that individuals may believe that there is little to be gained by reporting difficulties (Kitano, 1976).

HISPANIC COMMUNITIES IN THE UNITED STATES: HISTORICAL AND CULTURAL CONTEXT

As of the 1990 census, the Hispanic population was estimated to be over 22 million, or approximately 9 percent of the U.S. population (U.S. Bureau of the Census, 1992, 1993). The classification "Hispanic" obscures the diversity of this population. Individuals of Mexican heritage account for 64.3 percent of all Hispanics, while Puerto Ricans (10.6 percent), Cubans (4.7 percent), Central and South Americans (13.4 percent), and others (7 percent) comprise the remainder (Furino, 1992). Two-thirds of the Hispanic populations lives in urban areas (U.S. Bureau of the Census, 1990). The various subgroups have tended to settle in different geographic areas, with Mexicans living predominantly in California and Texas, Puerto Ricans in New York, and Cubans in Florida (Furino, 1991; Mendoza, 1994; U.S. Bureau of the Census, 1988).

[The U.S. Department of Commerce, Bureau of the Census, refers to all individuals with an ethnic origin from Spanish-speaking countries as "Hispanic." This includes, for instance, Spain, Puerto Rico, Cuba, and Central and South American countries. "Hispanic" is a more general term than "Latino," which is usually used to refer to persons whose ethnic origin is from a Spanish-speaking country in Latin America (Mendoza, 1994).]

In comparison with other groups, Hispanics have a higher fertility rate, give birth to children at a younger age, and have more children (U.S. Bureau of the Census, 1993). Although Mexican and Cuban families are likely to be headed by two parents, over 60 percent of children of parents of Puerto Rican descent are in single-parent-headed households, a situation strongly associated with poverty (Commonwealth Fund, 1995, cited in Guendelman, 1998). A recent study of mortality patterns among adult Hispanics suggests that older Hispanics experience lower overall mortality in comparison with non-Hispanic whites, but mortality among young and middle-aged Hispanics is similar to that of non-Hispanic whites (Liao, Cooper, Cao, Durazo-Arvizu, Kaufman, Luke, and McGee, 1998).

Of all Hispanic families, one third live below the U.S. poverty level (U.S. Bureau of the Census, 1993). Cuban Americans are the least likely of Hispanic groups to be living in poverty, while Puerto Ricans are the most likely to be poor (U.S. Bureau of the Census, 1990). Hispanics are more likely to be employed in service, agricultural, or blue collar jobs, where employers are less likely to provide health insurance benefits (Trevino, Moyer, Valdez, Stroup-Benham, 1991; U.S. Bureau of the Census, 1990), sick leave, parental leave, disability benefits, or retirement benefits (Bassford, 1995). A recent study found that among uninsured Hispanics, 60 percent of Cuban Americans, 53 percent of Mexican Americans and 46 percent of Puerto Ricans were employed (Trevino, Moyer, Valdez, Stroup-Benham, 1991). Mexican Americans are more likely to be employed than are Puerto Ricans, but are less likely to have health insurance, due to lack of employer-sponsored insurance and inability to afford private insurance premiums (Council on Scientific Affairs, 1991; Valdez, Morgenstern, Brown, Wyn, Wang, and Cumberland, 1993). Cuban Americans are more likely to have higher education and income levels and private health insurance. Puerto Ricans, however, who tend to have lower levels of both income and employment, are most likely to be insured by Medicaid (Lipton and Katz, 1989; Trevino and Moss, 1983). The less favorable occupational status and lower incomes are reflective of the lesser educational levels among Hispanics. For instance, only one-half of young adult Hispanics have a high school diploma (U.S. Bureau of the Census, 1993) and over 10 percent of Hispanics have less than 5 years of school (U.S. Bureau of the Census, 1988).

The Cultural Context

Language and Acculturation

As with Asians and Pacific Islanders, language may constitute a significant barrier to care. Research has demonstrated that Hispanic patients who speak English are more likely to have a regular source of care than those who speak only Spanish (Hu and Covell, 1986) and may be more willing to utilize available services (Trevino, Bruhn, and Bunce, 1979). Yet, English literacy is low in the Hispanic population in general. For instance, less than half of the Hispanic elderly are estimated to be fully literate in either English or Spanish (Cuellar, 1990).

Acculturation levels may vary across and within groups. Lower levels of acculturation have been associated with reduced likelihood of utilizing either inpatient or outpatient care (Wells, Golding, Hough, Burnam, and Karno, 1989), poorer oral health outcomes (Marcell, 1994), and more favorable prenatal health behaviors, including abstinence from alcohol, drug, and cigarette use during pregnancy (Moore and Devitt, 1989; Marin, Perez-Stables, and Marin, 1989; U.S. Department of Health and Human Services, 1996). Higher levels of acculturation have been associated with an increased likelihood of unplanned pregnancies, pregnancy complications, and delivery of preterm and low birthweight infants (Guendelman and English, 1995), as well as increased prenatal stress, less social support during pregnancy, higher medical risk, and greater drug and alcohol use (Zambrana, Scrimshaw, Collins, and Dunkel-Schetter, 1997). The relative lack of health providers who understand the cultural context of their Hispanic patients may exacerbate the provider-patient communication difficulties arising from differences in language (Council on Scientific Affairs, 1991).

Explanatory Models of Health

Individuals may interpret and respond to illness episodes using culture-specific explanatory models. These models have often been referred to as "folk illnesses" or "culture-bound syndromes," treatable through "folk practices" (Council on Scientific Affairs, 1991). These explanatory models are important because they may impact on individuals' decisions to seek care and/or to utilize a specific form of care.

Numerous explanatory models have been documented. These illnesses have been classified into three categories, based on the presumed underlying causative mechanisms. The first, "natural" illnesses, includes *aigre* or *mal aire* (bad air), *empacho* (intestinal obstruction), and *mollera caida* (fallen fontanelle). Magical diseases encompass *encono* (the festering of wounds), *mal ojo* (evil eye), and *maleficio* (witchcraft). *Melarchico* (melancholy), *susto* (fright), and *ataque de nervios* ("nervous attack") comprise the third category relating to psychological and interpersonal etiology (Scheper Hughes and Stewart, 1983). The complaints of symptoms may, in fact, be biologically based and require accurate diagnosis and treatment (DeLaCancela, Guarnaccia, and Carrillo, 1986; Hispanic Health Alliance, 1990; Trotter, 1985).

Many illnesses have been attributed to an imbalance of hot-cold in food or in climate. The vast literature addressing hot-cold syndromes and therapeutics can only be touched on here. Messer (1981: 133) has explained this paradigm:

[H]ot-cold syndromes...view health as a balance of opposing or complementary (hot-cold) qualities and illness as an imbalance or alteration in one quality. Where such terms are used, all body conditions, foods and medicines can be potentially classified as some degree of hot-cold...The general rule for health maintenance is avoidance of extremes of any one quality. In the event of imbalance (illness) the procedure is treatment by the principle of opposites. The particular body condition is analysed to be one or the other quality and is brought back into balance by introduction of quantities of the opposite quality.

The entrance of cold into the body has been said to cause the following syndromes: chest cramps, earaches, headaches, paralysis, pains due to sprains, stomach cramps, rheumatism, teething, and tuberculosis. An overabundance of heat is responsible for *algodoncillo* (whitening of the lips, tongue, and gums), *dispela* (outbreak of red spots on the extremities), dysentery, sore eyes, *fogazo* (red spots in the mouth and on the tongue), kidney ailments, *postemilla* (abscess in tooth), sore throats, warts, and rashes. Diarrhea, enteritis, and toothache can result from extremes of either hot or cold (Currier, 1966).

Treatment for maladies brought on by humoral imbalance includes the ingestion of teas (Kay and Yoder, 1987), herbal preparations (Foster, 1988), specific food preparations, or a combination of these remedies (Mathews, 1983). Illness can be prevented through the avoidance of exposures to heat or cold insults (Foster, 1984). In the case of unfamiliar maladies, the choice of a specific remedy often turns on precedent episodes of similar illness and a remembrance of the illness-remedy-outcome link (Mathews, 1983).

Reliance on humoral theory serves to (1) explain what has happened; (2) provide a prescription for what is to be done; and (3) afford individuals a degree of control over and an understanding of their own health (Foster, 1984). Additionally, the hot-cold paradigm provides a framework in which individuals can deal with anxieties and desires that cannot be addressed directly. Burgess and Dean (1962: 68) have said of the hot-cold framework:

> Other ways of attempting to deal with the internal stress of threats to life or to emotional security are to over-estimate external dangers, or to attribute internal threats almost entirely to external influences of various kinds; and, with this, to attempt magically to evade or appease an apparently external threat, or to balance one type of threat against another. The practice of giving "heating" or "cooling" foods in particular kinds of clinical conditions may be a form of this kind of balancing technique for evading what are regarded as threatening influences—not of a nutritional kind.

Humoral medicine, however, remains a subject of controversy. Despite the apparent widespread reliance on the hot-cold dichotomy, as evidenced by the studies noted above, various investigations have found that a significant proportion of the population under study was unaware of the classifications (Kay, 1977); that the categorization of terms often varies between urban and rural populations within the same area (Weller, 1983);

and that the interpretation and the application of the hot-cold distinction differs between groups (Browner, 1985). Logan (1977: 95), commenting on the deficiencies of humor-related research, stated:

> Most ethnographic accounts of humoral medicine are descriptive, in that no specific hypotheses or sets of relationships are central to the given research. It is of limited use simply to report that a given people classify certain items or conditions as hot and others as cold. For without explanation, that is, without relating the data to some fact of the group's culture, ecology, or biological adaptations, the data tell us little more than certain items and conditions are judged, by some informants, to be hot or cold.

Use or nonuse of traditional healing practices is closely related to health and illness beliefs; the beliefs may indicate the appropriateness of a particular source of care or form of treatment. The extent to which individuals adhere to cultural practices necessarily impacts on the extent to which they engage in self-diagnosis and self-prescription and the extent to which they are willing to consult with traditional healers or Western-style health care providers (Ludman et al., 1989).

Brandon (1991) found in his New York/New Jersey-based study of santeria that many of the Hispanics interviewed used home-grown plants to treat minor illnesses, such as inflammations, skin eruptions, muscle pains, and fevers. Healing rites, such as *rogacion de cabeza* (rogation of the head), were used to treat more serious maladies, such as depression, mental confusion, high blood pressure, and witchcraft. The cure requires that the patient recite a series of prayers and that the santero place a plant or animal preparation on the patient's head, to be worn for 24 hours. Unfortunately, Brandon did not explore how or why individuals chose between care from a santero or care from a medical provider.

Hispanic patients may seek assistance from traditional healers for a variety of conditions, including *aigre, empacho, mollera caida, encono, mal ojo, maleficio, melarchico,* or *susto.* Treatment may consist of herbal preparations, prayers, burning incense, or massages, depending upon the nature of the malady and the expertise of the healer (Martinez and Martin, 1966). Treatment may be sought from a folk healer (*curandero/a*), a masseuse/bonesetter (*sobadora*), or an herbalist (*albolaria*), depending upon the nature of the symptoms (Scheper Hughes and Stewart, 1983).

The selection of the medicinal substance to be used for healing is based on its metaphoric hot or cold quality (Foster, 1985; Browner, 1985). Once selected, these substances must be prepared for use, which often entails compounding multiple ingredients into the treatment, such as an ointment or infusion. The method of treatment administration depends not only on the symptoms or illness, but also on the humoral goals of the treatment. As an example, the extraction of heat may be accomplished through reliance on *emplastos*, a poultice consisting of grape leaves applied to the temples and cheeks with saliva. The expulsion of heat can be accomplished by purges or induced vomiting, brought about by a compound of cold ingredients such as salt, rose leaves and petals, and ash leaves (Foster, 1985).

The Historical Context

It is beyond the scope of this chapter to provide a summary of the historical context of each Hispanic group in the United States. Accordingly, a brief review is provided of the history of Mexicans and Puerto Ricans, the two largest Hispanic communities in the United States.

The Mexican American Context

The United States-Mexico border extends from the mouth of the Rio Grande River to the Pacific Ocean, a distance of almost 2,000 miles. The border was established as the result of the 1848 Treaty of Guadalupe Hidalgo, which ended the Mexican War, as it is referred to in the United States, or the American Intervention, as it is known in Mexico (Ehrlich, Bilderback, and Ehrlich, 1979). Tension from a variety of sources over time has characterized the border area and continues to do so: Mexican opposition to slavery in Texas and assistance to escaping slaves during the 1850s; the authorized incursion of U.S. troops into Mexico during the 1870s; the massacre of Americans at Santa Ysabel in 1916; the influx of American investors into Mexico in the 1920s; the expropriation of American-owned oil companies in Mexico by the Mexican government during the late 1930s; the introduction of U.S. agribusiness involvement in Mexican farming throughout the 1940s, 1950s, and 1960s, with disastrous economic consequences; the establishment and subsequent termination of the U.S. bracero program; the establishment of *maquiladoras* in border areas; and U.S. immigration policy (Ehrlich, Bilderback, and Ehrlich, 1979; Samora, 1971).

Mexican immigration to the U.S. gradually increased until the onset of the Depression. During the period from 1900 through 1904, Mexicans represented only .07 percent of the total immigrant influx to the U.S. However, that proportion had grown to 15.7 percent by the period from 1925 through 1929. Immigration decreased dramatically following the passage of the Deportation Act of March 4, 1929, which rendered some aliens deportable, and the May 4, 1929 law, which made it a felony for deported aliens to re-enter the U.S. illegally. The advent of the Depression further dampened Mexican immigration (Samora, 1971).

The need for agricultural labor during World War II, due in part to the forced relocation of Japanese Americans from the West Coast, prompted the establishment of the Bracero Program in 1942. That program was intended to provide agricultural labor to the U.S. in shortage areas. The desire of growers to obtain cheap labor after World War II led to the maintenance of the program until the early 1960s. Numerous researchers have traced the beginnings of the "illegal immigration problem" to the initiation of the Bracero Program and the growers' encouragement of migration—legal and illegal—to the U.S. (Ehrlich, Bilderback, and Ehrlich, 1979; Samora, 1971).

Access to health care is often impeded due to a lack of health insurance coverage. Latinos in general are more likely to be employed with smaller employers, who are less likely to offer health insurance coverage as a benefit. Many Latinos are employed in relatively low-paying industries, such as services industries, which are less likely to offer insurance, regardless of the size of the company (Quinn, 2000). Lack of legal status in the United States may also constitute a barrier to the receipt of care, due to both restrictions imposed by federal and/or state law on the receipt of publicly-funded care and individuals' fears of potential adverse immigration consequenes as a result of having sought medical care (Azevedo and Bogue, 2001; Fenton, Catalan, and Hargreaves, 1996).

The Puerto Rican Experience

Puerto Rico's population increased significantly during the 19th century, primarily due to the influx of Spanish royalists (Wagenheim and Jimenez de Wagenheim, 1994). Unlike other locales of the Caribbean, the lighter skinned population of Puerto Rico outnumbered those of darker skin color and slaves constituted a very small proportion of the total population. Despite the relatively small numbers of slaves, the abolition of the slave system was an integral part of Puerto Rico's struggle for autonomy.

That autonomy was to be short-lived. Spain granted Puerto Rico a charter in 1897, permitting a substantial degree of home rule. The new Puerto Rico government convened for the first time on February 11, 1898, only to be surrendered by Spain to the invading Americans on October 18, 1898, as compensation for the losses brought about by war. The Americans viewed Puerto Rico as a real estate venture even then, suitable as a naval base and for a winter vacation (Wagenheim and Jiminez de Wagenheim, 1994). U.S. military rule lasted only briefly, ending on April 12, 1900, with the appointment of a civilian governor by the president of the United States.

The American invasion brought with it economic changes, as well as political ones. Prior to the invasion, Puerto Rico had had a diversified subsistence economy with four basic export crops: tobacco, cattle, coffee, and sugar. That economy was essentially converted to a sugar crop economy, of which 60 percent was owned by absentee U.S. investors (Gonzalez, 1966; Steward, 1965).

The first rebellion against American rule occurred in 1909. Since that time, independence from the United States has remained an ongoing issue. Attempts to increase home rule during the early 1900s generally met with little sympathy, even as militant anti-American forces began to emerge in response to the high rates of starvation and disease occasioned by the later decline of the sugar cane-based economy and the control of the economy by absentee U.S. investors (Wagenheim and Jimenez de Wagenheim, 1994).

The Depression in the United States was felt in Puerto Rico. For instance, a 1933 study of the offshore municipality of Vieques Island found that the total population of 11,000 persons earned a total income of $500 per week, or less than 7 cents per person per day.

During the years following World War II, the sagging Puerto Rico economy was boosted through the implementation of "Operation Bootstrap," which promoted private investment instead of government development of industry. Liberal tax benefits and low wages were used to lure foreign investors (Rodriguez, 1994; Wagenheim and Jimenez de Wagenheim, 1994). However, these industries failed to provide sufficient employment and, as a result, surplus labor migrated to the mainland U.S. (Bonilla and Campos, 1981; Morales, 1986). Various benefits made possible through these ties with the mainland, such as citizenship, accessible air travel, and education systems, encouraged migration (Rodriguez, 1994).

The first phase of Puerto Rican migration occurred between 1900 and 1945 (Stevens-Arroyo and Diaz-Stevens, 1982). As of 1910, there were only 1,513 Puerto Ricans living throughout 39 states. By 1920, the mainland Puerto Rican community had increased to 11,811 islanders living in 45 states (Wagenheim and Jimenez de Wagenheim, 1994). The majority, however, settled in New York City (Rodriguez, 1994). Many of these immigrants were employed in working-class occupations (Chenault, 1970; Handlin, 1959).

The "great migration" occurred during the years from 1946 through 1964. Although the vast majority of migrants settled in New York, communities were also established in Connecticut, New Jersey, Chicago, and other areas (Stevens-Arroyo and Diaz-Stevens, 1982). Many of these migrants encountered intense racial prejudice in their new settlements, for which they were ill-prepared despite the efforts of the island government. Unable to pass as Americans, many Puerto Ricans attempted to dissociate themselves from the media-labeled "Puerto Rican problem" by calling themselves Hispanos or Latinos (Wagenheim and Jimenez de Wagenheim, 1994).

The migration period from 1965 through the present has been labeled "revolving door migration," reflecting the fluctuating in- and out-migration (Stevens-Arroyo and Diaz-Stevens, 1982). Although New York

City continues to attract the majority of the migrants, approximately 40 percent of those arriving from the island now settle outside of New York (Wagenheim and Jimenez de Wagenheim, 1994). The term "Neo-Rican" is now used to describe the "hybrid person" who speaks and thinks in both English and Spanish but feels a stranger in both cultures (Wagenheim and Jimenez de Wagenheim, 1994: 276).

Just as many African-Americans are familiar with the events associated with the Tuskegee syphilis study, discussed above, many Puerto Ricans recall either directly or indirectly events associated with the birth control trials conducted in Puerto Rico. The first series of these trials began in Puerto Rico in April 1956. Puerto Rico was chosen as a site because laws at that time prohibited the conduct of these trials in Massachusetts. Additionally, it was perceived that Puerto Rico was overpopulated at the time and in need of mechanisms to control reproduction. The relatively high rate of illiteracy would also allow researchers to examine the ability of an illiterate population to adhere to the prescription regimen (Ramirez and Seipp, 1983; McLaughlin, 1982; Vaughan, 1970).

The trial began with 100 volunteers from a housing project in Rio Piedras, a suburb of San Juan. Negative publicity soon discouraged some women from participating. The newspaper, *El Imparcial*, reported of the project's physician-director:

> A woman dressed as a nurse and who alleges to be working for the state government, is distributing between the house wives some pills to avoid conception and to counteract the increase in population in Puerto Rico . . . The Secretary of Health believes that it is a 'bad combination' that the public officials of the State offer themselves to be used in a Malthusian campaign, and he condemned also that the State Government is used as a bait for contraceptive campaigns of private agencies (Anon., April 21, 1956).

The trials have since been criticized as having failed to establish the long-term safety of the pill, thereby jeopardizing the health of the Puerto Rican research participants (Corea, 1985). It is unclear what long term effects, if any, this experience has had on the willingness of individuals of Puerto Rican ethnicity to participate as volunteers in research.

Substance Use and Health

Infectious Disease

HIV/AIDS. Although Hispanics comprise approximately 13 percent of the total U.S. population (Bureau of the Census, 1992, 1993), they account for 19 percent of all reported AIDS cases (Centers for Disease Control and Prevention, 2002f; Maldonado, 1998). The incidence of AIDS among Hispanics in the year 2000 was 22.5 per 100,000, a rate more than three times the rate for whites, but lower than the rate for African-Americans (Centers for Disease Control and Prevention, 2002c). In the same year, 31 percent of the AIDS cases among Hispanics were associated with injection drug use (Centers for Disease Control and Prevention, 2002a). Almost two-thirds of reported AIDS cases among men born in Central and South America, Cuba, and Mexico are attributed to male to male sex, while almost two-thirds of AIDS cases among Puerto Ricans are associated with injection drug use (Diaz, Buehler, Castro, and Ward, 1993; Selik, Castro, Pappaioanou, and Buehler, 1989).

Although Hispanic children account for only 13 percent of all U.S. children, 24 percent of childhood AIDS cases are among Hispanic children. Perinatal transmission accounts for 88 percent of Hispanic pediatric AIDS cases (Diaz, 1992). Limited knowledge of the transmission and prevention, as well as cultural norms that proscribe condom use, contributes to the transmission (Council on Scientific Affairs, 1991).

Syphilis.   For the year 2000, the incidence rate of syphilis among Hispanics was 1.8 per 100,000, a rate that is three times higher than that among non-Hispanic whites (Centers for Disease Control and Prevention, 2002f).

Tuberculosis.   Recent research has revealed a decrease in the rate of tuber-culosis for U.S.-born persons and an increase in the rates among the foreign-born (Anon, 1996a; Cantell, Snider, Cauthen, and Onorato, 1995). The rate of tuberculosis among Hispanics for the period 1991 to 2001 was 11.9 per 100,000, compared to 1.6 per 100,000 among non-Hispanic whites (Centers for Disease Control and Prevention, 2002g). The incidence of tuberculosis is substantially higher among Hispanics living in large urban areas, such as New York and Los Angeles, compared to those living else-where (Centers for Disease Control and Prevention, 1987).

Substance Use and Misuse

Hispanics have been found to have a slightly higher rate of heavy alcohol use compared with whites and African-Americans (United States Department of Health and Human Services, 1997). Alcoholism and cirrho-sis are prevalent among Mexican Americans and Puerto Ricans in particu-lar (Schinke, Moncher, Palleja, Zayas, and Schilling, 1988). Hispanic males have been reported to abstain from alcohol use for a period of time and then engage in binge drinking (Perez-Stable, Marin, and Marin, 1994). Hispanic youth have also been found to engage in extensive alcohol use. A recent study of 1500 high school students in San Francisco found that over one quarter of the Hispanic students used some type of alcohol at least once a week, while 13 percent drank to the point of intoxication on a daily basis (Morales, 1990).

Among adolescents, susceptibility to smoking has been found to be highest among Hispanics, compared to all other ethnic groups (Unger, palmer, Dent, Rohrbach, and Johnson, 2000). Significant factors related to susceptibility among migrant adolescents include age, gender, attitudes towards cigarettes, satisfaction with social support, and parent-child communication (Elder et al., 2000).

Compared to other groups, Hispanics are more likely to report smoke-free homes (Gilpin, White, Farkas, and Pierce, 1999). Puerto Ricans have been found to be more likely to be current smokers and ever smokers compared to Hispanics of Dominican, Colombian, and Ecuadorian ethnicity (Kerner, Breen, Tefft, and Silsby, 1998). Mexican-American women have been found to be less likely to use tobacco compared to non-Hispanic white women (Guendelman and Abrams, 1994). Research also indicates that the use of smokeless tobacco is lower among Hispanics as compared to non-Hispanic whites and African-Americans (Foreyt et al., 1993; Siegel, 1992).

Research indicates that Hispanics experience a disproportionate number of deaths due to narcotic use (Burge, Felts, Chenier, and Parrillo, 1995). Compared to other Hispanic groups, marijuana and cocaine use are more prevalent among Puerto Ricans (Vega, 1994). In general, however, Hispanics' rates of substance misuse are similar to those of whites and African-Americans (United States Department of Health and Human Services, 1997). A recent study of maternal drug use in New York City found that drug use was less common among foreign-born Hispanic mothers. Puerto Ricans had the highest percentage of reported drug use among island-born and mainland-born mothers, while Mexican mothers had the lowest rate of drug use among mainland-born mothers (Lederman and Sierra, 1994). Previous research has demonstrated low rates of maternal drug usage among Hispanic women compared to whites (Vega, Kolody, Hwang, and Noble, 1993). Young Hispanic males have rates of drug use similar to those of their white counterparts and somewhat higher in comparison with African-American youth. By contrast, Hispanic adolescent females use drugs at a rate lower than that of their white counterparts, but somewhat higher than African-American youth (Adams et al., 1995).

Suicide

Although Hispanics in general appear to have low rates of suicide, Cuban-born and Puerto Rican-born men have higher rates of suicide compared to non-Hispanic men, while the rates among Mexican American men are lower than among non-Hispanic men and higher than that among

merican men (Shai and Rosenwaike, 1988). Suicide rates are high-
₂ Puerto Rican and Cuban American men between the ages of
5 (Shai and Rosenwaike, 1988). High rates of suicide attempts
na₍ ₎ en documented. "Suicide fits" constitute one of the most prevalent socioemotional and behavioral mental health issues for Puerto Ricans
(Zavala-Martinez, 1994). Identified risk factors for suicidal ideation include stress, depression, low self esteem, family dysfunction, substance
abuse, and for youth, poor academic performance (Burge, Felts, Chenier,
and Parrillo, 1995). Immigrant status has also been linked to suicidal
ideation (Zavala-Martinez, 1994: Vega, Gil, and Warhelt, Aspospori, and
Zimmerman, 1993), with rates differing across various Hispanic ethnicities
(Vega, Gil, Warhelt, Aspospori, and Zimmerman, 1993).

NATIVE AMERICANS: HISTORICAL AND CULTURAL CONTEXT

Origin and Culture Areas

The term "Native American" refers to the indigenous population of
North America prior to the arrival of European settlers (Young, 1994).
The term includes American Indians, Eskimos (also known as Inuits), and
Aleuts (Young, 1994). The locale of origin of Native Americans is believed
to be Asiatic, although the date, duration, and point of entry of this migration remain in dispute (Dillehay and Meltzer, 1991; Greenberg, Turner,
and Zegura, 1986).

Prior to the arrival of European settlers, Native Americans' communities were distinguishable by "culture area," reflective of the varying cli-
matic and geographical conditions and individuals' attempts to adapt to
these varied conditions. These 13 culture areas included the Arctic, the
Sub-Arctic, the Northwest Coast, the Plateau, the Plains, the Prairies, the
East, California, the Great Basin, Baja California, the Southwest, Northeast
Mexico, and Meso-America (Driver, 1969).

The Arctic, encompassing portions of Alaska, Canada, and Greenland,
was generally characterized by its access to the sea. The Sub-Arctic included the interior portions of Canada and Alaska; moose and caribou
were the primary food sources. The Northwest Coast, which extended
from southeastern Alaska's panhandle to California's northwest corner,
is now known for its plank houses and totem poles. The Plateau region,
which includes portions of British Columbia, was plentiful in fish.

The Plains area, extending southward from central Alberta in Canada
to Mexico, is bounded by the Rocky Mountains and the Missouri River.
The Plains Indians are perhaps among the best-known because this culture

area included the Sioux, the Blackfoot, the Crow, and the Cheyenne. Unlike the predominantly nomadic Plains Indians, the Native Americans of the Prairies lived in villages near their farms, in areas that correspond to what is now the Midwest. Tribes of the Eastern culture area, which encompassed portions of New York, the Middle Atlantic states, and some portion of the southern states, included the Iroquois. The California culture area covered approximately two-thirds of what is now the state of California. The Great Basin area, which includes areas of California, Oregon, Idaho, Wyoming, and Colorado and all of Nevada and Utah, was characterized by extreme dryness. These Native American groups included the Ute, the Paiutes, and the Shoshone. Like the Great Basin, Baja California has large areas of desert, but also has areas of heavy rainfall. Most settlements in this area were located less than 50 miles from the ocean. Many were missionized by the Spanish. Both the Southwest and the Northwest Mexico areas are characterized by desert. The Southwest, which encompasses what is now Arizona, New Mexico, the Mexican states of Sonora and Sinaloa, and portions of Chihuahua and Durango, was home to the Hopi, the Zuni, the Navajo, the Apache, the Mohave, the Yuma, and the Yaqui. The Meso-American culture area, best known for the Aztecs and the Mayas, extends from southern Mexico through Guatemala, Honduras, El Salvador, and portions of Nicaragua (Driver, 1969).

Current Demographics

The 1990 census reported that there were 1,959,234 Native Americans, Eskimos, and Aleuts in the United States (Paisano, 1995), constituting almost 1 percent of the total population. This represents a 38 percent increase in the Native American population between 1980 and 1990 (McKenney and Bennett, 1994). This increase has been attributed to improvements in counting individuals on reservations, reliance on self-identification, and improved outreach programs and promotion campaigns in connection with the census (Paisano, 1995).

The 10 largest tribes included the Cherokee (19 percent of all Native Americans), Navajo (11.6 percent), Sioux (5.5 percent), Chippewa (5.5 percent), Choctaw (4.5 percent), Pueblo (2.9 percent), Apache (2.8 percent), Iroquois (2.7 percent), Lumbee (2.6 percent), and Creek (2.4 percent) (Bureau of the Census, 1994). A large proportion (27 percent) live on reservations, tribal trust lands, and in Alaskan Native villages (Bureau of the Census, 1993). Of those living on reservations, almost 20 percent of households disposed of sewage by means of other than public sewer, septic tank, or cesspool; almost 20 percent lacked complete plumbing facilities in their homes (Bureau of the Census, 1995). Over time, an increasing proportion of Native Americans have moved to urban areas (Young, 1994). The largest proportion of Native Americans live in Oklahoma, California, Arizona, New Mexico, Alaska, Washington, North Carolina, Texas, New York, and Michigan (Paisano, 1995).

Compared to the entire U.S. population, Native Americans are more likely to be younger, poorer, and less educated. The median age of the Native American population at the time of the 1990 census was 26 years, compared to a median age of 36 years for the entire U.S. (Paisano, 1995). Thirty-nine percent of the Native American population was under the age of 20, compared with 29 percent of the entire U.S. population. Thirty-one percent of Native Americans lived below the poverty level in 1989, compared with 13 percent among the entire U.S. population. The median family income of Native Americans, Eskimos, and Aleuts in 1990 was $21,750, compared to $35,225 for the entire U.S. population. Over half of Native Americans living on reservations and trust lands in 1989 were living below the poverty level (Bureau of the Census, 1993). And, although the educational attainment of Native Americans has improved significantly, as of 1990 only 9 percent of Native Americans had completed a bachelor's degree or higher, compared with 20 percent of the total U.S. population (Paisano, 1995).

The Cultural Context

Language

We know of a total of 221 mutually distinct Native American languages. The various culture areas correlate to a high degree with the areas in which specific languages are spoken. As one example, the Eskimo-Aleut language coincides with the culture areas of the Arctic (Driver, 1969).

Traditional Lifestyles

The culture areas were distinguished not only by language, but also by various aspects of health, such as nutritional status and patterns of health behaviors. In the Arctic culture area, for instance, Eskimos relied on sea mammals, such as the seal and the walrus, as their primary source of nutrition. Approximately half of their meat was eaten raw.

Sub-Arctic Native Americans relied primarily on caribou and small mammals, such as beaver, rabbit, and deer, for food. Their diet was supplemented with shellfish and fish. Eskimos and Native Americans in both the Arctic and Sub-Arctic areas used boiling in food preparation, by both direct-fire boiling and by placing heated stones in the liquid to be boiled (Driver, 1969).

Native Americans of the Northwest Coast relied predominantly on fish as a source of nutrition. Fish were preserved by burying them in pits and allowing them to decay or they were smoked. The addition of roots and berries supplemented the protein-rich diet with carbohydrates, sugar, iron, and copper.

The diet in the Plateau culture area included game, such as moose, elk, and deer, as well as wild plants and roots. Native Americans of the Plains relied heavily on the buffalo for sustenance, supplemented by elk, antelope, and bear, as well as by roots. In the Prairie culture area, Native Americans depended heavily on buffalo or deer, although maize, beans, squashes, and sunflowers were also cultivated. Food was often prepared by direct-boiling (Driver, 1969).

Famines in the East culture area were rare due to the diversity of the food sources, which included fish, hunted animals, and crops, such as beans, squashes, and corn. Similarly, small game was secondary to other sources of food in the California culture area. There, the diet was based primarily on the acorn and smaller seeds, although fish, small game, and invertebrates, such as grasshoppers and earthworms, also provided nutrition (Driver, 1969).

In contrast, wild plants served as the dominant food source in the Great Basin area. Deer and the mountain sheep were the most common animals, and rabbits and other game were hunted. Salt was obtained from the surface of the land in and around the lake beds. Native Americans in Northeast Mexico and Baja California similarly emphasized plants in their diet, including mesquite pods and cactus fruits. Although fish and shellfish were available to inhabitants near the coast, this was not true for those further inland, who often faced the possibility of famine and who suffered from chronic malnutrition (Driver, 1969).

The extent of farming varied across the Native American groups in the Southwest culture area. As much as 80 percent of the Pueblos' diet may have consisted of maize in its various forms. Meat was seldom available due to the scarcity of game, often resulting in protein deficiency. Reliance on wild plants, however, provided high fiber, carbohydrates, and micronutrients (Teufel, 1996). Famine and drought occurred not infrequently. The Navajo acquired farming from the Pueblos and by the nineteenth century were also relying on maize as the cornerstone of their diet. Farm crops also constituted an important part of the diet of the Mohave and the Yuma.

Maize was also an important crop to the Native Americans of the Meso-America culture area. Seeds were often dried and cooked by parching. Residents of this area were also able to rely on various animals as a source of nutrition, including turkeys, geese, ducks, and quail. Salt was obtained by evaporating salt water.

Explanatory Models of Health and Illness

Explanatory models of health and illness differed across the various culture areas. Depending upon the culture area and the specific type of disease in question, disease was believed to be caused by soul loss, natural origins, a supernatural being, contact with the dead, and violations of taboos (Driver, 1969). Cures often required the intervention of a shaman (Driver, 1969) and/or the application or ingestion of specific remedies, such as plants and teas (Chamberlin, 1909; Driver, 1969; Grinnell, 1905; Hridlicka, 1932; Landes, 1963; Vogel, 1970).

Despite the apparent success of some of the Native American curative remedies (Driver, 1969), the white settlers often displayed little regard for the abilities of the Native American medicine men and shamans. One writer characterized the medicine man as "an influence antagonistic to the rapid absorption of new ideas and the adoption of new customs" (Bourke, 1887: 451). Only by "thoroughly [routing] the medicine men from their intrenchments and [making] them the object of ridicule" could whites "bend and train the minds of our Indian wards in the direction of civilization" (Bourke, 887: 594).

The Historical Context

Leacock and Lurie (1971) have delineated four phases of Native American history following the arrival of the Europeans:

1. Early contact. This interchange, which was often on an equal footing, generally occurred through trade or missionaries.
2. Conflict-disruption. This phase was characterized by the large-scale settlement of the European settlers and resulting conflict, often due to the forcible displacement of Native American communities and the breach of treaty agreements.
3. Government controls. This phase is notable for the imposition of government controls and the establishment of reservations.
4. Cultural revival. This period reflects new forms of political organization in the context of industrial society.

Conflict and Disruption

These four periods are distinguishable in even the brief review of Native American history that follows. This synopsis begins with the 1600s, in what Leacock and Lurie would characterize as a period of conflict-disruption. Several continuing themes are easily apparent in this brief overview: settler's betrayal of negotiated agreements with various tribes; the decimation of tribes by disease and war; the settlers' disdain for Native

Americans, reflected in broken agreements, enslavement, corporal punishment for refusal to convert to Christianity, prohibitions against intermarriage, and in some cases, a policy of extermination.

In 1600, members of the Apache, Navajo, and Ute tribes were captured by Spaniards, with the assistance of the Pueblos, to be used as slave labor and household servants. These kidnapping raids by the Spanish continued into the 1900s (Nies, 1996). In 1609, British settlers in Jamestown, Virginia burned Powhatan villages and captured the Powhatan as slaves. In 1614, English sea captain Thomas Hunt captured 24 New England coastal Indians and sold them as slaves in Spain (Nies, 1996).

New England Indians, from Massachusetts to Maine, suffered a smallpox epidemic from 1616 to 1619. The infection was believed to be transmitted from European fishermen on the coast. Lacking immunity to the disease, entire tribes died from starvation and malnutrition. Various tribes would be decimated by other epidemics in later years. For instance, over 190,000 Huron died between 1633 and 1635 due to a smallpox epidemic. Indian oral history tells us that during this epidemic, French Jesuit missionaries advised the Huron that those who were baptized as Catholics would be spared. The missionaries gave the unbaptized blankets from smallpox victims, resulting in transmission of the infection.

By 1660, approximately 1,000 British settlers per year were arriving in Massachusetts Bay. The Indians interpreted the gifts that they received from the British as a rental fee for land use; the British believed that these exchanges represented the purchase price to a tract of land which was private property. This misunderstanding constituted the source of much conflict to follow.

In 1622, after years of conflict over land and other issues, the Powhatan attacked the Jamestown Colony. The royal British Virginia Company ordered that the Powhatan be exterminated and prohibited all peace negotiations. In 1623, the English invited the Powhatan leaders to a peace conference, where the Powhatan were served poisoned wine. Those who survived were shot. The Powhatan-British conflicts continued for at least a decade (Nies, 1996).

Numerous other attempts by Native Americans to negotiate peace with the European settlers also met with failure. In 1641, the Five Nations of the Iroquois attempted to reach a settlement with the French. Their efforts were rebuffed because the French believed that such an agreement would not further their economic interests. In 1649, Virginia settlers disregarded the terms of an agreement with the Powhatan and encroached further onto lands guaranteed to the Powhatan.

By the mid- to late-1600s, numerous Native American rebellions occurred against the British, French, and Spanish settlers. These rebellions were often provoked by settlers' kidnapping raids, infringements on

Native American lands, breaches of agreements, and physical punishment of Native American leaders for "idolatry" (Nies, 1996). In 1691, Virginia banished all English who married Indians, blacks, or anyone with mixed ancestry (Nies, 1996).

The 1700s were characterized by continuing conflict between Native American tribes and various European groups and between Native American tribes with differing loyalties to the European settlers. French, British and Spanish colonists continued to appropriate land as their own. The British, in particular, were known for their continuing kidnapping raids to capture Native Americans for sale as slaves (Francis, 1996). The sale of alcohol to Native Americans had become an issue; the Powhatan leader Anne complained of this practice to the Virginia legislature in 1715, to no avail. Sir Jeffrey Amherst, a British commander, became known for his genocidal policy towards the Indians: "Could it not be contrived to send the smallpox among the disaffected tribes of Indians? We must on this occasion [smallpox outbreak] use every stratagem in our power to reduce them" (Nies, 1996: 191). Amherst had blankets taken from smallpox victims and given to healthy Indians, ensuring the transmission of the epidemic.

Life under the new United States appeared to be no better for Native Americans than it had been under the colonists and European powers. Large numbers of Great Lakes Indians died during a smallpox epidemic from 1780 to 1782 (Nies, 1996). Numerous tribes and confederacies, such as the Iroquois Six Nations, were forced to cede their lands. The new government respected negotiated agreements no more than the previous authorities had (Francis, 1996; Nies, 1996).

Contact with the Indians continued to be regulated. The third Trade and Intercourse Act, passed in 1799, provided for the appointment of federal agents to tribes and restricted those without a license from trading with Indians.

Government Controls

The 1800s witnessed the imposition of further government controls on Native Americans. The new government continued to breach agreements, often due to a desire for increased amounts of land. Conflicts between the settlers and the Indians continued as a result. Federal policy towards Native Americans was clearly one of assimilation and removal. The government prohibited traditional religious observances and required that Indian children attend boarding schools, cut their hair, learn English, and convert to Christianity. The Indian Allotment Act of 1887 dissolved the previously established reservation system and tribal landholding, converting much reservation land into large parcels in an attempt to make Indians individual landowners and to promote their assimilation (Nies, 1996).

Cultural Revival

The 1900s have been called an Indian renaissance. The release of the Meriam Report of 1928 harshly criticized the allotment policy and recommended reforms in land management and support for communally held tribal lands. The allotment policy had resulted in the reduction of Indian-held lands from 155 million acres in 1881 to approximately 69 million acres in 1934, when the government officially abandoned the policy. Additionally, there was almost a complete lack of health, education, and employment facilities available to Native Americans.

Following the federal termination of 13 tribes between 1948 and 1960, resulting in their loss of federal recognition, annuities, and services, numerous Indian groups organized programs and actions to renegotiate land deals and address numerous problems on the reservations (Nies, 1996). Native American publications were established in various communities (Francis, 1996).

Substance Use and Health

Numerous theories have been advanced in an attempt to explain the decline in the Native American population over time. One of the better known theories posits the decline of the Native American population as the result of disease transmission resulting from contact with infected and infectious European settlers (Ashburn, 1947). Others have argued, however, that low population levels among some groups resulted from periods of starvation and the practice of female infanticide (Helm, 1980). Johansson (1982) has delineated four phases in the mortality of Native Americans. The first phase, which predated contact with European settlers, was characterized by a birth rate slightly greater than the death rate. During the initial contact period, the birth rate declined and the mortality rate increased. The birth rate eventually exceeded the death rate towards the end of the nineteenth century. Finally, during the twentieth century, the mortality rate and the birth rate have declined.

Compared to all groups in the U.S., Native Americans have a higher rate of potential years of life lost due to injuries, and a lower rate due to chronic diseases such as cancer or circulatory problems (USDHHS, 1990). Native Americans experience a higher rate of restricted activity days compared to all U.S. groups (USDHHS, 1990). During the period from October 1994 through January 1995, almost one third of all Indians and Alaska

Natives aged 15 and older reported having a disability; of those over the age of 65, 1 in every 2 reported having a disability (U.S. Census Bureau, 1997).

Infectious Disease

Sexually Transmitted Diseases.   National rates of sexually transmitted disease, such as syphilis and gonorrhea, tend to be lower among Native American populations compared to other U.S. groups (Young, 1994), although the Native American rates may be higher in certain geographic areas (Toomey, Oberschelp, and Greenspan, 1989; Rice, Roberts, Handsfield, and Holmes, 1991). Although few cases of AIDS have been reported among Native Americans, the majority of reported cases have been attributable to unprotected sexual intercourse (Metler, Conway, and Stehr-Green, 1991). At least one writer has identified a number of potential vulnerabilities to HIV transmission among the Navajo, including refusal to officially acknowledge homosexuality within the Navajo, the use of alcohol and marijuana which serve as disinhibitors and lead to greater risk-taking, and the high rate of suicidality (Sulivan, 1991).

Hepatitis.   In comparison to non-Native Americans, Native Americans experience a high prevalence of both hepatitis A and hepatitis B (Williams, 1986; Schreeder, Bender, McMahon, Moser et al., 1983). Hepatitis A infection results from both the consumption of contaminated water and foods and from person-to-person transmission via the oral-fecal route (Benenson, 1995). In contrast, infection with hepatitis B results from person-to-person transmission through sexual transmission or contact with contaminated blood or blood products, such as blood transfusions, contact with blood through shared use of injection equipment, or hemodialysis (Benenson, 1995).

Tuberculosis.   Although tuberculosis has been documented among Native Americans prior to the arrival of the European settlers (Paulsen, 1987), it is believed that both the incidence and the virulence of tuberculosis among Native Americans increased in the postcontact period (Clark, Kelley, Grange, and Hill, 1987). Various recent studies have documented high rates of tuberculosis among specific Native American populations. Breault and Hoffman (1997) found in their study of the Oglala Sioux on the Pine Ridge reservation in South Dakota that the relative risk of tuberculosis for a Pine Ridge Native American was 18.9 compared to the South Dakota population. The age-specific relative risk for the Pine Ridge population age 65 and older was 65.7. Tuberculin tests were positive in 70 percent of the diabetic patients on the reservation. For the year 2001, American Indian and Alaskan Natives experienced an incidence rate of 11.0 cases per 100,000 and accounted for 233 of the reported 15,989 cases (Centers for Disease Control and Prevention, 2002g).

Mental Health: Adolescents

Little research has been conducted to examine the prevalence or nature of eating disorders among Native American groups (Davis and Yager, 1992). One of the few studies to do so found that compared to Hispanics and non-Hispanic whites, Native American high school students displayed a higher prevalence of disturbed eating behaviors and attitudes (Smith and Krejci, 1991).

Among adolescents in the U.S., rates of suicide are highest among Native Americans. The 1988 Indian Health Service Adolescent Health Survey, administered to 7,254 students in grades 6 through 12, found that nearly 15 percent of the respondents had tried to commit suicide at least once (Grossman, Milligan, and Deyo, 1991). The following factors were associated with a suicide attempts: a history of mental problems, a feeling of alienation from family and community, having a friend who attempted suicide, weekly consumption of hard liquor, a family history of suicide or a suicide attempt, a poor self-perception of health, a history of physical abuse, being female, and sexual abuse.

Alcohol Use

Alcohol misuse has taken its toll on Native American communities. Alcohol has been associated with as much as 90 percent of all homicides involving Native Americans and has been implicated as a factor in many suicides, accidental-injury deaths (Bachman, 1991; Gallaher, Fleming, Berger, and Sewell, 1992), and vehicular safety issues (Chang, Lapham, and Barton, 1996). Children of parents who misuse alcohol are at higher risk of abuse and neglect (Berger and Kitzes, 1989; Lujan, DeBruyn, May, and Bird, 1989).

It appears that initially, at least, the colonists provided alcohol to Native Americans in much the same way that they offered it to each other, as a welcome or as a gift (Mancall, 1995). Later, however, the sale of alcohol to Native Americans was prohibited due to the perceived adverse effects of alcohol on Native Americans, such as accidents, and the colonial perception that drinking by Native Americans was a threat to society. Both the Dutch and the English imposed monetary penalties and/or corporal punishment on those found selling alcohol to Native Americans. Despite these prohibitions, Native Americans were able to obtain alcohol during this temperance period (Mancall, 1995). Native American use of alcohol continued, both because Native Americans wanted the alcohol and because the colonists were ambivalent about the alcohol trade. However, the sale of alcohol served a need much deeper than mere commercial benefit. As Mancall (1995: 170) notes,

> [Alcohol] became, especially in the last decades of the colonial period, crucial to the way colonists and Indians understood each other. Indians' responses to liquor reinforced colonists' notions about their cultural and racial inferiority; colonists' desire to maintain the trade despite its all too apparent costs reinforced Indians' notions about the deeply rooted problems of colonial culture...
>
> The liquor trade joined with the growing colonial population and recurring epidemics to destabilize Indian villages, and perhaps contributed to the decision of countless Indians to sell their land to colonists and move westward, beyond colonial settlements...
>
> The alcohol trade plagued relations between Indians and colonists precisely because each group interpreted its existence as a sign of the other's failings.

Numerous theories have been advanced in an attempt to explain the prevalence of alcohol misuse among Native Americans. One theory posits that the availability of alcohol is determinative, noting the increased use of alcohol among Native Americans living near urban areas and the increased usage among those who are more "acculturated" to non-Native American society (Levy and Kunitz, 1974). Others have argued that alcohol is an escape from problems, including the forcible relocation of many Native American communities, the loss of a traditional way of life, and the attempted imposition of new spiritual beliefs by the missionaries (Dozier, 1966). Others have suggested that, in addition, drinking serves to release repressed aggression and to solidify group bonds (Littman, 1970).

Whether there exists a genetic basis for alcohol misuse remains undetermined and controversial. Study results have yielded conflicting findings, some indicating that Native Americans actually metabolize ethanol more quickly than Caucasians (Segal and Duffy, 1992; May, 1994), while at least one study observed a slower rate of disappearance of blood alcohol (Fenna, Mix, Schaefer, and Gilbert, 1971). Additionally, these studies are difficult to interpret due to reliance on varying definitions and measurements (Schaefer, 1981).

Chapter 5

Considering the Historical and Cultural Context
Sex and Sexual Orientation

WOMEN

Some might assert that a separate chapter devoted to women is superfluous. Yet, this focus is critical for a variety of reasons. First, biological sex and societally constructed and imposed gender roles have often been inextricably intertwined throughout history, resulting in the construction of specified spheres of acceptable activity for women. An understanding of women and their needs in the context of treatment requires an examination of this relationship (Clarke, 1990).

Second, various health concerns that may arise in the context of addressing substance use may impact women to a far greater degree than men, such as relationship violence. Third, various issues relating to access to care and the quality of that care are critical to women, including the greater reliance on psychoactive medications for the treatment of women's complaints as compared to those of men (Ogur, 1986). Finally, women and men differ biologically and with respect to health indicators. Sex differences have been attributed to one or more of the following factors, all of which are relevant in the research context: (1) biological factors, such as hormones, (2) acquired risks through work and leisure activities, (3) psychosocial aspects of symptoms and care, (4) health reporting behavior, and (5) the effect of previous health care on future health (Verbrugge, 1990).

This chapter begins with an overview of the role of biological sex in the determination of gender role and the impact of that relationship on women's health care and health research generally; these have implications for substance use treatment and research.

Cultural and Historical Context: Sex and Gender

Prior to the late 18th century, women in the United States were viewed as fundamentally similar to men, but inferior, due to the underdevelopment of their reproductive organs. Beginning with the late 18th century, women were seen as biologically different from men, but still inferior, as evidence by their smaller skulls and resulting smaller brain capacity (Fee, 1979). A division of labor by biological sex, it was argued, was justified and necessary because women's lives were tyrannized and controlled by their reproductive systems, from menstruation, through childbearing and childrearing, through menopause. Consequently, women were not only debilitated but disabled and unsuited for larger societal roles (Smith-Rosenberg, 1973).

Unlike men who, it was believed in the 19th century, had the power to indulge or repress their sexual impulses (Skene, 1989 cited in Smith-Rosenberg, 1973), women were subject to cyclical periods of pain, weakness, irritability, and insanity (Wiltbank, 1854, cited in Smith-Rosenberg, 1973). Puberty represented a precipitous crossing into womanhood, fraught with danger of disease should there be either an "excess or a deficiency of the proper influence of these organs [ovaries] over the other parts of the system" (Kellogg, 1895: 371, cited in Smith-Rosenberg, 1973). The preservation of health, then, demanded full attention to the development of healthy reproductive organs, which could be accomplished by adherence to a regimen of rest, a simple diet, and an unchallenging routine of domestic tasks (Smith-Rosenberg, 1973). Menopause was similarly ominous, resulting in numerous diseases including diarrhea, vaginal inflammation, paralysis, tuberculosis, diabetes, depression, hysteria, and insanity, due to the cessation of menstruation and the "violation of the physiological and social laws dictated by [a woman's] ovarian system" (Smith-Rosenberg, 1973: 192). Such violations included education, attempts at birth control or abortion, a failure to adequately attend to the needs of one's husband or children, an overly indulgent lifestyle, and engaging in sexual intercourse during or after menopause (Smith-Rosenberg, 1973).

Hysteria, in particular, was believed to be an affliction specific to women. Hysteria was brought on by feelings of depression, nervousness, or crying and could manifest in the form of an hysterical "fit" similar to an epileptic seizure. Gradually, the seizure was eliminated as a diagnostic criterion of the illness, so that hysteria could be diagnosed on the basis of any number of symptoms, including loss of sensation, nausea, headache, pain, or contracture or paralysis of an extremity (Smith-Rosenberg, 1973). The onset of hysteria was attributed to "the indolent, vapid and unconstructive life of the fashionable middle- and upper-class woman, or by the ignorant, exhausting, and sensual life of the lower- or working-class woman" (Smith-Rosenberg, 1985: 205).

It has been postulated that the diagnosis of hysteria, defined by the medical profession as a disease, enabled women to assume a sick role and, concomitantly, to renegotiate their roles within their families. The restructuring of domestic activities to accommodate the illness essentially permitted a woman to opt out of her traditional role, without provoking the disapproval and confrontation that a more overt rejection of role would have entailed (Smith-Rosenberg, 1973).

The emergence, then, in the late 1800s and through the mid-1900s of the "New Woman" clearly violated existing taboos. "New Women" abandoned the domestic setting, seeking an education not equal, but identical, to that received by men (Smith-Rosenberg, 1973). It was predicted that such women would disrupt a delicate psychological balance through the emphasis on the mind rather than the ovaries. Within men, however, the brain and heart were dominant, permitting them to pursue such intellectual activities. One physician predicted:

> The nervous force, so necessary at puberty for the establishment of the menstrual function, is wasted on what may be compared as trifles to perfect health, for what use are they without health? The poor sufferer only adds another to the great army of neurasthenics and sexual incompetents, which furnish neurologists and gynecologists with so much of their material . . . Bright eyes have been dulled by the brain-fag and sweet temper transformed into irritability, crossness and hysteria, while the womanhood of the land is deteriorating physically.
>
> She may be highly cultured and accomplished and shine in society, but her future husband will discover too late that he has married a large outfit of headaches, backaches and spine aches, instead of a woman fitted to take up the duties of life (Darnall, 1901: 490).

Men who stimulated their sexual organs through masturbation rather than their brains through intellectual pursuits would meet a similar fate (Smith-Rosenberg, 1978).

The late 19th century medical view of women and their role, then, rested on four assumptions: (1) a closed energy system, whereby the use of the brain resulted, essentially, in the theft of energy from the ovaries; (2) a hierarchy of bodily functions which, as indicated, placed the ovary in a position superior to that of the brain; (3) the physiological fragility of the female; and (4) the dichotomization or polarization of male (brain/mind) and female (body/ovaries) function (Smith-Rosenberg,

1973). Women who rejected these premises and engaged in violative behaviors were characterized by physicians as an "intermediate sex," fusing the female and male to become the "Mannish lesbian" (Smith-Rosenberg, 1985: 265).

Medical discourse which had previously focused on homosexuality in men to the almost complete exclusion of women now began to address female homosexuality. Von Krafft-Ebing delineated four categories of homosexual women. Those in the first category were not recognizable as lesbians based on their physical characteristics, but would respond to the overtures of more masculine-behaving women. The second category encompassed those lesbians who preferred to wear male garments. Those in the third category were "inverted," having assumed a masculine role. Women in the fourth category, "gynandry," had reached the epitome of degenerative homosexuality:

> The woman of this type possesses of the feminine qualities only the genital organs; thought, sentiment, action, even external appearance are those of a man. Often enough one does come across in life such characters whose frame, pelvis, gait, appearance, coarse masculine features, rough, deep voice, etc. betrayed rather the man than the woman (Von Krafft-Ebing, 1908: 333–336).

Such women, Von Krafft-Ebing reported, avoided the women's fashion and pursued, instead, male sports. Additionally, the desire for privileges and power traditionally associated with men exceeded a sexual desire for other women (Von Krafft-Ebing, 1908). Women who rejected traditional female gender norms were, in essence, abnormal.

Unlike Von Krafft-Ebing, the sexologist Ellis attributed "inversion" to biological and hereditary factors, concluding that it was irreversible. He distinguished between those women who were congenitally inverted and those with a genetic disposition, for whom homosexuality was an acquired, preventable, and curable trait (Ellis, 1895). Definitions of masculinity and femininity arose directly from the biological basis for sex. Like Krafft-Ebing, Ellis concluded that departures from socially determined roles were abnormal. Those who were congenitally inverted were not only sexually active, unlike normal women, but also competed aggressively with men for their sexual partners (Ellis, 1895–1896). By the 1920s, charges of lesbianism became a common strategy to discredit female professionals and reformers (Smith-Rosenberg, 1985).

The women's health movement was to have a lasting impact on women's health and health care and, not surprisingly, their social roles as well. Eagan (1994) has traced the beginning of the movement to 1970, when women protested over their exclusion from congressional hearings on the use of birth control pills. Numerous events converged to alert women to the dangers of relying on physicians as their only source of information in making health care decisions. The first printing of *Our Bodies, Ourselves* was released in 1971, providing women with a basic source of information. Abortion was legalized in 1973 with the decision in *Roe v. Wade*. In 1971, it was revealed that DES, used by millions of women to prevent miscarriage, was linked to a rare form of vaginal cancer in the daughters of women who had ingested the drug (Herbst, Ulfelder, and Poskanzer, 1971). The publication of *Why Me?* challenged medicine's reliance on the Halsted radical mastectomy to treat breast cancer (Kushner, 1975). That procedure had required the removal of the entire breast, the axillary lymph nodes, and the underlying chest wall muscle.

Substance Use and Health

Infectious Disease

Human Immunodeficiency Virus (HIV). In 1988, seven years after the HIV epidemic was first recognized, the proportion of AIDS cases attributable to women was 10 percent. By 2003, that figure had risen to 30 percent. Although African-American and Hispanic women comprise 21 percent of the U.S. population, 78 percent of cumulative AIDS cases in women are attributable to these groups (Centers for Disease Control and Protection, 2002d). In 1992, AIDS became the fourth leading cause of death among women aged 25 to 44 years, but had been the leading cause of death among African-American women since 1987 (Guinan and Leviton, 1995). In the year 2000, 38 percent of AIDS cases among women resulted from heterosexual intercourse and an additional 25 percent were attributable to injection drug use (Centers for Disease Control and Prevention, 2002d).

Cancer

Lung cancer deaths among women have been increasing since the 1960s and it is now the leading cause of cancer deaths among white and African-American women (Centers for Disease Control, 1993). Cigarette smoking is the leading cause of lung cancer deaths among women in the United States; approximately 90 percent of all lung cancer deaths among U.S. women smokers are attributable to smoking (Centers for Disease Control and Prevention, 2001). Not surprisingly, cancer has been found to be the most feared disease among women due to its perceived incurability and associated suffering (Gordon, Venturini, Del Tucco, Palli, and Paci, 1991; Murray and McMillan, 1993). Smoking has also been found to be a major cause of cancers of the oropharynx and bladder among women, and has been associated with an increased risk for cervical cancer (Centers for Disease Control and Prevention, 2001).

Cardiovascular Disease

Smoking is a major cause of coronary heart disease among women and has been associated with an increased risk of ischemic stroke and peripheral vascular atherosclerosis. The risk of coronary heart disease is reduced substantially approximately 1 to 2 years after ceasing smoking. The increased risk of stroke that is associated with smoking approaches that of an individual who never smoked approximately 10 to 15 years after ceasing smoking (Centers for Disease Control and Prevention, 2001).

Reproductive Health

Reproductive health has often focused on issues relating to birth control and contraception. Although numerous methods had been used throughout time to prevent pregnancy, it was not until the mid-19th century that birth control gained public attention. In part a response to growing concern with falling birth rates among middle- and upper-class whites, Congress in 1863 passed the Comstock Law. This law defined contraception as obscene and prohibited distribution of birth control information through the mail (Poirier, 1990).

Margaret Sanger championed efforts of women to control their bodies throughout the control of contraception. She was arrested twice, once in 1912 for the distribution of information through the mail and again in 1916, following the opening of a clinic that fitted women with diaphragms (Sanger, 1938). Ultimately, Sanger advocated laws that permitted only physicians to prescribe and fit diaphragms; the reasons for her position remain subject to debate (Kennedy, 1970; Reed, 1978).

The federal Comstock Law was not overturned until 1938. In the interim, though, many states had implemented legislation prohibiting birth control. It was not until the 1965 Supreme Court decision in *Griswold v. Connecticut* that women were permitted access to birth control information, subsumed under a right to privacy (Dienes, 1972). The contraceptive pill was released on the U.S. market in the 1960s.

The testing and use of birth control has raised numerous ethical issues. The first anovulatory drugs were tested on poor Puerto Rican women in Puerto Rico. At least one author has raised concerns regarding the nature of the informed consent, given the economic and political context (Gordon, 1976). U.S. government-sponsored family programs emerged during the Depression and often targeted its sterilization efforts towards poor women.

Numerous reports have documented the involuntary sterilizations of poor women and women of color (Davis, 1981; Dreifus, 1977; Larson, 1995; Rodrigues-Trias, 1978). The use among poor women of Depo-Provera, a long-term contraceptive injection, has raised similar ethical concerns (Cassidy, 1980; Levine, 1980).

It was not until the mid-1880s that most states made most abortions illegal, including abortions performed by physicians. Prior to that time, many states permitted abortion until "quickening" (Smith-Rosenberg, 1985). It was in response to the lobbying of the American Medical Association that harsh anti-abortion laws were enacted. As chairman of an AMA committee formed to ascertain the number of abortions performed in the United States, Horatio Stover opined against the availability of abortions to married middle- and upper-class women, who "prefer to devastate with poison and with steel their wombs rather than . . . forego the gaieties of a winter's balls, parties, and plays, or the pleasure of a summer's trips and amusements" (Stover and Heard, 1865: 72). The efforts of Stover and the AMA, together with the Protestant clergy and Roman Catholic church, effectively ended the availability of legal abortion until the 1970s. The anti-abortion rhetoric and efforts were supported through the Comstock Law which, as noted above, prohibited the distribution of birth control information through the mail. In 1964 alone, 10,000 women were admitted to New York City hospitals for treatment of severe complications resulting from criminal abortions.

At least one author has asserted that the intensity of this anti-abortion movement was a direct outgrowth of obstetricians' and gynecologists' concern over their low professional status, public reputation, and relative lack of knowledge and their perceived lack of financial power at the hands of the bourgeois matrons who sought their services (Smith-Rosenberg, 1985). The husbands and fathers of the unborn child were exonerated from all responsibility in the decision to abort. Speaking of the women seeking an abortion, an AMA committee observed:

> She becomes unmindful of the course marked out for her by Providence, she overlooks the duties imposed on her by the marriage contract. She yields to the pleasures—but shrinks from the pains and responsibilities of maternity; and, destitute of all delicacy and refinement, resigns herself, body and soul, into the hands of unscrupulous and wicked men. Let not the husband of such a wife flatter himself that he possesses her affection (Atlee and O'Donnell, 1871: 241).

During the 1960s, various groups lobbied for relaxed abortion laws. The 1973 Supreme Court decision in *Roe v. Wade* relegated first trimester abortion decisions to a woman and her physician; only after the first trimester could the state regulate or prohibit abortion. Later court decisions restricted the case's impact. For instance, *Maher v. Roe* resulted in a prohibition against the use of federal funds to perform abortions (Poirier, 1990).

Intentional Violence

Domestic Violence. Because definitions vary across studies, it becomes difficult to compare incidence and prevalence rates. The proportion of women reporting severe domestic violence in a one year period (being kicked, bitten, hit, choked, threatened by a gun, or wounded by a gun or knife) ranges from .27 percent in a probability sample of 60,000 women (Klaus and Rand, 1984) to 5 percent in a nonprobability sample of 304 women (Meredith, Abbott, and Adams, 1986). Total domestic violence, including severe domestic violence, has ranged in a one year period from 8.4 percent in a stratified random sample of 1,324 women (Plitcha and Weisman, 1995) to 22 percent in the nonprobability sample noted above (Meredith, Abbott, and Adams, 1986). Lifetime prevalence of severe domestic violence has been reported to range from 9 percent of 602 women in a stratified random sample (Petersen, 1980) to 12.6 percent of 2,143 women in a stratified random sample (Straus, Gelles, and Steinmetz, 1980). Lifetime prevalence of total domestic violence has ranged from 7.3 percent (McFarlane, Christoffel, Batemen, Miller, and Bullock, 1991) to 30 percent (Straus and Gelles, 1990; Teske and Parker, 1983). Domestic violence has been found to be more prevalent among younger persons (Straus, Gelles, and Steinmetz, 1980; Straus and Gelles, 1990; Teske and Parker, 1983) and among those with lower incomes (Stark and Flitcraft, 1988). Domestic violence has also been associated with alcohol use (Eberle, 1982; Teske and Parker, 1983).

Injuries resulting from domestic violence include bruises, cuts, concussions, broken bones, miscarriages, loss of hearing or vision, and scars from burns, bites, or knife wounds (Council on Scientific Affairs, 1992). Reactions to domestic violence include shock, denial, withdrawal, confusion, psychological numbing, and fear. Long-term effects include fear, anxiety, fatigue, sleeping and eating disturbances, depression, and suicidal thoughts or attempts (Stark and Flitcraft, 1988).

Rape. Epidemiological data indicate that the prevalence of rape is high; at least 20 percent of adult women, 15 percent of college women, and 12 percent of adolescent girls have experienced sexual abuse and assault during their lifetimes (Koss, 1988). Reports indicate that rape victims may initially experience shock, numbness, withdrawal, and denial. Longer term effects include chronic anxiety, nightmares, sexual dysfunction, physical distress

(Koss and Harvey, 1991), phobias, depression, hostility (Resick, Calhoun, Atkeson, and Ellis, 1981), and suicidal thoughts (Kilpatrick, Veronen, and Best, 1985; Resick, Jordan, Girelli, Hutter, and Marhoefer-Dvorak, 1989).

Substance Use

The prevalence of smoking among women has decreased in recent years from 33.9 percent in 1965 to 22.0 percent in 1998. The prevalence of smoking is higher among women with 9 to 11 years of education (32.9 percent), compared to those with 16 or more years of education (11.2 percent). It is also higher among women who are living below poverty levels (29.6 percent), compared to those who are not (21.6 percent) (Centers for Disease Control and Prevention, 2001). The prevalence of smoking among various groups for the period 1997 through 1998 was 34.5 percent among American Indian and Alaska Native women, 23.5 percent among non-Hispanic white women, 21.9 percent of African-American women, 13.8 percent of Hispanic women, and 11.2 percent of Asian and Pacific Islander women. More than one-quarter of all women of reproductive age are smokers. Compared to other ethnic/racial groups, non-Hispanic white women have a higher prevalence of smoking during pregnancy (Centers for Disease Control and Prevention, 2001).

The prevalence of cigar smoking among women has increased dramatically during the last few years, although adolescent girls are more likely to smoke cigars than are adult women. Women and girls are much less likely than males to use either pipes or smokeless tobacco (Centers for Disease Control and Prevention, 2001).

Among individuals who smoke heavily, women are more likely than men to report being dependent on cigarettes. Smoking cessation programs that include elements of peer support or family support are more likely to be successful among adolescent girls in comparison to adolescent boys (Centers for Disease Control and Prevention, 2001).

QUEER COMMUNITIES

It is believed that between 2 and 10 percent of the U.S. population is gay or lesbian (Gadpaille, 1995). However, relatively little is known about the demographic characteristics of those who identify themselves as gay, lesbian, or bisexual. Some data are available from the National Lesbian Health Care Survey, which involved 1,917 volunteers recruited primarily through lesbian and gay health organizations and practitioners and through publicity furnished by numerous professional organizations (Ryan and

Bradford, 1988). Survey findings indicated that respondents were 17 years of age and older; that over one-quarter had completed college and more than one-third held an advanced degree; and that over one-half were employed in a professional capacity on a full-time basis. The majority of respondents self-identified as white, non-Hispanic with no religious affiliation.

Relatively little research has been devoted to an examination of the health issues confronting non-heterosexuals and transsexuals. Numerous methodological problems have been identified in the research conducted to date. For instance, there exists no consensus among clinicians and behavioral scientists regarding the definition of "homosexuality" (Friedman, 1988) and multiple definitions of the labels "bisexual," "gay," and "lesbian" exist (Francoeur, Perper, and Scherzer, 1991). Only a minority of researchers define the population being investigated and the methods of identifying eligible respondents vary considerably across studies (Sell and Petrulio, 1996). Researchers often fail to recognize the distinction between sexual identity (I am a gay/lesbian), sexual behavior (I have sex with men/women), and community participation (I am a member of a gay/lesbian community) (Golden, 1987; Rothblum, 1994). Second, probability sampling is rarely used to assemble study participants, often resulting in selection bias (Platzer and James, 1997; Sell and Petrulio, 1996). Instead, participants are often recruited from gay or lesbian organizations or are recruited based on their self-identity as gay/lesbian or their involvement in same-sex sexual activity. These three dimensions, while somewhat overlapping, are not synonymous and emphasis on the inappropriate dimension in recruitment efforts will impact the ability to address the research question at issue (Rothblum, 1994). Third, individuals' self-identity may change over time and context (Rothblum, 1994). It is important to reflect on these issues in evaluating the summary that follows.

Cultural and Historical Context

U.S. society's displeasure with homosexuality and lesbianism is evident from its earliest beginnings. Thomas Jefferson, for instance, proposed in 1779 that "Whoever shall be guilty of sodomy shall be punished if a man by castration, if a woman by cutting through the cartilage of her nose a hole one-half inch in diameter" (Quoted in Abramson, 1980: 187).

By the end of the 19th century, homosexuality and lesbianism had become a medical concern rather than only a moral or theological one. Von Krafft-Ebing attributed homosexuality to degeneracy, as did Westphal and Charcot (Bullough, 1976; Miller, 1995; Schmidt, 1984). Others, however, were more sympathetic. Ulrichs, a German lawyer, conceived of homosexuals as a third sex, whose gender characteristics and choice of sexual object were inverted due to developments in the uterus (Miller, 1995). Ellis, a British sexologist, also believed that homosexuality was inherited and rejected its characterization as a sign of moral degeneracy. He further rejected the stereotyping of homosexuals (Miller, 1995).

Freud's psychoanalytic model of homosexuality, however, came to dominate American medical thought. Freud initially postulated that all individuals are essentially bisexual and that homosexuality was neither an illness nor a form of degeneracy. He characterized homosexuality as an arrested stage of development (Miller, 1995). American psychoanalysts, rejecting Freud's observation that homosexuals generally functioned well and ignoring his skepticism regarding its curability, often depicted homosexuality as a disease and a form of moral corruption (Berg and Allen, 1958; Bergler, 1957; Chideckel, 1935; Rado, 1933; Stekel, 1946). Lesbians, for instance, were characterized as hostile (Bene, 1965), fearful of pregnancy and childbirth (Rado, 1933), aggressive and domineering (Bene, 1965; Caprio, 1954; Fenichel, 1945), sadistic (Socarides, 1968), homicidal (Caprio, 1954), fearful of disappointment, and guilt-ridden. Their specific "condition" was said to result from rape, incest, tomboyish behavior, seduction by an older woman, masturbation, and fear of dominance (Rosen, 1974). Numerous strategies were adopted in an effort to cure individuals of their homosexuality, including castration, hormone therapy, and hypnosis (Miller, 1995).

During the 1910s and 1920s, despite these views, Greenwich Village in New York provided a relatively tolerant environment, which permitted same-sex relationships and homosexuality (Miller, 1995). By the 1920s, gay balls had become an accepted event in the Village. Police crackdowns, however, were quite common during the 1920s. These raids abated somewhat during the 1930s, when the New York police permitted gays to socialize in public so long as they didn't draw attention to themselves. That tolerance, however, was somewhat short-lived (Miller, 1995).

The notion of homosexuals as sick became entrenched through the work of Rado, Bieber, Wilbur, and Socarides. Rado (1933) attributed homosexuality to fears of the opposite sex, while Bieber (1965) characterized homosexuality as resulting from life with a detached and hostile father and a seductive mother. Socarides (1968) insisted that the majority of homosexuals were either neurotic or psychotic. The apparent consensus viewing homosexuality as a pathology resulted in the inclusion of homosexuality as a sociopathic personality disturbance in the 1952 edition of the American Psychiatric Association's *Diagnostic and Statistical Manual of Mental Disorders* (DSM).

Military recruits in the U.S. were asked about their sexual orientation during World War II recruitment efforts. Homosexual men and women were labeled "sexual psychopaths" (Berube, 1990). Gradually, the military toughened its policies against homosexuals. Concurrently, various agencies and individuals within the federal government, including the Federal Bureau of Investigation and the infamous attorney Roy Cohn, embarked on a campaign to eliminate homosexuals from government service (Miller, 1995). "Sexual perversion" became a sufficient basis for the exclusion of an individual from federal employment.

The pathological nature of homosexuality was put into question as a result of Kinsey and colleagues' studies (1948, 1953) which indicated that homosexual behavior was more widespread than had been thought. The 1968 edition of *Diagnostic and Statistical Manual of Mental Disorders* (DSM) reclassified homosexuality as an "other non-psychotic mental disorder," together with fetishism, pedophilia, voyeurism, exhibitionism, sadism, and masochism (Miller, 1995). The July 17, 1969 raid of the Stonewall Inn in Greenwich Village in New York City marked the commencement of what was to become the gay and lesbian liberation movement (Miller, 1995). Instead of leaving, the bar patrons resisted the police raid, creating "the Boston Tea Party of the Gay Movement" (Altman, 1973). This movement constituted a transformation of approach within the gay communities, from one of reconciliation and adjustment (gay people can fit into American society) to one of self-acknowledgement and assertiveness (American society needs to change). The impact of this movement is reflected in the 1973 de-classification of homosexuality as a mental disorder following the vote of the American Psychiatric Association membership to remove homosexuality per se from the nosology (Miller, 1995).

Despite these milestones, state laws continued to prohibit homosexual behavior. Although there were many monogamous gay couples, urban male culture of the 1970s was characterized by anonymous sexual encounters with multiple partners. The emergence of what was to become known as AIDS provoked marked changes in individual behaviors, including the adoption of safe sex practices, and in community values, such as the initiation of benefit coverage for domestic partners and the implementation by the Food and Drug Administration of procedures to expedite the approval of drug treatments (Miller, 1995).

Substance Use and Health

Access to Care

Access to health care that is both necessary and sensitive has been identified as a major issue confronting gay, lesbian, bisexual, and transsexual patients. The majority of lesbians often do not reveal their sexual orientation to health care providers (Cochran and Mays, 1988; Reagan, 1981) due to the perceived or actual risk of hostility, neglect, denial of care, condescension, or other negative response from the health care provider (Bradford and Ryan, 1987; Denenberg, 1992; Perrin and Kulkin, 1996; Raymond, 1988; Steven and Hall, 1988; Stevens, 1995; Trippet and Bain, 1992).

These fears are far from misplaced. A recent study of 278 nursing students' attitudes towards lesbian patients found that a large proportion of the nursing students (38 percent) believed that lesbians seek to seduce heterosexual women; that lesbians can be identified on the basis of their relatively masculine appearance (31 percent); and that lesbians provide a negative role model for children (11 percent) (Eliason, Donelan, and Randall, 1992). Randall (1989) found in her survey of 100 nursing educators that 24 percent believed that lesbian behavior is wrong, 23 percent believed that lesbianism is immoral, and 15 percent indicated that lesbians are perverted. Almost one fifth of the respondents (19 percent) indicated that state laws punishing lesbians for their sexual behavior should be preserved. Heterosexist and homophobic attitudes have also been noted among social workers (Berkman and Zinberg, 1997) and physicians (Douglas, Kalman, and Kalman, 1985; Mathews, Booth, Turner, and Kessler, 1986; Oriel, Madlon-Kay, Govaker, and Mersy, 1996). Such attitudes have been found to affect both the quality of the care provided (Schatz and O'Hanlan, 1994; Wise and Bowman, 1997) and the perception by heterosexual physicians of the competency of their homosexual colleagues (Oriel et al., 1996). They may extend so far as to interfere with the ability of gay or lesbian parents to obtain pediatric care for their children (Perrin and Kulkin, 1996). Such attitudes and practices are not, unfortunately, surprising in view of the scant training provided to either medical school students (Robinson and Cohen, 1996; Townsend, Wallick, Pleak, and Cambre, 1997; Wallick, Cambre, and Townsend, 1992) or to nursing students (Leifer and Young, 1997) on the topics of homosexuality and bisexuality.

In response to such attitudes, lesbian patients may adopt any number of protective strategies, including rallying support, screening providers, seeking mirrors of their experience, maintaining vigilance, controlling information, bringing a witness, challenging mistreatment, and escaping perceived danger (Hitchcock and Wilson, 1992; Stevens, 1993; Stevens, 1994).

Various additional barriers to accessing health care by gay men and lesbian women have been identified, including lack of insurance (Stevens, 1993), ceilings on coverage, exclusions due to pre-existing conditions, "gatekeepers" at health maintenance organizations (Stevens, 1993), lack of financial resources (Bradford and Ryan, 1989; Stevens, 1993), and providers' lack of attention to preventive care and education (Trippet and Bain, 1992).

Infectious Disease

Sexually Transmitted Disease. Sexually transmitted diseases appear to be less common among lesbian women than among heterosexual men or women or homosexual men (White and Levinson, 1995). The reasons for this are unclear. Accordingly, women who are sexually active with women experience lower incidence rates of gonorrhea and syphilis than all other groups except those who have never been sexually active (Degan and Waitkevicz, 1982). Various other infections are also uncommon among women who are sexually active only with other women. These include chlamydia, herpes virus, and human papillomavirus (Johnson, Guenther, Laube, and Keettel, 1981; Johnson, Smith, and Guenther, 1987). Female-to-female transmission of human immunodeficiency virus also appears relatively uncommon (Chu, Buehler, Fleming, and Berkelman, 1990; Harris, Thiede, McGough, and Gordon, 1993; Marmor, Weiss, Lydon, Weiss, Saxinger, Spira, and Feorino, 1986; Monzon and Capellon, 1987; Sabatini, Patel, and Hirschman, 1984). However, bacterial vaginosis, candidiasis and *Trichomonas vaginalis* appear to be common (Degan and Waitkevicz, 1982; Johnson and Palermo, 1984; Johnson, Smith, and Guenther, 1987; Sivakumar, DeSilva, and Roy, 1989; Trippet and Bain, 1993). Despite the apparently low risk of transmission of many of these infections, it is clear that they are transmissible between women (Berger, Kolton, Zenilman, Cummings, Feldman, and McCormack, 1995; Edwards and Thin, 1990; Simkin, 1993; Sivakumar, DeSilva, and Roy, 1989; Walters and Rector, 1986). Further, many lesbians may have had some heterosexual sexual contact and may continue to be sexually active with men on a regular or intermittent basis, while identifying as lesbian (Einhorn and Polgar, 1994; Rankow, 1997).

Various strategies have been suggested to reduce the risk of STD transmission, including HIV, between female sexual partners. These include the use of female condoms, gloves, and dental dams (Kahn, 1987; White and Levinson, 1995); the avoidance of cervical and vaginal secretions, menstrual blood, and blood from vaginal and rectal trauma in partners (White and Levinson, 1995); the avoidance of fresh semen when undergoing artificial insemination (Chiasson, Stoneburner, and Joseph, 1990; Eskenazi, Pies, Newstetter, Shepard, and Pearson, 1989); and refraining from sharing sex toys (Rankow, 1997).

Men who have sex with men continue to account for the largest proportion of individuals reported with AIDS each year, and the largest proportion (70 percent) of new HIV infections each year. In the year 2000, men who have sex with men accounted for 13,562 of reported AIDS cases. In the same year, 50 percent of reported HIV infections among adolescent males ages 15 to 19 and 53 percent of reported HIV cases among men ages 20 to 24 were attributable to male-to-male sexual contact (Centers for Disease Control and Prevention, 2002e).

Gastrointestinal Infections. Gay men are at increased risk of specific gastrointestinal infections due to transmission through receptive anal intercourse and oral-anal sexual contact. These infections include *Giardia lamblia, Entamoeba histolytica,* Shigella species, *campylobacter,* and hepatitis A (Rompalo, 1990). They are also at increased risk for transmission of hepatitis B virus, STDs, and HIV due to unprotected anogenital intercourse (de Wit, van Griensven, Kok, and Sandfort, 1993; Harrison and Silenzio, 1996).

"Coming Out"

Gay men and women must often address issues related to "coming out," the process of discovering one's homosexuality and revealing it to others. This process, which may begin at any age, is often associated with considerable emotional distress (Schneider, 1989). The process involves a shift in core identity and occurs in four phases: (1) awareness of homosexual feelings, (2) testing and exploration, (3) identity acceptance, and (4) identity integration and disclosure to others (Faderman, 1985; Walpin, 1997). The coming out process appears to differ between males and females in that the process appears to be more abrupt in males and more likely to be associated with depression or suicide attempts (Gonsiorek, 1988). Prevailing social attitudes can impact the experience of coming out (Savin-Williams, 1998; Schneider, 1989; Faderman, 1985). Ethnic minority gays and lesbians may be minorities within minorities and may consequently face additional multiple levels of discrimination (Greene, 1994).

Adolescents may be particularly vulnerable during this process. Confusion about sexual orientation may result in depression, poor school performance, substance misuse, acting out, and suicidal ideation (Feinleib, 1989). Coming out may provoke negative responses from others, including family conflict and rejection (Kreiss and Patterson, 1997), loss of friendship with peers (Nelson, 1997), and verbal abuse from teachers (Uribe and Harbeck, 1992), resulting in the exacerbation of feelings of confusion and isolation (Kreiss and Patterson, 1997; Nelson, 1997).

Substance Use

Significant research has been conducted on the use of alcohol among gays and lesbians. Fifeld (1975) found in a study of individuals frequenting bars that the lesbian and gay respondents drank an average of 6 drinks per bar visit and frequented bars, on average, 19 times per month. McKirnan and Peterson (1989a, 1989b) found from their survey of 748 lesbians and 2,652 gay men that a higher proportion of gays and lesbians used alcohol, marijuana, and cocaine compared to the general population. Bradford, Ryan, and Rothblum (1994) found in their study of the health of 1,925 lesbians that almost one-third used tobacco on a daily basis, 30 percent drank alcohol more than once a week, and 6 percent used alcohol on a daily basis. Nearly half of the women reported that they used marijuana at least occasionally, while almost one-fifth reported having used cocaine. Other researchers have reported increased use of alcohol and drug use in lesbians compared with heterosexual women and women in the general population (Bradford, Ryan, and Rothblum, 1994; Lewis, Saghir, and Robins, 1982; Milman and Su, 1973; Roberts and Sorenson, 1994, cited in Roberts and Sorenson, 1995). Research findings also indicate that lesbians and bisexual women under the age of 50 are more likely than heterosexual women to smoke (Gruskin, Hart, Gordon, and Ackerson, 2001).

Various explanations have been advanced in an attempt to understand the extensive use of alcohol and other substances: (1) dysfunctional families of origin (Gardner-Loulan, 1983; Glaus, 1988; Hepburn and Gutierrez, 1988; Swallow, 1983), (2) societal oppression (Cantu, 1983; Glaus, 1988; Martin and Lyon, 1972; Weathers, 1980; Willowroot, 1983), and (3) past trauma including incest (Bass and Davis, 1988; Bradford, Ryan, and Rothblum, 1994; Covington and Kohen, 1984; Evans and Schaefer, 1987; Perry, 1995). Earlier medical writings postulated that the high use of alcohol among lesbians was related to masculinity (Knight, 1937), guilt (Weijl, 1944), and the need to contain sexual drives (Clark, 1919; Stekel, 1946). However, more recent research findings suggest that participation in the "bar culture" as a primary means of socialization, particularly among younger lesbian and bisexual women, may explain the higher rates of alcohol use (Heffernan, 1998). Additional explanatory factors include stress, depression, external and internalized homophobia and heteosexism (Abbott, 1998; Heffernan, 1998; Hughes and Wilsnack, 1997). Numerous approaches have been utilized to address excessive alcohol use among gays and lesbians, including psychotherapy, 12-step programs, and Alcoholics Anonymous (Hall, 1993).

Suicide

Numerous studies have documented high rates of suicidal behavior among gays and lesbians in comparison with heterosexuals. A 1977 study by Jay and Young of over 5,100 lesbians and gay men found that 40 percent of the gay men and 39 percent of the lesbians had attempted or seriously considered suicide. Bell and Weinberg (1987) reported from their study of 979 gays and lesbians that significantly higher percentages of gays than heterosexuals had attempted or seriously contemplated suicide. Saunders and Valente (1987) concluded that lesbians had 2.5 times more suicidal behavior than heterosexuals. Bradford, Ryan, and Rothblum (1994) found in their study involving 1,925 lesbians that 19 percent had thought about suicide sometimes and 2 percent had thought about it often. Eighteen percent of the respondents had attempted suicide, often through the use of drugs, razor blades, alcohol, weapons, gas, or a car.

Gay, lesbian, and bisexual youth may be at especially high risk of suicide (Gibson, 1989; Proctor and Groze, 1994; Remafedi, 1990). Proctor and Groze (1994) found in their study of 221 gay, lesbian, and bisexual youth that over 40 percent had attempted suicide. Gibson (1989) has found in his study that 20 to 35 percent of gay youths interviewed had attempted suicide and 50 percent had experienced suicidal ideation. Saghir and Robins (1973) found that five out of six homosexual men who attempted suicide did so before they reached the age of 20. Numerous factors associated with suicide and suicide attempts have been identified, including depression (Remafedi, Farrow, and Deisher, 1991), social isolation, anger, feelings of inadequacy (Sears, 1991), paternal alcoholism, familial physical abuse, familial suicide attempts (Schneider, Farberow, and Kruks, 1989), violence directed against gays (Hunter, 1990), lack of support (Gonsiorek, 1988), and sexual experience before the age of 14 (Jay and Young, 1979).

Physical and Sexual Abuse

Relatively few studies have been conducted on the use of physical or sexual violence within same sex relationships. Those that have, have consistently noted such violence among a high proportion of study respondents. Studies of battering among both gay men and lesbian women have consistently found an association between heavy substance abuse and victimization (Burke and Follingstad, 1999; Cruz and Firestone, 1998; Stermac, Sheridan, Davidson, and Dunn, 1996).

One of the earlier studies, conducted by Brand and Kidd (1986), found that 30 percent of the 55 lesbian respondents reported ever having been "physically abused." Later studies found even higher proportions. Bologna, Waterman, and Dawson (1987) utilized the Conflict Tactics Scale (Straus, Gelles, and Steinmetz, 1980) in their survey of 70 lesbian women and gay men. Fifty-six percent of the lesbian women and 25 percent of the gay male respondents reported abuse by their current or most recent partner. Over one half of the 1,099 lesbians participating in Lie and Gentlewarrior's (1991) survey reported physical abuse by their current partner. Lie, Schilit, Bush, Montagne, and Reyes (1991), utilizing the Conflict Tactics Scale (Straus, Gelles, and Steinmetz, 1980), found that 25 percent of the 174 lesbian respondents were experiencing abuse by their then-current partner and 75 percent had ever experienced abuse.

A more recent study by Lockhart, White, Causby, and Isaac (1994), which also utilized the Conflict Tactics Scale (Straus, Gelles, and Steinmetz, 1980), found that almost one-third of the 284 lesbian respondents had been physically abused during the previous year. Similar findings have been noted by Schilit, Lie, and Montagne (1990). A high prevalence of abuse was also noted by Waldner-Haugrud, Gratch, and Magruder (1997) among their 283 gay and lesbian participants. Results indicated that 47.5 percent of the lesbians and 29.7 percent of the gay men had been victimized by a same sex partner at some time. Lesbians reported an overall prevalence rate for violence of 38 percent, compared to a rate of 21.8 percent for gay men. Both lesbians and gay men most frequently reported pushing, receiving threats, and slapping as the primary forms of abuse. Thirty-eight percent of the lesbians and 21.8 percent of the gay men reported using violence against their partners. The National Lesbian Health Care Survey results indicated that 15 percent of the 1,925 respondents suffered physical and/or sexual abuse as an adult (Bradford, Ryan, and Rothblum, 1994). More than half of the women reporting abuse as adults identified their lover (53 percent, gender unspecified) or their husbands (27 percent) as the perpetrator (Bradford, Ryan, and Rothblum, 1994).

Despite the apparently high prevalence of physical abuse, lesbian victims have been found less likely to seek help in shelters or from counselors (Morrow and Hawxhurst, 1989). Dissatisfaction has been reported with several sources of assistance: the clergy, police, and private physicians (Bradford, Ryan, and Rothblum, 1994).

Chapter 6

Diversity Issues in Treatment

The previous chapters examined concepts of diversity and the historical and cultural contexts that give rise to both the experiences of various groups and to our understandings of diversity. Chapters 6 and 7 focus on the application of these understandings and the integration of the diverse experiences of various groups into the development and conduct of treatment programs and research endeavors.

INTEGRATING DIVERSITY INTO TREATMENT: GENERAL CONSIDERATIONS

Diversity and Service Delivery

Attention to diversity can be integrated into various aspects of service delivery in the context of substance use treatment: the identification of the target population that is to be served; the development of a value base that emphasizes the importance and the reasons for the importance of services attuned to diversity considerations; flexibility in service design and delivery that recognizes and accounts for differences within and between groups; the involvement of the community in the development of services; and the development of evaluation strategies and tools that reflect a multi-cultural perspective (Mason, 1994). Five specific elements have been identified as being critical to this integration: multiculturalism, resilience and strengths, skills and knowledge, the development of community capacity and empowerment, and community participation (Delgado, 1998).

The operationalization of multiculturalism encompasses several key principles. First, the services must be available in the language that is preferred by the client. This refers not only to the language itself, such as Spanish or English or Vietnamese, but to the level of that language as well. For instance, if a client communicates in two and three syllable words, it is not helpful for a counselor to use five and six syllable words that may be beyond the educational level and understanding of the client. In addition, "language" encompasses a familiarity with nonverbal cues appropriate to the individual's background.

Second, it may be critical to many clients to have staff of the program reflect their own characteristics. However, in small, insular communities, some clients may wish to forego this sense of familiarity due to concerns that their privacy will be somewhat limited because of intra-community familiarity. In addition, the services and service providers must respect cultural values and reinforce a sense of pride (Delgado, 1998).

Involving Community

It is also important that organizations providing substance abuse services understand the strengths that exist in the community they are serving, engage and involve that community in the development and planning of the services, and establish collaborative relationships (Delgado, 1998). This helps to avoid the development of and reliance on a deficit paradigm, whereby only outsiders and experts are deemed to have adequate knowledge and expertise to address the substance abuse issues. Efforts to address substance abuse may, as a result, be more successful because they will develop and capitalize on the strengths of individuals, families, and communities through, for instance, individuals' participation on organizational boards and committees and through the establishment of collaborations through both formal and informal channels (Delgado, 1998).

First, however, the community to be engaged must be identified. This process may be more complex than it appears at first, in part due to individuals' simultaneous memberships in multiple communities. *Webster's Third New International Dictionary* (1993) has defined a community as

(1) a body of individuals organized into a unit or manifesting usually with awareness some unifying trait: a. state, commonwealth; b. people living in a particular place or region; c. a monastic body or other unified religious body; d. an interacting population of different kinds of individuals constituting a society or association or simply an aggregation of mutually related individuals in a given location; e. a group of people marked by a common characteristics but living within a larger society that does not share that characteristic... (2) society at large ... (3) common or joint ownership, tenure experience, or pertinence.

The concept of community, however, may reflect much more. Wilkinson (1986, cited in Chekki, 1990: 1) has characterized community as the "active ingredient in all of social life, a factor to be taken into account in attempting to understand whatever social processes and structures one finds in a given setting." The community, then, may be indispensable to the solution when addressing substance abuse. In a given context, the community may be defined geographically; by shared characteristics or attributes, such as ethnicity, age, sexual orientation, or behavior; and/or by a form of sustained social interaction (Sinnika Dixon, 1989).

As an example, researchers asked African-Americans in Durham, North Carolina, gay men in San Francisco, California, injection drug users in Philadelphia, Pennsylvania, and HIV vaccine researchers across the United States to indicate what the word "community" signified to them (MacQueen, McLellan, Metzger, Kegeles, Strauss, Scotti, Blanchard, and Trotter, 2001). The groups shared a common understanding of "community" as a group of individuals with diverse characteristics, linked by social ties, common perspectives, and efforts to engage in joint action in geographical locations. However, significant differences also existed. The gay men in San Francisco emphasized a shared history and perspective as being critical to a sense of community, as well as a sense of identity with a specific location. In contrast, the African-American participants in Durham and the injection drug users in Philadelphia identified locus as the key element of community, followed by joint action and social ties.

In formulating services to address issues of diversity, then, it is critical that providers understand not only how they are defining the community of interest, but also how their clients define their own communities of interest and how they rank their various memberships within multiple communities.

BARRIERS TO TREATMENT

Documentation of Need

Services tend to be available to populations whose need for those services has been well-documented. For some populations, however, adequate data are not available and, as a result, adequate services may be lacking.

Consider, for example, the availability of data relating to substance use among Asians and Pacific Islanders. Most of the national surveys on substance use, such as the National Household Survey on Drug Abuse, conducted during 1988 and 1989, targeted African-American and Hispanic respondents (National Institute on Drug Abuse, 1990). Data relating to Asians and Pacific Islanders, however, were incorporated into a category "Other" due to the relatively small sample size. In addition, the survey excluded Hawaii and Alaska. This strategy renders it more difficult to understand the incidence and prevalence of substance use in these communities, data which are critical to program development and planning.

A number of studies have indicated that there is a low incidence of substance abuse in Asian and Pacific Islander populations. (See chapter 4 for a discussion of some of these studies.) However, many of these studies did not target the groups that may be at highest risk of substance use, such as adolescents and immigrants. Many recent studies have also focused on an examination of genetic factors that may contribute to less substance abuse, potentially resulting in the obfuscation of cultural and social factors that underlie the occurrence of abuse and dependence. As a result of this focus and the resulting lack of data, inadequate data exist to support the need for treatment services for these communities (Ja and Aoki, 1993).

A separate issue, but one that relates to the failure to document the need for services, is the relative infrequency with which physicians screen their patients for substance use and the inadequacy of mechanisms available for such screening in primary care settings. A survey of primary care physicians in two cities in Maryland, for example, found that only 41 percent routinely screened for alcohol-related problems and even fewer, 20 percent, screened for other drug problems (Duszynski, Nieto, and Valente, 1995). Although the American Medical Association and the United States Preventive Services Task Force (1989) have recommended that physicians screen patients for drug abuse, they have not identified an instrument to be used for this purpose. Many of those currently in existence are lengthy and time-consuming (McPherson and Hersch, 2000), rendering them unwieldy in the context of the brief consultations permitted in managed care practices. Many of the forms that are available, regardless of their length, have not been translated or validated in other languages and, those that have been are often difficult to locate. Practitioners may confront additional problems in attempts to screen adolescents for substance use, such as issues related to confidentiality and privacy (McPherson and Hersch, 2000). Because substance abuse screening is frequently nonexistent or insufficient, the data available through record reviews are, as a result, inadequate as a basis for an accurate assessment of need.

Lack of Culturally Specific Models of Treatment

Unfortunately, many treatment programs regard ethnic groups as monolithic entities with similar patterns of substance use, similar cultures, and similar concerns. However, this is an inaccurate portrayal. For instance, the classification "Asian" in the United States census encompasses more than 29 subgroups, while the term "Pacific Islander" refers to more than 20 additional groups. These groups together speak more than 100 diverse languages (Loue, Lloyd, and Loh, 1996). A similar situation exists with respect to the designation "Hispanic," which encompasses individuals from over 20 diverse subgroups (see Therrien and Ramirez, 2000). And, although Spanish is often a common language for individuals who self-designate as Hispanic, some individuals may not speak Spanish at all and among those who do, significant variations in language may exist.

Most treatment programs assume a "one-size-fits-all" approach and assume that a program will address cultural concerns and nuances adequately through the use of translations and ethnic- and linguistic-specific staff (Ja and Aoki, 1993). However, some approaches may, in fact, be antithetical to specific cultural approaches. For instance, the public admission of substance use that is required as a part of the 12-Step approach may be rejected by individuals who are concerned about the shame that such a confession will bring to themselves and to their family members and communities.

Legal Risks

Criminal Prosecution

There has been significant controversy surrounding the existence of a woman's legal, as opposed to moral, obligation to refrain from substance use during pregnancy. In a 1992 survey of 81 obstetric and pediatric programs, 92 percent of the respondents surveyed agreed that a woman has an *ethical* obligation to the health of the fetus, while only 31 percent agreed that she has a *legal* obligation (Pelham and DeJong, 1992).

Regardless of the nature of the obligation to refrain from substance use during pregnancy, a woman's attempts to obtain treatment during pregnancy may well prove futile. A report of the United States General Accounting Office concluded that women seeking substance abuse treatment confront a "lack of adequate treatment capacity and appropriate services among programs that will treat pregnant women and mothers with young children. The demand for drug treatment uniquely designed for pregnant women far exceeds the supply" (United States General Accounting Office, 1991: 20). A 1989 study of 95 percent of the drug treatment programs in New York City found that 54 percent refused to treat any pregnant women, 67 percent refused to accept pregnant women receiving Medicaid, and 87 percent refused to treat crack-using pregnant women who received Medicaid (Chavkin, 1990). Programs may be wary of admitting pregnant women due to fears of fetal injury resulting from treatment (Wilkins, 1990). Those programs that do offer treatment to pregnant women are often insensitive to concerns that are critical to the women, such as prenatal care and child care (Wilkins, 1990). At least one court has ruled on the basis of applicable state law that a hospital's policy denying treatment in its substance abuse recovery program to pregnant addicts could constitute sex discrimination for which the hospital could be liable (*Elaine W. v. Joint Diseases North General Hospital*, 1993). (This case highlights the possibility that a provider's refusal to address adequately issues of diversity, such as in its admission policies, could potentially result in liability for failure to do so.)

Despite this apparent reluctance to hold a woman legally responsible for the use of illicit substances during pregnancy, and the difficulties inherent in attempting to obtain treatment, during the last 25 years, women who have ingested illegal substances during pregnancy have been prosecuted for child abuse and neglect, child endangerment, drug trafficking, assault with a deadly weapon, manslaughter, and homicide (*Ferguson v. Charleston*, 2001; *State v. Deborah J.Z.*, 1999; *Nevada v. Encoe*, 1994; *Commonwealth v. Welch*, 1993; *Johnson v. State*, 1992; *People v. Morabito*, 1992; *State v. Gray*, 1992; *State v. Gethers*, 1991; *People v. Stewart*, 1987; *Reyes v. Superior Court*, 1977). Women, unlike men, risk criminal prosecution and termination of their parental rights if they are substance-dependent during pregnancy and do not seek treatment. However, they face the same potential risks if they seek do substance abuse treatment during pregnancy.

A number of states have amended their statutes to specifically permit such prosecutions. As an example, Wisconsin in 1998 amended its child abuse laws to provide that mandatory reporters, such as physicians, social workers, counselors, and various other professionals, who have "reason to suspect that an unborn child has been abused [or] to believe that an unborn child is at substantial risk of abuse" must report such suspicions to a law enforcement or child welfare agency (Wisconsin Statutes, 1998). The patient's right to keep confidential all information regarding her condition no longer applies when "the examination of the expectant mother of an unborn child was caused by the habitual lack of self-control of the expectant mother of the unborn child in the use of alcohol beverages, controlled substances or controlled substance analogs, exhibited to a severe degree." Child welfare and law enforcement personnel are instructed to determine if the unborn child is in immediate danger and to take any necessary action, which may include confinement without a hearing for up to 48 hours. A court may order treatment and impose restrictions on travel (Wisconsin Statutes, 1998).

Additionally, the focus of the prosecution is not on the woman's use of an illegal substance, but rather on the child's status as addicted or injured. This is rendered even more draconian in view of the arbitrary distinctions that are drawn between legal and illegal activities. For instance, under the Wisconsin statute, although alcohol may be legally ingested by individuals over a specified age, a woman's use of alcohol during pregnancy may potentially subject her to involuntary confinement. And, the reach of the statute may be extended to encompass even legal behaviors that could be perceived as potentially injurious to the fetus, such as the use of cigarettes or the consumption of caffeine. One writer explained how it has come to be that women, rather than men and women, have become the focus of these concerns:

> The addiction field has adopted the stereotypical images of women that characterize them as diseased, neurotic, pathological, and polluted. Within our drug using culture, men learn to drink, while women simply do not. Women with addiction are automatically labeled "bad mothers" as a result of their deviance and the resultant implication of "destability" in the family.... "[A]ddiction" dependency is socially unacceptable when it interferes with a woman's social role as a housewife, mother, or dutiful daughter, while "subordinate" dependency is highly valued when it involves being dependent on a husband or male protection, in fact, the latter is viewed as the central operating principle in her life. Women who may be facing criminal prosecution for prenatal drug exposure have engaged in the unacceptable type of dependency. Furthermore, many of these poor women may also fail to satisfy the subordinate type of dependency, as many are left by their husbands or boyfriends after the pregnancy has been discovered, forcing her to support herself and the child (Richer, 2000: 1144).

Although fathers and other male figures may be involved in providing the woman with drugs or in exposing the unborn child to environmental hazards of drug use, they have not been subjected to criminal prosecution in such circumstances. One writer noted,

> Future fathers...also have a duty to safeguard the interests of the child to be born. Fathers and other men sometimes play a central role in encouraging or assisting in drug use by pregnant women and are arguably culpable in other damage caused to future children. Domestic violence during pregnancy endangers both mother and future child. In addition, secondhand exposure to crack cocaine, marihuana, and tobacco smoke may present at least marginal potential dangers to pregnant women and their fetuses. The pregnant woman's actions may frequently pose a greater immediate risk of harm, but that is not always the case (De Ville and Kopelman, 1999).

Numerous states now permit the removal of the newborn child from a mother who has ingested substances during pregnancy. A study of foster care in three states found that the number of children 36 months of age and younger that had been placed in foster care increased 110 percent during the period 1986 to 1991. (United States General Accounting Office, 1994). A random sample of foster care case files revealed that the proportion of young children deemed to be at risk from substance abuse during this period increased from 29 to 62 percent. In some instances, a woman's parental rights have been terminated due to her use of substances during pregnancy (*In re A.W.*, 1990).

Research has demonstrated that pregnant women who fear prosecution and the loss of their children due to substance use are less likely to seek treatment and are also less likely to seek prenatal care (United States General Accounting Office, 1991). The American Society of Addiction Medicine (1989: 47) has cautioned that the "[c]riminal prosecution of chemically dependent women will have the overall result of deterring such women from seeking both prenatal care and chemical dependency treatment, thereby increasing, rather than preventing, harm to children and society as a whole."

This disparate treatment of women seeking substance abuse treatment, as compared with men in the same situation, poses a direct threat to the ethical principle of justice, which emphasizes the allocation of benefits and burdens across all groups. Our punitive approach to substance-abusing pregnant women disproportionately imposes on them significant handicaps without also affording them the positive opportunities available to non-pregnant individuals.

Immigration Consequences

The estimated foreign-born population of the United States in March 2000 was 28.4 million, or roughly 10.4 percent of the United States population (Schmidley, 2001). The immigration laws are not kind to individuals who are not citizens of the United States and who have engaged in the use of illicit substances. The immigration law provides for the inadmissibility of non-U.S. citizens who are drug abusers or addicts (8 U.S.C §1182). In addition, individuals who are legally present in the United States, but who are not citizens, may be deported if at any time after admission they have been a drug abuser or addict or have been involved in the trafficking of a controlled substance. They may also be deported if they have been confined to jail or prison for a specified period of time, which may be in conjunction with a drug offense, including simple possession (8 U.S.C §§1101, 1227). These provisions apply even to permanent residents ("green card" holders) who may have spent most of their lives in the United States but who have not received U.S. citizenship. Consequently, individuals born outside of the United States who have not naturalized as citizens bear a substantial risk in seeking substance abuse treatment because if their participation in a treatment program were to become known to immigration authorities, they and/or their family members could potentially be deported.

DEVELOPING CULTURE-CENTRIC APPROACHES

African-American Communities

Significant objections have been raised against syringe exchange programs, both within and outside of African-American communities. Harm reduction is premised on the idea that injection drug users can reduce the potential for drug-related harm while continuing to engage in drug use (Strang and Farrell, 1992). Accordingly, harm reduction requires that the user acknowledge these potential risks, such as crime, disease transmission, and impaired health, and assume responsibility for the reduction of such risks to themselves and to others (Koutroulis, 2000; Kane, 1993). Within the harm reduction framework, abstinence may be tolerated, accepted, and/or legitimated as a treatment objective (Marlatt, 1996; Strang and Farrell, 1992). This approach stands in sharp contrast to that of many withdrawal treatment services, which are often oriented towards facilitating abstinence from drug use. Those clients who fail to achieve complete abstinence are perceived as having failed in some way (Keene and Raynor, 1993).

It is precisely because of the failure of harm reduction to embrace abstinence as its single goal that many African-American communities have rejected its usefulness as a potential treatment modality. The Reverend Cleveland B. Sparrow argued vociferously against Washington, D.C.'s proposed needle exchange program, claiming that needle exchange advocates were committing genocide against the black race (Thomas and Quinn, 1993). Garcia (1992: 37), noting the high prevalence of single-parent households in African-American communities, has stressed that "forces which would further erode family life or parental authority must be strenuously resisted." The allowance or endorsement of a syringe exchange program or harm reduction approach may be perceived in African-American communities as undermining "efforts of parents and churches to inculcate virtues of self-restraint" and permitting drug abusers to focus on changing their needles rather than changing their lives to improve their health (Garcia, 1992: 41). This perspective may well be reflected in utilization rates of syringe exchange programs. A study of the success of New Haven, Connecticut's syringe exchange program found that, although the program served as a successful conduit to bring injectors and noninjectors into substance abuse treatment programs, the injectors who utilized the exchange were significantly less likely to be African-American (Heimer, 1998).

Asian and Pacific Islander Communities

It is important to remember that cultural factors differ across Asian and Pacific Islander ethnicities, social classes, and religions. Consequently, although generalizations may be made in an attempt to understand differences and similarities, such generalizations may not be relevant to specific individuals or to all groups.

Among some groups, substance use may not be seen as an issue that is problematic. For instance, recall the traditional use of opium among Hmong populations in Southeast Asia. Many Hmong have immigrated to the United States; it is not inconceivable that a number of these individuals have either used opium themselves or have relatives who have used opium, in an ear in which it was legal, or tolerated, in their native countries. Consequently, their view towards the continued use of opium or similar drugs may be at variance with the legal restrictions and penalties imposed in the United States.

In many traditional Asian and Pacific Islander cultures, the family, rather than the individual, is critical. The concept of family, however, often differs from the view of family as a nuclear entity that is embodied in the United States census. Instead, the family may be conceived of as a superorganic structure that extends into the past and future. The needs of this superorganic family, which includes attention to the maintenance of health and prosperity in subsequent generations, are paramount; the needs of individual family members are subsidiary. Because mental illness threatens the health of subsequent generations and is believed to be genetic on origin, many families may conceal any indication of its existence and, as a result, are reluctant to seek assistance from outside of the family (Fugita, Ito, Abe, and Takeuchi, 1991). Such may be the case, as well, for substance use.

This orientation to the group also extends to the community. It has been found, for instance, that Asian and Pacific Islander Americans tend to be more sensitive towards and more concerned about others in social situations than are non-Hispanic white Americans (Johnson and Marsella, 1978) and often strive to maintain harmony and equilibrium in their interactions with others (Johnson, Marsella, and Johnson, 1974). A revelation of undesirable conduct to outsiders causes the individual, his or her family, and potentially the community, to "lose face," thereby bringing shame to its members (Loue, Lane, Lloyd, and Loh, 1999).

Religious beliefs may also play a critical role in how individuals, families, and communities approach various situations. Buddhism teaches, for instances, that all life is subject to suffering and that escape from suffering can be achieved through the path of right belief, right thought, right speech, right action, right livelihood, right effort, right mindfulness, and right concentration (Pedersen, 1991). An admission of substance use necessarily indicates a violation of these basic precepts. Similar concepts of suffering are reflected in various Japanese beliefs such as *gaman* (to endure) and *shikata ga nai* (whatever has happened cannot be helped). One must endure suffering in order to avoid *hazu kashii* (ridicule and embarrassment) (Fugita, Ito, Abe, and Takeuchi, 1991; Mokuau, 1990).

Many individuals may also attribute events to *karma*, a widely-held belief that one's framework and experiences are defined by previous deeds and misdeeds and future destinies. A popular interpretation of *karma* holds that one's misfortunes in this lifetime are the consequence of misdeeds during the present or a previous lifetime. The suffering engendered by substance abuse, then, may be taken to represent the inevitable imposition of suffering as a result of one's previous missteps.

It is not surprising, then, that in many Asian and Pacific Islander families and communities, substance abuse is not an issue that is easily discussed. An acknowledgement of substance use may bring shame on both the individual involved and on his or her family members. As a result, denial of substance use is not uncommon. Data from the California Statewide Alcohol Needs Assessment indicate that denial may constitute the primary barrier to substance abuse treatment among individuals of Chinese, Japanese, Korean, and Filipino ethnicity; similar findings relate to individuals of various Southeast Asian and Pacific Islander ethnicities (Morales, 1991).

An ideology of self-reliance may prevail in many Asian and Pacific Islander communities. In part, this reluctance to seek assistance from outside of the community may have developed in order to avoid exposing vulnerabilities to others, resulting in shame and a loss of face. However, the historical legacy of maltreatment of individuals of Asian and Pacific Islander ethnicities has also fostered a sense of mistrust in dealing with "white" institutions (Yamashiro and Matsuoka, 1999).

Hispanic/Latino Communities

Various researchers have argued that substance abuse treatment for Latinos must be culturally appropriate in order to be effective; cultural appropriateness demands the recognition of various aspects of Latino life (Caudle, 1993) and the difficulties encountered in the process of acculturation (Markides, Ray, and Stroup-Benham, 1990). Despite the many differences that exist across Latino cultures, several common themes are notable.

First, treatment must address, minimally, the relevance of the family in Latino life and the traditional roles assigned to men and women within these cultures. Many Latina women are raised in patriarchal and authoritarian environments that, reinforced by the values of organized religion, expect that women will aspire to marriage and motherhood and nurture and care for others (Falicov, 1982). These expectations are epitomized in the concept of *marianismo*.

Although *marianismo* derives from the Virgin Mary, it is not confined to only Catholic Latinas. Women are considered to be men's spiritual superiors. Consequently, they are more able to endure the suffering that is inflicted upon them (Stevens, 1973). Accordingly, Latinas may internalize the expectation that they nurture others and attempt to maintain family unity and connections, even in the face of unhappiness (Vasquez, 1994). The "ten commandments of *marianismo*" have been enumerated as follows:

1. Do not forget a woman's place.
2. Do not forsake tradition.
3. Do not be single, self-supporting, or independent-minded.
4. Do not put your own needs first.
5. Do not wish for more in life than being a housewife.
6. Do not forget that sex is for making babies—not for pleasure.
7. Do not be unhappy with your man or criticize him for infidelity, gambling, verbal and physical abuse, alcohol or drug abuse.
8. Do not ask for help.
9. Do not discuss personal problems outside of the home.
10. Do not change those things which make you unhappy that you can realistically change (Gil and Vasquez, 1996: 8).

Women who fulfill these expectations of a "good" woman can expect to be protected, while those who are "bad," such as those who have sex outside of marriage, can be expected to be labeled as such (Stolen, 1991).

Such role expectations render it extraordinarily difficult to seek help for substance use for oneself or one's family member. These difficulties may be exacerbated by corresponding role expectations of males and obligations to the family.

The concept of *machismo* encompasses men's roles as providers and protectors of their families, responsible for upholding family honor and maintaining the integrity of the family unit (Gutman, 1996; Obeso and Bordatto, 1979). Consequently, *machismo* prohibits a showing of weakness, potentially precluding help seeking or health seeking attempts (Quesada, 1976). Anaya (1996: 93) has described what it means to grow up *macho* in the Mexican American culture:

> The male child observes and learns to be the king, how to act as numero uno, how to act around men and women. In a community that is poor and often oppressed there is much suffering, so he is taught aguantar: to grin and bear it. "Aguantate," the men around him say. A macho man doesn't cry in front of men. A macho doesn't show weakness. Grit your teeth, take the pain, bear it alone. Be tough. You feel like letting it out? Well, then let's get drunk with our compadres, and with the grito that comes from within, we can express our emotions...
>
> The macho learns many games while learning to be numero uno. Drinking buddies who have a contest to see who can consume the most beer, or the most shots of tequila, are trying to prove their maleness. From the pissing contest to drinking, the wish to prove his manliness becomes antisocial, dangerous. The drunk macho driving home from the contest he won can become a murderer.

Consequently, the traditional approach used by Alcoholics Anonymous, whereby individuals acknowledge their powerlessness over alcohol and surrender themselves to a higher power, may be anathema to some Latino men (Alvarez, 2001). To address, various Alcoholics Anonymous groups for Latinos in the Los Angeles area have adapted their meetings to permit participants to simultaneously express male assertiveness (*machismo*) and to surrender to a higher power (Hoffman, 1994).

Traditional values such as *respeto*, respect towards elder males, *humilidad*, humility, and *familismo*, the promotion of loyalty to and from the family, may also impact on an individual's ability and/or willingness to seek substance use treatment or to discuss a family member's substance use with others. The concept of *familismo* has not been well understood by providers who are unfamiliar with Latino cultures and, consequently, Latino families may have erroneously been diagnosed as enmeshed or codependent (Santiago-Rivera, Arredondo, and Gallardo-Cooper, 2002). Conversely, *familismo* can be seen as a strength. Not infrequently, for instance, *compadres* (godparents) may be older individuals who play an important role in the life of the family and/or the community. As such, they may be instrumental at the level of the family or the community in helping to address issues related to substance use.

The concept of *personalismo* may also be relevant to individuals' (non)acceptance of various treatment environments. Warm, friendly, personal, and positive relationships are highly valued. Environments that appear sterile and impersonal may dissuade individuals and their families from participating in a program or from returning for a subsequent visit

(Flaskerud, 1986). Programs that utilize a confrontational style may have difficulty retaining Latino clients in their programs because the behavior may be interpreted as an affront to one's dignity (Alvarez, 2001).

Immigrant Communities

Individuals who have left their country for another may undergo various stages of the migration process. The first stage is that of preparation, in which individuals decide whether or not to emigrate from the country of origin and say their farewells to family members and friends. The second stage consists of the actual act of migration and the quality of that experience. The third stage is a period of overcompensation, during which individuals may adhere rigidly to traditions and customs as a means of preserving a sense of connectedness and stability. The fourth period is one of decompensation, during which they may face family crises, including role conflicts. Ultimately, immigrants may also experience a transgenerational impact due to immigration, meaning a divergence in values and behaviors between the younger and older generations that may lead to additional conflicts within the family (Zúñiga, 1992). The second and third stages of migration may bring with them feelings of relief at one's initial admission to the new culture; feelings of disenchantment and disillusion, as a result of unmet expectations within the new culture; and, ultimately, acceptance of the negative and the positive elements within the new host culture (Arredondo-Dowd, 1981).

The stage at which an individual is ensconced in the immigration process may be highly relevant to his or her willingness and ability to participate in treatment, how he or she presents for treatment, and the delivery of that treatment if it is to be effective. Consider, for example, a situation in which an individual immigrates to the United States after having witnessed the execution of family members in his or her home country. He comes to the attention of a service provider after having been arrested for driving while intoxicated. The individual is having difficulty sleeping and tries to forget what he has seen, but cannot. He is unable to concentrate on any task for any extended period of time. In addition, he is using alcohol to sleep at night. Initially, it may seem that the alcohol use is a direct result of the trauma that was experienced and that he continues to experience. Further discussion, however, may reveal that the gentleman's use of alcohol has always been excessive. However, he does not perceive that he is abusing alcohol and does not identify it as a problem. It may be critical to the success of his treatment to acknowledge and address the recent trauma that he has suffered, before moving on to address his use of alcohol.

Varying levels of acculturation have been found to be associated with varying levels of substance use. (See chapter 4 for additional discussion.) Acculturation has been defined as

> [a] process of attitudinal and behavioral change undergone . . . by individuals who reside in multicultural societies (e.g., the United States, Israel, Canada, and Spain), or who come in contact with a new culture due to colonization, invasion, or other political changes (Marin, 1992: 236).

The process of acculturation is related to the extent of the individual's identification with his or her culture of origin, the importance placed on having contact with people from other cultures, and the "numerical balance" between the individuals who comprise the majority culture and those of a particular subgroup (Marin, 1992). The process of acculturation is extraordinarily complex, involving multiple dimensions, including language preference, ethnic identity, family dynamics, cognitive style, coping style, affective behaviors, interpersonal behaviors, and sociopolitical behaviors. In each domain, individuals may choose to reject the newer culture that they have encountered, assimilate completely so as to reject their culture of origin and embrace their newfound culture, or combine aspects of the host culture and the native culture to produce a hybrid (Gallardo-Cooper, 1999; Falicov, 1998).

In order to be effective, a treatment program must acknowledge and address the varying levels of acculturation that may exist within its client population. For instance, the decision to provide counseling sessions in English or in another language is directly tied to individuals' ability not only to understand English when it is spoken or written, but to use English as an expressive form for issues relevant to the counseling. A new entrant to the United States who does not have English as his or her primary language, for instance, may be able to give directions in English, but may not be able to explain his or her frustrations and fears in English.

Native American Communities

It has been said that "the history of Native Americans is marked by the grief, anger, and loss of spirit of many peoples (Lowery, 1999: 477) and, as a consequence, substance abuse treatment must acknowledge and address this pain: "The primary cause of alcoholism is not physical but spiritual and the cure must also be of the spirit" (Napoleon, 1991: 2). It is not surprising, then, that Indian women in a chemical dependency project in Minnesota reported that their decision to stop using drugs or alcohol was the result of a spiritual experience, such as a dream or a vision (Hawkins, Day, and Suagee, 1993). Factors that have been found to be particularly helpful to American Indian/Alaska Native women in recovery include the presence of other American Indian/Alaska Native women in the program and the incorporation of spiritual and cultural elements into the recovery program (Center for Reproductive Health Policy Research, 1995).

A culture-centric treatment approach has been found to be critical to the success of treatment programs. A review of more than 50 Native American substance abuse treatment programs conducted over a 10-year period found that the most successful shared 4 characteristics: they were initiated by individuals in the communities; they had charismatic role models, who provided program direction; they involved the recovering individuals in therapy and interaction with the group, both as client and healer; and they perceived themselves as a social alternative to the drinking culture. Tribal-centric programs included, depending upon the particular tribe, the traditional purification sweat, vision quest, the Sun Dance ritual, the peyote ritual, the peacemaking process, and the American Indian Alcoholics Anonymous programs (Weibel-Orlando, 1989).

The values of the harmony ethos, as reflected in the American Indian Alcoholics Anonymous (AI-AA) programs, can be contrasted with the attitudes reflected in traditional Alcoholics Anonymous (AA) programs. AI-AA programs stress cooperation, sharing, silence, simplicity, tradition, spiritual values, natural medicine, unity with others, acceptance of others as they are, and the honoring of elders. In contrast, AA emphasizes competition, ownership, verbalism, complexity, innovation, material values, synthetic drugs, separateness from nature, efforts to change others, and the honoring of oneself. An additional example can be found in the incorporation of the following steps, among others, into traditional AA programs:

> We come to believe that a Power greater than ourselves can restore us to sanity.
> We admit to God, to ourselves, and to another human being, the exact nature of our wrongs.
> Make a list of all persons we have harmed and become willing to make amends to them all.

In comparison, the corollary steps in the AI-AA programs state:

> We come to believe that the power of the Pipe is greater than ourselves and can restore us to our Culture and Heritage.
> We acknowledge to the Great Spirit, to ourselves, and to the Native American Brotherhood, our struggles against the tide and its manifest destiny.
> Make a list of all the harm that come to our people from Demon Alcohol, and become willing to make amends to them all (French, 2000: 90).

A lack of familiarity with the traditional harmony ethos, which has been found to be a critical element of treatment programs, may lead to erroneous diagnoses of psychopathology (French, 2000). Traditional healing processes also encompass the elements of humor, patience, the use of silence as a therapeutic tool, the use of descriptive statements rather than direct questions, the use of metaphors and imagery, and self-disclosure through oral history (Garrett and Garrett, 1994).

Women

Women may face unique challenges in their attempts to obtain care. First, treatment slots may be unavailable for women or, if they do exist, there may be significantly fewer reserved for women as compared with men (Sterk, Dolan, and Hatch, 1999). Many inpatient treatment programs may fail to consider and incorporate issues of relevance to women. For instance, there may be inadequate attention paid to day care issues and the treatment plan itself may fail to address issues related to the parent-child relationship. Many programs utilize confrontational approaches, more commonly acceptable to male clients, rather than a nurturing approach (Hatch, 1996). Sterk and colleagues (1999: 2066) reported the comments of one of their study participants:

> I really wanted to be in the program. I was ready to quit, but I knew I couldn't do it by myself. Every day we had to be at meetings, and the counselors would have the women talk about everything and scream at each other. It was worse than on the street. . . . I needed a shoulder to lean on, not someone to make me feel like a slut.

Queer Communities

Various theories have been advanced to explain the origin of the relatively high rates of drinking and drug use that are seen in some segments of queer communities. Some researchers have posited that excessive substance use among gay men may be associated with issues relating to dependency, power, and masculinity (Siegel and Lowe, 1994). Others have hypothesized that some gay men who were perceived as less masculine while they were growing up later use alcohol and/or drugs as a compensatory mechanism that allows them to feel more in control, more sexually assertive, and more physically and verbally aggressive (Nicoloff and Stiglitz, 1987). Others may experience social anxiety and fear, particularly in dating situations, and alcohol offers a means by which they can reduce their levels of anxiety (McKirnan and Peterson, 1989b). In many segments of the gay male community, there is a marked emphasis on sexuality and physicality, and drugs and alcohol may be an integral component of that social scene, rendering it that much more difficult for individuals to reduce or cease usage (Hicks, 2000). Some lesbian women may rely on alcohol to reduce sex role conflict (Ritter and Terndrup, 2002). In addition, a number of lesbian women and gay men may use substances to reduce or mask feelings of internalized homophobia, guilt, and shame (Hicks, 2000).

It is clear that substance use may be integrally related to issues relating to sexuality, sexual orientation, and treatment by others due to one's sexual orientation. These issues may not be addressed at all in most substance use treatment programs and, if they are, it is most often in a heterosexist context (Niesen and Sandall, 1990). Consequently, it may be uncomfortable for nonheterosexuals to discuss significant issues whose resolution is critical to their own recovery (Kus and Latcovich, 1995). Accordingly, a number of authors have recommended the establishment of specialized recovery programs specific to gay men and lesbian women (Hicks, 2000; Kus and Latcovich, 1995).

Specialized programs present a number of advantages in addition to providing a safe forum in which to address issues of sexuality that may be related to one's substance use. First, they offer a setting in which the likelihood of harassment due to sexual orientation is significantly reduced (Ritter and Terndrup, 2002). Second, participation in a treatment program with like-minded individuals who are also trying to address their substance use present an opportunity to establish a new and healthier support system (Kus and Latcovich, 1995). Third, the treatment program can not only help participants to address issues related to internalized homophobia, but also can assist them to formulate constructive strategies for dealing with societal sexism and heterosexism without relying on substances (Cabaj, 1995; Crawford, 1990). Fourth, gay and lesbian individuals may have to address numerous ancillary issues, such as partner violence and parent-child conflicts, whose contexts differ significantly from those experienced by their heterosexual counterparts. Specialized treatment programs permit individuals the opportunity to address such issues without fear of judgment (Anderson, 1996; Cabaj, 1996; Cabaj, 1995).

Many gay and lesbian women may be uncomfortable with treatment programs premised on a belief in God or a higher power as a result of their denunciation and outright rejection by various religious groups (Hicks, 2000; Kus and Latcovich, 1995). Lesbians, in particular, may be offended by the patriarchal portrayal of God, the antifeminist conception of a higher power, and the admonition to surrender one's personal power that characterize many 12-step programs (Razzano, Hamilton, and Hughes, 2000; MacEwan, 1994). It is critical that a treatment program both acknowledge that such sentiments and experience exist and provide an opportunity to explore and address aspects of spirituality that may be critical to recovery.

Diversity Issues in Addiction and Treatment Research

INTEGRATING DIVERSITY ISSUES IN RESEARCH: GENERAL CONSIDERATIONS

As in the context of treatment, the concept of diversity is strongly linked to the ethical principle of justice, which demands that there be an equitable sharing of the benefits and the burdens of research. This prohibits, then, the exclusion from the research of persons from specified groups, absent a strong scientific justification for doing so. Various international documents that have been formulated to guide research reflect this concern. The *International Ethical Guidelines for Biomedical Research Involving Human Subjects* (Council for International Organizations of Medical Sciences, 2002: 12) speaks to the equitable distribution of burdens and benefits and the recruitment process:

> **Justice** refers to the ethical obligation to treat each person in accordance with what is morally right and proper, to give each person what is due to him or her. In the ethics of research involving human subjects the principle refers primarily to **distributive justice**, which requires the equitable distribution of both the burdens and the benefits of participation in research. Differences in distribution of burdens and benefits are justifiable only if they are based on morally relevant distinctions between persons; one such distinction is vulnerability. "Vulnerability" refers to a substantial incapacity to protect one's own interests owing to such impediments as a lack of capability to give informed consent, lack of alternative means of obtaining medical care or other expensive necessities, or being a junior or subordinate member of a hierarchical group. Accordingly, special provision must be made for the protection

of the rights and welfare of vulnerable persons. ...In general, the research project should leave low-resource countries or communities better off than previously or, at least, no worse off. It should be responsive to their health needs and priorities in that any product developed is made reasonably available to them, and as far as possible leave the population in a better position to obtain effective health care and protect its own health.

Justice requires also that the research be responsive to the health conditions or needs of vulnerable subjects. The subjects selected should be the least vulnerable necessary to accomplish the purposes of the research. Risk to vulnerable subjects is most easily justified when it arises from interventions or procedures that hold out for them the prospect of direct health-related benefit. Risk that does not hold out such prospect must be justified by the anticipated benefit to the population of which the individual research subject is representative. (Bold in original.)

Similarly, the *International Guidelines for Ethical Review of Epidemiological Studies* (CIOMS, 1991: 11) explains that

Justice requires that cases considered alike be treated alike and the cases considered to be treated different be treated in ways that acknowledge the difference. When the principle of justice is applied to dependent or vulnerable subjects, its main concern is with the rules of *distributive justice*. Studies should be designed to obtain knowledge that benefits the class of persons of which the subjects are representative: the class of persons bearing the burden should receive an appropriate benefit, and the class primarily intended to benefit should bear a fair proportion of the risks and burdens of the study.

The rules of distributive justice are applicable within and among communities. Weaker members of communities should not bear disproportionate burdens of studies from which all members of the community are intended to benefit, and more dependent communities and countries should not bear disproportionate burdens of studies from which all communities or countries are intended to benefit. (Italics in original.)

The document explains further:

Epidemiological studies are intended to benefit populations, but individual subjects are expected to accept any risks associated with studies. When research is intended to benefit mostly the better off or healthier members of a population, it is particularly important in selecting subjects to avoid inequity on the basis of age, socioeconomic status, disability or other variables. Potential benefits and harm should be distributed equitably within and among communities that differ on grounds of age, gender, race, or culture, or otherwise (Council for International Organizations of Medical Sciences, 1991: 21).

The National Commission for the Protection of Human Subjects of Biomedical and Behavioral Research (1978: 9–10) advised that:

> The selection of research subjects needs to be scrutinized in order to determine whether some classes (e.g., welfare patients, particular racial and ethnic minorities, or persons confined to institutions) are being systematically selected simply because of their easy availability, their compromised position, or their manipulability, rather than for reasons directly related to the problem being studied. Finally, whenever research supported by public funds leads to the development of therapeutic devices and procedures, justice demands both that these not provide advantages only to those who can afford them and that such research should not unduly involve persons from groups unlikely to be among the beneficiaries of subsequent applications of the research.

The *Institutional Review Board Guidebook* (Penslar, no date) cautions that subjects

> should not be selected either because they are favored by the researcher or because they are held in disdain (*e.g.*, involving "undesirable persons" in risky research). Further, "social justice" indicates that an order of preference in the selection of classes of subjects (*e.g.*, adults before children) and that some classes of subjects (*e.g.*, the institutionalized mentally infirm or prisoners) may be involved as research subjects, if at all, only on certain conditions.

BARRIERS TO RECRUITMENT

History and Its Legacy

Previous chapters discussed in some detail a number of studies that have been conducted in the United States with members of specific communities. These include, for instance, the experiments on African-Americans during slavery and the Tuskegee syphilis study. These undertakings essentially disregarded the rights of the research participants. As a result, they have left a lasting impression on many communities and have resulted in a distrust of health researchers and an unwillingness to participate in research. For instance, The Tuskegee syphilis study, serves as evidence to many of the government's indifference to persons with black skin. A survey of 220 African-Americans found that 43 percent believed that research in the United States is ethical, 11 percent believed that it is unethical, and 46 percent wanted more information but indicated that they were somewhat wary of research (Million-Underwood, Sanders, and Davis, 1993). Interviews with 1,882 patients in 5 geographic areas found that being African-American was associated with the belief that medical research usually or always involves unreasonable risk and that patients usually or always are pressured into participating in research (Sugarman, Kass, Goodman, Parentesis, Fernandes, and Faden, 1998). Not surprisingly, some communities view AIDS as yet another genocidal effort directed at blacks (Cantwell, 1993; Guinan, 1993; Thomas and Quinn, 1991). A survey of 520 African-Americans found that 27 percent agreed or somewhat agreed with the statement, "HIV/AIDS is a man-made virus that the federal government made to kill and wipe out black people" (Klonoff and Landrine, 1999). An additional 23 percent neither agreed nor disagreed. Those who believed that AIDS is a genocidal conspiracy were more likely to be male college graduates who had experienced some frequent racial discrimination (Klonoff and Landrine, 1999).

Other communities have also been subjected to research endeavors that have, or could have, unjustifiably subjected their members to inordinate risks. As a result, members of these communities may be distrustful of research and of efforts to enlist their cooperation.

The "Tearoom Trade" study has become well-known throughout many gay communities as a symbol of deception. This study, conducted by Humphreys, a doctoral candidate in sociology at the University of Washington, sought to identify the characteristics of men who sought quick and impersonal sexual gratification from other men. At the time that it was conducted, the public and police often subscribed to stereotypes regarding homosexuality.

Humphreys served as the "watchqueen" at various "tearooms," stationing himself near the men participating in sex so that he could keep watch and cough at the approach of a police car or a stranger. He eventually revealed his identity and his motivation for serving in this role. Many of the better-educated clientele agreed to speak with him about their practices. Humphreys was concerned, however, about the potential for bias that might result from a sample that was weighted heavily towards those of higher socioeconomic status. He secretly followed some of the other men and recorded their license plate numbers. He then matched these numbers with the records of the department of motor vehicles. Approximately one year later, Humphreys visited these men and, representing himself as a health service interviewer, obtained extensive data regarding their marital status and sexual behaviors.

As a result of Humphreys' findings, it was learned that many of the men seeking anonymous sexual gratification with other men identified themselves neither as homosexual nor bisexual. Over one-half of them were married and living with their wives. Many of the men were Catholic and, often due to family planning concerns, had infrequent sexual relations with their wives. Approximately 14 percent of the individuals interviewed were interested primarily in homosexual relations (Humphreys, 1970).

Although many social scientists later praised Humphreys' research, it subjected the men to numerous legal risks. Humphreys' data could have been accessed by law enforcement agencies through subpoenas, thereby compromising the men's confidentiality and privacy and subjecting them to the risk of prosecution and conviction and their consequences, such as the loss of employment or marital relationships.

Gay men have been suspicious of government efforts to combat HIV as a result of the initial characterization of the disease as affecting only gay men, the labeling of the disease as Gay Related Immune Disorder (GRID), and the perceived unwillingness of the federal government to fund adequately HIV research and prevention efforts (Cantwell, 1993). Injecting drug users may also question researchers' motives, believing that the government continues to prohibit needle exchange programs, despite mounting evidence in support of their usefulness in reducing HIV transmission, and to underfund drug treatment programs as part of a systematic effort to eliminate injecting drug users through their deaths.

Women have also been subjected to research without their knowledge and consent, resulting in serious harm. Consider, for instance, the history surrounding the development of diethylstilbesterol (DES).

Diethylstilbesterol is a synthetic estrogen. It was developed in London in 1938 and was prescribed during the period from 1945 to 1971 to prevent spontaneous abortions. Initial studies of the drug's efficacy were conducted at Harvard University in the late 1940s. Although the investigators did not have a control group against which to compare the results, they concluded from their findings that the use of DES would result in a healthier maternal environment (Weitzner and Hirsch, 1981). A later study at Tulane University, however, found that the women who had been treated with DES had more miscarriages and premature births as compared with the mothers who had not been given DES.

Pregnant women at the Lying-in Hospital of the University of Chicago were randomized to a clinical trial, with one-half of the women receiving DES and the other half receiving placebo. The researchers found that the women receiving DES were more likely to have miscarriages and small babies than those who received placebo. None of the women were informed that they were participating in research, none were told what drug they were taking, and none were asked for consent to participate. In 1951, the Food and Drug Administration concluded that DES was safe for use in pregnancy. The drug continued to be used for 20 years. By 1971, it was estimated that 1.5 million babies had been exposed to DES. In 1971 alone, approximately 30,000 had been exposed (Weitzner and Hirsch, 1981).

Researchers reported in 1971 that between 1966 and 1971, 7 cases of clear-cell adenocarcinoma had been found in teenage girls (Herbst, Ulfelder, and Poskanzer, 1971). The one element that appeared to be common to these rare cases of cancer was ingestion of DES by the girls' mothers during their pregnancies. Injuries to female babies of DES mothers have included vaginal and cervical dysplasia, adenosis, uterine structural abnormalities, infertility, menstrual irregularities, fetal death and premature birth, and breast and reproductive-tract cancers (Weitzner and Hirsch, 1981). Injuries to male babies have also been reported, including penile bleeding, testicular masses, hypoplastic testes, and sterility (Weitzner and Hirsch, 1981).

Numerous lawsuits were filed against the University of Chicago for the injuries alleged to have resulted from this experiment. In at least two cases, the lawsuits were settled prior to trial.

Distrust of public health professionals has also resulted from what has been perceived as an attempt to exclude particular groups, such as women, injecting drug users, and persons of color, from participating in research that appears to be promising (Levine, 1989; Steinbrook, 1989). Non-English speakers have often been excluded because of the logistical difficulties and increased costs associated with the translation of forms and the interpretation of interviews. Females have been systematically excluded because of reproductive considerations and the fear of liability should injury to the woman, the fetus, or the potential fetus occur (Merton, 1993).

Stigmatization, Ostracism, and Violence

Recruitment for some studies may be hindered due to fear of ostracism, stigmatization, or violence if an individual's disease status were to become known in his or her community. These fears may be more frequent in some subgroups than others. For instance, in some cultures, a fatal disease may be associated with witchcraft and sorcery, resulting in ostracism of the individual from his or her family (Schoepf, 1991). Women who have disclosed their HIV status may become the targets of partner violence (Gielen, O'Campo, Faden, and Eke, 1997). Gay men's HIV status has also been found to be associated with increased rates of partner violence (Greenwood, Relf, Huang, Pollack, Canchola, and Catania, 2002). Association with a study related to a particular disease may give rise to an assumption that the individual actually has the disease, with the subsequent exclusion of the individual from his or her community.

Economic Factors

Individuals' economic status may be a consideration in the decision to participate in research (Ballard, Nash, Raiford, and Harrell, 1993; El-Sadr and Capps, 1992). Individuals who are poorer, who will not have to expend a great deal of money to participate, such as in the form of transportation costs, and who will receive monetary incentives could be more willing to participate. The recruitment of women, for instance, may be particularly difficult if the study does not adequately compensate participants for the costs of child care and does not consider the competing demands on the parent's time and income (Vollmer, Hertert, and Allison, 1992; Smeltzer, 1992).

Legal Difficulties

As in the context of treatment, some individuals may be at risk for adverse legal consequences if their substance use becomes known. This includes, in particular, pregnant women, who risk criminal prosecution and the loss of their children, and immigrants, who face possible removability as a result of their substance use. (These risks are explored in detail in the context of treatment, discussed in chapter 6.) As a result, recruitment from these groups may be difficult. The strict maintenance of confidentiality and privacy is critical to reduce the potential risks to study participants.

DEVELOPING CULTURE-CENTRIC APPROACHES

Tailoring the Recruitment Efforts

Various strategies have been suggested to increase the likelihood that participants from specified communities will participate in the research. The following strategies, for instance, have been found to be successful in recruiting members of African-American communities: (1) making a commitment to the recruitment of African-American participants, (2) striving to enhance the study's credibility through outreach programs, (3) involving churches and other organizations, (4) developing publicity campaigns that target African-Americans, (5) attending to individuals' concerns, such as the location and time of their participation, (6) using incentives, (7) relying on African-American role models, (8) being flexible in adjusting the study design, (9) relying on lay health workers, and (10) making door-to-door recruitment efforts (Shavers-Hornaday, Lynch, Burmeister, and Torner, 1997).

Reducing Risks of Participation

The potential for adverse legal consequences to participants in substance use-related research can be reduced through the use of a certificate
of confidentiality. The Public Health Service Act authorizes the Secretary
of the United States Department of Health and Human to issue such a
certificate:

> Protection of privacy of individuals who are research subjects. The Secretary
> may authorize persons engaged in biomedical, behavioral, clinical, or other
> research (including research on mental health including research on the use
> and effect of alcohol and other psychoactive drugs) to protect the privacy
> of individuals who are the subject of such research by withholding from
> all persons not connected with the conduct of such research the names or
> other identifying characteristics of such individuals. Persons so authorized to
> protect the privacy of such individuals may not be compelled in any Federal,
> State, or local, civil, criminal, administrative, legislative, or other proceedings
> to identify such individuals (42 U.S.C. §241(d)).

Although there is little law related to the enforcement of this provision,
the confidentiality protections have been upheld by a New York Court
of Appeals against an attempt to learn the identity of a substance abuse
treatment patient (*People v. Newman*, 1973).

In order for these provisions to apply, the researcher must apply for a
certificate of confidentiality in order to have the records protected under
the relevant provision. In order to do this, the researcher must first verify that the research that he or she is conducting and for which he or she
is seeking a certificate of confidentiality is encompassed within the statu-
tory provision relating to research on mental health, including the use and
effects of alcohol and other drugs. Second, the researcher must file an application for a certificate with the designated official of the National Institutes
of Health. The research need not be funded by the National Institutes of
Health to be eligible for coverage by a certificate of confidentiality. A separate application must be filed for each research project for which a certificate is requested. The application must contain the following information:
the name and address of the investigator responsible for the research; the
name of the sponsor or institution with which the investigator is affili-
ated; the location(s) of the research; a description of the research facilities;
the names and addresses of all personnel who will have major responsibility for the conduct of the research; a description of these individuals'
experience, an outline of the research protocol; the date on which the research will begin and the projected date of completion; a specific request
signed by both the individual responsible for the research and an institutional official for the authority to withhold the names and other identifying

information related to the research participants; the reasons for the request of such authority; and assurances that the persons applying for the certificate will comply with federal regulations relating to the protection of human subjects, that a grant of authority will not be represented as an endorsement of the research, and that specified information will be provided to the research participants.

References

Abbott, L.J. (1998). The use of alcohol by lesbians: A review and research agenda. *Substance Use and Misuse, 33,* 2647–2663.

Abel, E.L. (1998). *Fetal Alcohol Abuse Syndrome.* New York: Plenum Press.

Abramson, H.A. (1980). The historical and cultural spectra of homosexuality and their relationship to the fear of being lesbian. *Journal of Asthma Research, 17,* 177–188.

Action on Smoking and Health v. Harris. (1980). 655 F.2d 236 (D.C. Cir.).

Adams, P., Schoenhorn, C., Moss, A., Warren, C., & Kann, L. (1995). Health-risk behaviors among our nation's youth: United States, 1992. *Vital and Health Statistics, Series 10, Data from the National Health Interview Survey, 192,* 1–51.

Adovasio, J.M. & Fry, G.S. (1976). Prehistoric psychotropic drug use in northeastern Mexico and trans-Pecos Texas. *Economic Botany, 30,* cited in PT. Furst. (1976). *Hallucinogens and Culture.* Novato, California: Chandler & Sharp Publishers, Inc.

Agbayani-Siewert, P. (1994). Filipino American culture and family: Guidelines for practitioners. *Journal of Contemporary Human Services, September,* 429–438.

Akers, R.L. (1977). *Deviant Behavior: A Social Learning Approach.* Belmont, California: Wadsworth.

Akutsu, P.D., Sue, S., Zane, N.W., & Nakamura, C.Y. (1989). Ethnic differences in alcohol consumption among Asians and Caucasians in the United States: An investigation of cultural and physiological factors. *Journal of Studies on Alcohol, 50,* 261–267.

Alaniz, M.L. & Wilkes, C. (1998). Pro-drinking messages and message environments for young adults: The case of alcohol industry advertising in African American, Latino, and Native American communities. *Journal of Public Health Policy, 19,* 447–472.

Albrecht, G.L., Levy, J.A., Sugrue, N.M., Prohaska, T.R., & Ostrow, D.G. (1989). Who hasn't heard about AIDS? *AIDS Education and Prevention, 1,* 261–267.

Aldrich, M.S. (1998). Effects of alcohol on sleep. In E.S.L. Gomberg, A.M. Hegedus, & R.A. Zucker (Eds.). *Alcohol Problems and Aging* (pp. 281–300). Bethesda, Maryland: United States Department of Health and Health Services.

Allport, G.W. (1979). *The Nature of Prejudice.* Cambridge, Massachusetts: Perseus Books Publishing.

Altman, D. (1973). *Homosexual Oppression and Liberation.* New York: Avon Books.

Alvarez, L.R. (2001). Substance abuse in the Hispanic population. In A.L. López & E. Carrillo (Eds.). *The Latino Psychiatric Patient: Assessment and Treatment* (pp. 193–217). Washington, D.C.: American Psychiatric Publishing, Inc.

American Medical Association. (1993). *Factors Contributing to Mental Health Care Cost Problem.* Chicago, Illinois: American Medical Association.

American Psychiatric Association. (2000). *Diagnostic and Statistical Manual of Mental Disorders, Fourth Edition, Text Revision.* Washington, D.C.: American Psychiatric Association.

American Society of Addiction Medicine, Board of Directors. (1989). Public Policy Statement on Chemically Dependent Women and Pregnancy, Sept. 25.

Anaya, R. (1996). "I'm the king: The macho image. In R. Gonzalez (Ed.). *Muy Macho: Latino Men Confront Their Manhood* (pp. 57–73). New York: Doubleday.

Anderson, S.C. (1996). Addressing heterosexist bias in the treatment of lesbian couples with chemical dependency. In J. Laird & R.J. Green (Eds.). *Lesbian and Gay Couples and Families: A Handbook for Therapists* (pp. 316–340). San Francisco: Jossey-Bass.

Anderson, S.K., McPhee, D., & Govan, D. (2000). Infusion of multicultural issues in curricula: A student perspective. *Innovative Higher Education, 25,* 37–57.

Anglin, M.D. (1988). The efficacy of civil commitment in treating narcotic addiction. In *Compulsory Treatment of Drug Abuse: Research and Clinical Practice* (pp. 8–34). [National Institute on Drug Abuse Research Monograph No. 86].

Anonymous. (1965). AMA reaffirms effort to end discrimination. *Journal of the National Medical Association, 57,* 105.

Anonymous. (1956). Pills are distributed against the birth rate. *El Imparcial,* April 21. Cited in Watkins, E.S. (1998). *On the Pill: A Social History of Oral Contraceptives, 1950–1970.* Baltimore, Maryland: Johns Hopkins University Press.

Anonymous. (2001a). State-specific prevalence of current smoking among adults, and policies and attitudes about secondhand smoke—United States, 2000. *Morbidity and Mortality Weekly Report, 50,* 1101–1106.

Anonymous. (1996a). Tuberculosis morbidity—United States, 1995. *Morbidity and Mortality Weekly Report, 45,* 365–370.

Anonymous. (2001b). Youth tobacco surveillance—United States, 2000. *Morbidity and Mortality Weekly Report, 50,* 1–84.

Anthony, J.C., Warner, L.A., & Kessler, R.C. (1994). Comparative epidemiology of dependence on tobacco, alcohol, controlled substances, and inhalants: Basic findings from the National Comorbidity Survey. *Experimental and Clinical Psychopharmacology, 2,* 244–268.

Appleyard, J., Messeri, P., Haviland, M.L. (2001). Smoking among Asian American and Hawaiian/Pacific islander youth: Data from the 2000 National Youth Tobacco Survey. *Asian American and Pacific Islander Journal of Health, 9,* 5–14.

Arbes, S.J., Agustsdottir, H., & Slade, G.D. (2001). Environmental tobacco smoke and periodontal disease in the United States. *American Journal of Public Health, 91,* 253–257.

Arizona Revised Statutes Annotated §§36–3701 to 36–3716 (West Supp. 1999).

Arnold, C.L., Davis, T.C., Berkel, H.J., Jackson, R.H., Nandy, I., & London, S. (2001). Smoking status, reading level, and knowledge of tobacco effects among low-income pregnant women. *Preventive Medicine, 32,* 313–320.

Arredondo-Dowd, P. (1981). Personal loss and grief as a result of immigration. *Personnel and Guidance Journal, 59,* 376–378.

Ashburn, P.M. (1947). *The Ranks of Death: A Medical History of the Conquest of the Americas.* New York: Coward-McCann.

Atlee, W.L. & O'Donnell, D.A. (1871). Report of the Committee on Criminal Abortion. *Transactions of the American Medical Association, 22.*

Attias, B. (1998). History of opium, http://www.csun.edu. Cited in H. Fernandez. (1998). Heroin. Center City, Minnesota: Hazelden.

Azevedo, K. & Bogue, H.O. (2001). Health and occupational risks of Latinos living in rural America. In M. Aguirre-Molina, C.W. Molina, & R.E. Zambrana (Eds.). *Health Issues in the Latino Community* (pp. 359–380). San Francisco: John Wiley & Sons, Inc.

Bachman, J.G., Wallace, J.M., Jr, O"Malley, P.M., Johnston, L.D., Kurth, C.L., & Neighbors, H.W. (1991). Racial/ethnic differences in smoking, drinking, and illicit drug use among American high school seniors, 1976–1989. *American Journal of Public Health, 81*, 372–377.

Bachman, R. (1991). The social causes of American Indian homicide as revealed by the life experiences of thirty offenders. *American Indian Quarterly, 15*, 471–487.

Baker, R., Burton, P., & Smith, R. (1995). *Drag: A History of Female Impersonation in the Performing Arts*. New York: New York University Press.

Bakker, A., van Kesteren, F.J.M., Gooren, L.J.G., & Bezemer, P.D. (1993). The prevalence of transsexualism in the Netherlands. *Acta Psychiatrica Scandinavia, 87*, 237–238.

Ballard, E.L., Nash, F., Raiford, K., & Harrell, L.E. (1993). Recruitment of black elderly for clinical research studies of dementia: The CERAD experience. *Gerontologist, 33*, 561–565.

Barr, A. (1999). *Drink: A Social History of America*. New York: Carroll and Graf.

Barr, B., Sterling, E., & Williams, J. (2001). The war on drugs: Fighting crime or wasting time? *American Criminal Law Review, 38*, 1537–1564.

Barrett, W.P. (Trans.). (1931). *The Trial of Jeanne d'Arc*. London: Routledge.

Bass, E. & Davis, L. *The Courage to Heal: A Guide for Women Survivors of Child Sexual Abuse*. New York: Perennial Library.

Bassford, T.L. (1995). Health status of Hispanic elders. *Clinics in Geriatric Medicine, 11*, 25–38.

Baumeister, L., Marchi, K., Pearl, M., Williams, R., & Braveman, P. (2000). The validity of information on "race" and "Hispanic ethnicity" in California birth certificate data. *Health Services Research, 35*, 869–883.

Bell, A.P. & Weinberg, M.S. (1987). *Homosexualities: A Study of Diversity Among Men and Women*. New York: Simon & Schuster.

Bene, E. (1965). On the genesis of female sexuality. *British Journal of Psychiatry, 111*, 815–821.

Benenson, A.S. (Ed.). (1995). *Control of Communicable Disease Manual* (16th ed.). Washington, D.C.: American Public Health Association.

Bennett, W. (1998). Should drugs be legalized? In J.A. Schaler (Ed.). *Drugs: Should We Legalize, Decriminalize, or Deregulate?* (pp. 63–67). Amherst, New York: Prometheus Books.

Berg, C. & Allen, C. (1958). *The Problem of Homosexuality*. New York: Citadel.

Berger, B.J., Kolton, S., Zenilman, J.M., Cummings, M.C., Feldman, J., & McCormack, W.M. (1995). Bacterial vaginosis in lesbians: A sexually transmitted disease. *Clinics of Infectious Disease, 21*, 1402–1405.

Berger, L.R. & Kitzes, J. (1989). Injuries to children in a Native American community. *Pediatrics, 84*, 152–156.

Bergler, E. (1957). *Homosexuality: Disease or Way of Life*. New York: Hill & Wang.

Bergstrom, A.L. (1997). Medical use of marijuana: A look at federal and state responses to California's Compassionate Use Act. *DePaul Journal of Health Care Law, 2*, 155–182.

Berkman, C.S. & Zinberg, G. (1997). Homophobia and heterosexism in social workers. *Social Work, 42*, 319–332.

Berube, A. (1990). *Coming Out Under Fire*. New York: Free Press.

Bieber, I. (1965). Clinical aspects of male homosexuality. In J. Marmor (Ed.). *Sexual Inversion*. New York: Basic Books.

Billy, J.O.G., Tanfer, K., Grady, W.R., & Klepinger, D.H. (1993). The sexual behavior of men in the United States. *Family Planning Perspectives, 25*, 52–60.

Blassingame, J.W. (Ed.). (1977). *Slave Testimony: Two Centuries of Letters, Speeches, Interviews, and Autobiographies*. Baton Rouge, Louisiana: Louisiana State University Press.

Bloomquist, E.R. (1971). *Marijuana: The Second Trip*. Beverly Hills, California: Glencoe Press.

Boas, F. (1940). *Race, Language, and Culture*. New York: Free Press.

Boggs Act of 1951, Pub. L. 82–255, 65 Stat. 767.

Bolin, A. (1992). Coming of age among transsexuals. In T.L. Whitehead & B.V. Reid (Eds.). *Gender Constructs and Social Issues* (pp. 13–39). Chicago: University of Chicago Press.

Bolin, A. (1994). Transcending and transgendering: Male-to-female transsexuals, dichotomy and diversity. In G. Herdt (Ed.). *Third Sex, Third Gender: Beyond Sexual Dimorphism in Culture and History* (pp. 447–485). New York: Zone Books.

Bologna, M.J., Waterman, C.K., & Dawson, L.J. (1987, July). Violence in gay male and lesbian relationships: Implications for practitioners and policy makers. Paper presented at the Third National Conference for Family Violence Researchers, Durham, New Hampshire.

Bonilla, F. & Campos, R. (1981). A wealth of poor: Puerto Ricans in the new economic order. *Daedalus, 110*, 133–176.

Bonnie, R.J. & Whitebread, C.H. II. (1999). *The Marijuana Conviction: A History of Marijuana Prohibition in the United States.* New York: Lindesmith Center.

Bourgois, P. (1997). In search of Horatio Alger: Culture and ideology in the crack economy. In C. Reinarman & H.G. Levine (Eds.). *Crack in America: Demon Drugs and Social Justice* (pp. 57–76). Berkeley, California: University of California Press.

Bonacini, M., Groshen, M.D., Yu, M.C., Govindarajan, S., & Lindsay, K.L. (2001). Chronic hepatitis C in ethnic minority patients evaluated in Los Angeles County. *American Journal of Gastroenterology, 96*, 2438–2441.

Bourke, J. (1887–88). The medicine men of the Apache. *Ninth Annual Report, Bureau of American Ethnology, 1887–88.* Cited in V.J. Vogel. (1970). American Indian Medicine. Oklahoma City, Oklahoma: University of Oklahoma Press.

Bradford, J. & Ryan, C. (1987). *The National Lesbian Health Care Survey.* Washington, D.C.: National Lesbian and Gay Health Foundation.

Bradford, J. & Ryan, C. (1989). *The National Lesbian Health Care Survey: Final Report.* Washington, D.C.: National Lesbian and Gay Health Foundation.

Bradford, J., Ryan, C., & Rothblum, E.D. (1994). National Lesbian Health Care Survey: Implications for mental health care. *Journal of Consulting and Clinical Psychology, 62*, 228–242.

Brand, P.A. & Kidd, A.H. (1986). Frequency of physical aggression in heterosexual and female homosexual dyads. *Psychological Reports, 59*, 1307–1313.

Brandon, G. (1991). The uses of plants in healing in an Afro-Cuban religion, Santeria. *Journal of Black Studies, 22*, 55–76.

Brandt, A.M. (1985). Racism and research: The case of the Tuskegee syphilis study. In J.W. Leavitt & R.L. Numbers (Eds.). *Sickness and Health in America: Readings in the History of Medicine and Public Health* (pp. 331–343). Madison, Wisconsin: University of Wisconsin Press.

Breakwell, G.M. (1986).*Threatened Identities.* New York: Methuen.

Breault, J.L. & Hoffman, M.G. (1997). A strategy for reducing tuberculosis among Oglala Sioux Native Americans. *American Journal of Preventive Medicine, 13*, 182–188.

Brennan, L.M. (1998). Drug courts: A new beginning for nonviolent drug-addicted offenders—An end to cruel and unusual punishment. *Hamline Law Review, 22*, 355–412.

Breslau, N., Johnson, E.O., Hiripi, E., & Kessler, R. (2001). Nicotine dependence in the United States: Prevalence, trends, and smoking persistence. *Archives of General Psychiatry, 58*, 810–816.

Brewer, D.D., Fleming, C.B., Haggerty, K.P., & Catalano, R.F. (1998). Drug use predictors of partner violence in opiate-dependent women. *Violence and Victims, 13*, 107–115.

Brook, J.S., Whiteman, M., Gordon, A.S., & Cohen, P. (1986). Dynamics of childhood and adolescent personality traits and adolescent drug use. *Developmental Psychology, 22*, 403–414.

Brown, T.N., Schulenberg, J., Bachman, J.G., O'Malley, P.M., & Johnston, L.D. (2001). Are risk and protective factors for substance use consistent across historical time?: National data from high school classes of 1976 through 1997. *Prevention Science, 2,* 29–44.

Brown, W.J. (1992). Culture and AIDS education: Reaching high-risk heterosexuals in Asian-American communities. *Journal of Applied Communication Research, August,* 275–291.

Browne, E., Prager, J., Lee, H.Y., & Ramsey, R.G. (1992). CNS complications of cocaine abuse: Prevalence, pathophysiology, and neuroradiology. *American Journal of Roentgenology, 159,* 137–147.

Browner, C.H. (1985). Criteria for selecting herbal remedies. *Ethnology, 24,* 13–32.

Bullough, V.L. (1976). Homosexuality and its confusion with the 'secret sin' in pre-Freudian America. In V.L. Bullough (Ed.). *Sex, Society, and History* (pp. 112–124). New York: Science History.

Burch, G.I. & Pendell, E. (1947). *Human Breeding and Survival.* New York: Penguin.

Bureau of the Census. (1994). *1990 Census of Population.* Washington, D.C: Government Printing Office.

Bureau of the Census, U.S. Department of Commerce, Economics and Statistics Administration. (1993). *We the . . . First Americans.*

Bureau of the Census, U.S Department of Commerce, Economics and Statistics Administration. (1995). *Bureau of the Census Statistical Brief: Housing of American Indians on Reservations—Plumbing* [SB/95-9].

Bureau of the Census, U.S. Department of Commerce, Economics and Statistics Administration. (1997, October 31). Census Bureau Fact Sheet for Native American Month. Available at http://www.census.gov/Press-release/fs97-11.html.

Burge, V., Felts, M., Chenier, T., & Parrillo, A. (1995). Drug use, sexual activity, and suicidal behavior in U.S. high school students. *Journal of School Health, 65,* 222–227.

Burgess, A. & Dean, R.F.A. (1962). *Malnutrition and Food Habits.* London: Tavistock.

Burke, L.K. & Follingstad, D.R. (1999). Violence in lesbian and gay relationships: Theory, prevalence, and correlational factors. *Clinical Psychology Review, 19,* 487–512.

Burnham, J.C. (1993). *Bad Habits: Drinking, Smoking, Taking Drugs, Gambling, Sexual Misbehavior, and Swearing in American History.* New York: New York University Press.

Burr, J.A. & Mutchler, J.E. (1993). Nativity, acculturation, and economic status: Explanations of Asian American living arrangements in later life. *Journal of Gerontology, 48,* S55–S63.

Burris, S., Finucane, D., Gallagher, H., & Grace, J. (1996). The legal strategies used in operating syringe exchange programs in the United States. *American Journal of Public Health, 86,* 1161–1166.

Byers, T., Graham, S., Rzepka, T., & Marshall, J. (1985). Lactation and breast cancer—Evidence for a negative association in premenopausal women. *American Journal of Epidemiology, 121,* 664–674.

Byrd, W.M. & Clayton, L.A. (1992). An American health dilemma: A history of blacks in the health system. *Journal of the National Medical Association, 84,* 189–200.

Cabaj, R.P. (1995). Sexual orientation and the addictions. *Journal of Gay and Lesbian Psychotherapy, 2,* 97–117.

Cabaj, R.P. (1996). Substance abuse in gay men, lesbians, and bisexuals. In R.P. Cabaj & T.S. Stein (Eds.). *Textbook of Homosexuality and Mental Health* (pp. 783–799). Washington, D.C.: American Psychiatric Press.

California Welfare and Institution Code Annotated §§6600–6609.3 (West 1998 & Supp. 2000).

Callender, C. & Kochems, L.M. (1986). Men and not-men: Male gender-mixing and homosexuality. *Anthropology and Homosexual Behavior.*

Campbell, R.J. (1981). *Psychiatric Dictionary,* 5th ed. London: Oxford University Press.

Cancer and Steroid Hormone Study of the Centers for Disease Control and the National Institute of Child Health and Human Development. (1987). The reduction in risk of ovarian cancer associated with oral contraceptive use. *New England Journal of Medicine, 316*, 650–655.

Cantell, M., Snider, D., Cauthen, G., & Onorato, I. (1995). Epidemiology of tuberculosis in the United States, 1985–1992. *Journal of the American Medical Association, 272*, 535–539.

Cantu, C. (1983). In sobriety you get life. In J. Swallow. (1983). (Ed.). *Out from Under: Sober Dykes and Our Friends*. San Francisco: Spinsters/Aunt Lute.

Cantwell, A., Jr. (1993). *Queer Blood: The Secret AIDS Genocide Plot*. Los Angeles: Aries Rising Press.

Cao, L. & Novas, H. (1996). *Everything You Need to Know About Asian-American History*. New York: Penguin Books.

Capps, L.L. (1994). Change and continuity in the medical culture of the Hmong in Kansas City. *Medical Anthropology Quarterly, 8*, 161–177.

Caprio, F.S. (1954). *Female Homosexuality: A Psychodynamic Study of Lesbianism*. New York: Citadel.

Carlson, E.B. & Rosser-Hogan, R. (1993). Mental health status of Cambodian refugees ten years after leaving their homes. *American Journal of Orthopsychiatry, 63*, 223–231.

Carter, D.J. & Wilson, R. (1991). *Ninth Annual Status Report: Minorities in Higher Education*. Washington, D.C.: American Council on Education.

Cartwright, S. (1851). Diseases and peculiarities of the Negro race: Presented at the medical convention in Louisiana. *DeBow's Review, 11*, 64–69, 331–336.

Cartwright, W.S. (1999). Cost of drug abuse to society. *Journal of Mental Health Policy and Economics, 2*, 133–134.

Cassidy, M.M. (1980). Depo-Provera and sterilization overview. In H.B. Holmes, B.B. Hoskins, & M. Gross. (Eds.). *Birth Control and Controlling Birth*. Clifton, New Jersey: Humana Press.

Caudle, P. (1993). Providing culturally sensitive health care to Hispanic clients. *Nurse Practitioner, 18*, 43–46, 50–51.

Cellar, D.F., Nelson, Z.C., & Yorke, C.M. (2000). The five-factor model and driving behavior: Personality and involvement in vehicular accidents. *Psychological Reports, 86*, 454–456.

Centers for Disease Control. (1993). Mortality trends for selected smoking-related cancers and breast cancer—United States, 1950–1990. *Morbidity and Mortality Weekly Report, 42*, 857, 863–866.

Centers for Disease Control and Prevention. (2002a). Drug-Associated HIV Transmission Continues in the United States. Available at http://www.cdc.gov/hiv/pub/facts/idu.htm. Accessed 1/21/2003.

Centers for Disease Control and Prevention. (2001). Health consequence of tobacco use among women—Fact sheet. Women and Smoking: A Report of the Surgeon General—2001. Available at http://www.cdc.gov/tobacco/sgr/sgr_forwomen/factsheet.htm. Accessed 2/10/2003.

Centers for Disease Control and Prevention. (2002b). HIV/AIDS among African Americans. Available at http://www.cdc.gov/hiv/pubs/facts/afm.htm. Accessed 1/21/2003.

Centers for Disease Control and Prevention. (2002c). HIV/AIDS among Hispanics in the United States. Available at http://www.cdc.gov/hiv/pub/facts/hispanic.htm. Accessed 1/21/2003.

Centers for Disease Control and Prevention. (1997). *HIV/AIDS Surveillance Report, 9*, 1–43.

Centers for Disease Control and Prevention. (2002d). HIV/AIDS among U.S. Women: Minority and Young Women at Continuing Risk. Available at http://www.cdc.gov/hiv/pub/facts/women.htm. Accessed 2/10/2003.

Centers for Disease Control and Prevention. (2002e). Need for Sustained HIV Prevention among Men Who Have Sex with Men. Available at http://www.cdc.gov. Accessed 2/10/2003.

Centers for Disease Control and Prevention. (2002f). STD Surveillance 2000. Available at http://www.cdc.gov/std/stats00/TOC2000.htm. Accessed 1/21/2003.

Centers for Disease Control and Prevention. (2002g). Surveillance Reports: Reported Tuberculosis in the United States, 2001. Available at http://www.cdc.gov/nchstp/tb/surv/surv2001/default.htm. Accessed 1/21/2003.

Centers for Disease Control and Prevention. (1987). *Tuberculosis in the United States*. Washington, D.C: Department of Health and Human Services [DHHS Publ. No. (CDC) 89-8322].

Center for Reproductive Health Policy Research. (1995). *Evaluating the Effectiveness of Alcohol and Substance Abuse Services for American Indian/Alaska Native Women*. San Francisco, California: University of California, Institute for Health Policy Studies.

Chamberlin, R.V. (1909). Some plant names of the Ute Indians. *American Anthropologist, 11*, 27–40.

Chang, I., Lapham, S.C., & Barton, K.J. (1996). Drinking environment and sociodemographic factors among DWI offenders. *Journal of Studies of Alcohol, 57*, 659–669.

Charatz-Litt, C. (1992). A chronicle of racism: The effect of the white medical community on black health. *Journal of the National Medical Association, 84*, 717–725.

Charness, M.E., Simon, R.P., & Greenberg, D.A. (1989). Ethanol and the nervous system. *New England Journal of Medicine, 321*, 442–454.

Chavkin, W. (1990). Drug addiction and pregnancy: Policy crossroads. *American Journal of Public Health, 80*, 483–487.

Chekki, D.A. (1990). Introduction: Main currents and new directions in community sociology. In D.A. Chekki (Ed.). *Research in Community Sociology, Vol. I: Contemporary Community Change and Challenge* (pp. 1–22). Greenwich, Connecticut: Jai Press.

Chen, X., Cruz, T.B., Schuster, D.V., Unger, J.B., & Johnson, C.A. (2002). Receptivity to pro-tobacco media and its impact on cigarette smoking among ethnic minority youth in California. *Journal of Health Communication, 7*, 95–111.

Chen, X., Unger, J.B., Cruz, T.B., & Johnson, L.A. (1999). Smoking patterns of Asian-American youth in California and their relationship with acculturation. *Journal of Adolescent Health, 24*, 321–328.

Chenault, L. (1970). *The Puerto Rican Migrant in New York City*. New York: Columbia University Press.

Cheung, F. & Dobkin de Rios, M.F. (1982). Recent trends in the study of mental health of Chinese immigrants to the United States. *Research in Race Relations, 3*, 145–163.

Chi, I., Wibben, J.E., & Kitano, H.H. (1989). Differences in drinking behavior among three Asian-American groups. *Journal of Studies on Alcohol, 50*, 15–23.

Chiasson, M.A., Stoneburner, R.L., & Joseph, S.C. (1990). Human immunodeficiency virus transmission through artificial insemination. *Journal of Acquired Immune Deficiency Syndromes, 3*, 69–72.

Chideckel, M. (1935). *Female Sex Perversion: The Sexually Aberrated Woman As She Is*. New York: Eugenics.

Chilcoat, H.D. & Schutz, C.G. (1996). Age-specific patterns of hallucinogen use in the U.S. population: An analysis using generalized additive models. *Drug and Alcohol Dependence, 43*, 143–153.

Christie, N. (1986). The ideal victim. In E.A. Fattah, (Ed.). *From Crime Policy to Victim Policy* (pp. 17–30). New York: St. Martin's Press.

Chu, S.Y., Buehler, J.W., Fleming, P.L., & Berkelman, R.L. (1990). Epidemiology of reported cases of AIDS in lesbians, United States 1980–89. *American Journal of Public Health, 80,* 1380–1381.

Clark, E.G. & Danbolt, N. (1955). The Oslo study of the natural history of untreated syphilis. *Journal of Chronic Disease, 2,* 311–344.

Clark, G.A., Kelley, M.A., Grange, J.M., & Hill, M.C. (1987). The evolution of mycobacterial disease in human populations. *Current Anthropology, 28,* 45–62.

Clark, L.P. (1919). Some psychological aspects of alcoholism. *New York Medical Journal, 109,* 930–933.

Clarke, A.F. (1990). Women's health: Life cycle issues. In R.D. Apple (Ed.). *Women, Health, and Medicine in America: A Historical Handbook* (pp. 3–39). New York: Garland Publishing, Inc.

Clarke, G., Sack, W.H., & Goff, B. (1993). Three forms of stress in Cambodian adolescent refugees. *Journal of Abnormal Child Psychology, 21,* 65–77.

Cochran, S.D. & Mays, V.M. (1988). Disclosure of sexual preference to physicians by black lesbian and bisexual women. *Western Journal of Medicine, 149,* 616–619.

Cochran, S.D., Mays, V.M., & Leung, L. (1991). Sexual practices of heterosexual Asian-American young adults: Implications for risk of HIV infection. *Archives of Sexual Behavior, 20,* 381–391.

Cohen, D.A., Mason, K., & Scribner, R. (2001). The population consumption model, alcohol control practices, and alcohol-related traffic fatalities. *Preventive Medicine, 34,* 187–197.

Cohen, P., Brook, J., Cohen, J., Velez, C.N., & Garcia, M. (1990). Common and uncommon pathways to adolescent psychopathology and problem behavior. In L.N. Robins & M. Rutter (Eds.). *Straight and Devious Pathways from Childhood to Adulthood* (pp. 242–258). New York: Cambridge University Press.

Collins, R.L., Ellickson, P.L., & Bell, R.M. (1998). Simultaneous polydrug use among teens: Prevalence and predictors. *Journal of Substance Abuse, 10,* 233–253.

Comings, D.E. (1998). The molecular genetics of pathological gambling. *CNS Spectrums, 3,* 20–37.

Comings, D.E., Rosenthal, R.J., & Lesieur, H.R. (1996). A study of the dopamine D_2 receptor gene in pathological gambling. *Pharmacogenetics, 6,* 223–234.

Commander, M.J., Odell, S.O., Williams, K.J., Sashidharan, S.P., & Surtees, P.G. (1999). Pathways to care for alcohol use disorders. *Journal of Public Health Medicine, 21,* 65–69.

Commission on Wartime Relocation and Internment of Civilians. (1997). *Personal Justice Denied.* Washington, D.C.: Civil Liberties Public Education Fund.

Commonwealth Fund. (1995). *National Comparative Survey of Minority Health Care.* Commonwealth Fund. Unpublished manuscript. Cited in S. Guendelman (1998). Health and disease among Hispanics. In S. Loue (Ed.). *Handbook of Immigrant Health* (pp. 277–301). New York: Plenum.

Commonwealth v. Welch. (1993). 864 S.W.2d 280 (Ky.).

Compassionate Use Act of 1996, California Health & Safety Code §11362.5 (Deering 2002).

Conant v. McCaffrey. (2000). 2000 U.S. Dist. LEXIS 13024 (N.D. Cal.).

Conigliaro, J., Maisto, S.A., McNeil, M., Kraemer, K., Kelley, M.E., Conigliaro, R., & O'Connor, M. (2000). Does race make a difference among primary care patients with alcohol problems who agree to enroll in a study of brief interventions? *American Journal on Addictions, 9,* 321–330.

Controlled Substances Act of 1970, 84 Stat. 1274, codified at 21 U.S.C. §841.

Cooper, J.R., Bloom, F.E., & Roth, R.H. (1996). Cellular foundation of neuropharmacology. In J.R. Cooper, F.E. Bloom, & R.H. Roth (Eds.). *The Biochemical Basis of Neuropharmacology,* 7th ed. (pp. 9–48). New York: Oxford University Press.

Cooper, R.S. (1994). A case study in the use of race and ethnicity in public health surveillance. *Public Health Reports, 109,* 46–52.

Corea, G. (1985). *The Hidden Malpractice: How American Medicine Mistreats Women*. New York: Harper Colophon Books.

Corti, C. (1931). A History of Smoking (trans. P. England). London: George G. Harrap & Co., Ltd.

Council for International Organizations of Medical Sciences. (2002). *International Ethical Guidelines for Biomedical Research Involving Human Subjects*. Geneva: Author.

Council for International Organizations of Medical Sciences. (1991). *International Guidelines for Ethical Review of Epidemiological Studies*. Geneva: Author.

Council on Scientific Affairs. (1991). Hispanic health in the United States. *Journal of the American Medical Association, 265*, 248–252.

Council on Scientific Affairs. (1992). Violence against women: Relevance for medical practitioners. *Journal of the American Medical Association, 267*, 3184–3189.

Courtwright, D.T. (1998). Should we legalize drugs? History answers... No. In J.A. Schaler (Ed.). *Drugs: Should We Legalize, Decriminalize, or Deregulate?* (pp. 83–91). Amherst, New York: Prometheus Books.

Covington, S.S. & Kohen, J. (1984). Women, alcohol, and sexuality. *Advances in Alcohol and Substance Abuse, 4*, 41–56.

Crawford, D. (1990). *Easing the Ache: Gay Men Recovering from Compulsive Behaviors*. New York: Plume.

Cregler, T.J. & Mark, H. (1986). Medical complications of cocaine abuse. *New England Journal of Medicine, 315*, 1495–1500.

Crichton, D. (1992). Gender reassignment surgery for male primary transsexuals. *South African Medical Journal, 83*, 347–349.

Cross, J.C., Johnson, B.D., Davis, W.R., & Liberty, H.J. (2001). Supporting the habit: Income generation activities of frequent crack users compared with frequent users of other hard drugs. *Drug and Alcohol Dependence, 64*, 191–201.

Crowley, T.J., McDonald, M.J., Whitmore, E.A., & Mikulich, S.K. (1998). Cannabis dependence, withdrawal, and reinforcing effects among adolescents with conduct symptoms and substance use disorders. *Drug and Alcohol Dependence, 50*, 27–37.

Crum, R.M. & Anthony, J.C. (2000). Educational level and risk for alcohol abuse and dependence: Differences by race-ethnicity. *Ethnicity and Disease, 10*, 39–52.

Cruz, J.M. & Firestone, J.M. (1998). Exploring violence and abuse in gay male relationships. *Violence and Victims, 13*, 159–173.

Cuellar, J.B. (1990). Hispanic-American aging: Geriatric education curriculum developed for selected health professionals. In M.S. Harper (Ed.). *Minority Aging: Essential Curricula Content for Selected Health and Allied Health Professionals* (pp. 365–413). Washington, D.C.: U.S. Government Printing Office [DHHS Pub. No. HRS P-DV-90-4].

Cummings, H.S. (1929). Preliminary Report on Indian Hemp and Peyote, 1929. Cited in R.J. Bonnie & C.H. Whitebread II. (1999). *The Marijuana Conviction: A History of Marijuana Prohibition in the United States*. New York: Lindesmith Center.

Currier, R.L. (1966). The hot-cold syndrome and symbolic balance in Mexican and Spanish-American folk medicine. *Ethnology, 5*, 251–263.

Daniels, R. (1962). *The Politics of Prejudice*. Berkeley, California: University of California Press.

Danziger, G. & Kuhn, J.A. (1999). Drug treatment courts: Evolution, evaluation, and future directions. *Journal of Health Care, Law, and Policy, 3*, 166–188.

Darnall, W.E. (1901). The pubescent schoolgirl. *American Gynecological and Obstetrical Journal, 18*, 488–493.

Davis, A.Y. (1981). Racism, birth control, and reproductive rights. In A.Y. Davis (Ed.). *Women, Race, and Class* (pp. 202–221). New York: Random House.

Davis, C. & Yager, J. (1992). Transcultural aspects of eating disorders: A critical literature review. *Culture, Medicine, & Psychiatry, 16*, 377–394.

Davis, J.F. (1991). *Who Is Black? One Nation's Definition*. University Park, Pennsylvania: Pennsylvania State University Press.

De Ville, K.A. & Kopelman, L.M. (1999). Fetal protection in Wisconsin's revised child abuse law: Right goal, wrong remedy. *Journal of Law, Medicine & Ethics, 27*, 332–342.

de Wit, J.B.F., van Griensven, G.J.P., Kok, G., & Sandfort, T.G.M. (1993). Why do homosexual men relapse into unsafe sex? Predictors of resumption of unprotected anogenital intercourse with casual partners. *AIDS, 7*, 1113–1118.

Dee, T.S. (2001). Alcohol abuse and economic conditions: Evidence from repeated cross-sections of individual-level data. *Health Economics, 10*, 257–270.

Degen, K. & Waitkevicz, H.J. (1982). Lesbian health issues. *British Journal of Sexual Medicine, May*, 40–47.

Deibert, A.V. & Bruyere, M.C. (1946). Untreated syphilis in the male Negro. III. Evidence of cardiovascular abnormalities and other forms of morbidity. *Journal of Venereal Disease Information, 27*, 301–314.

Delgado, M. (1998). Setting the context. In M. Delgado (Ed.). *Alcohol Use/Abuse Among Latinos: Issues and Examples of Culturally Competent Services* (pp. 5–19). New York: Haworth Press, Inc.

Demleitner, N.V. (2002). "Collateral damage": No re-entry for drug offenders. *Villanova Law Review, 47*, 1027–1065.

Dienes, C.T. (1972). *Law, Politics, and Birth Control*. Urbana, Illinois: University of Illinois Press.

DeLaCancela, V., Guarnaccia, P.J., & Carillo, E. (1986). Psychosocial distress among Latinos: A critical analysis of *ataques de nervios. Humanity and Society, 10*, 431–447.

DeLucia, A.J. (2001). Tobacco abuse and its treatment. Turning old and new issues into opportunities for the occupational health nurse. *AAOHN, Official Journal of the American Association of Occupational Health Nurses, 49*, 243–259.

Denenberg, R. (1992). Invisible women. Lesbians and health care. *Health PAC Bulletin, 22*, 14–21.

Department of Health and Human Services. (1991). *Drug Abuse and Drug Abuse Research: Third Triennial Report to Congress*. Washington, D.C.: Author.

Di Chiara, G. & Imperato, A. (1988). Drugs abused by humans preferentially increase synaptic dopamine concentrations in the mesolimbic system of freely moving rats. *Proceedings of the National Academy of Sciences of the United States of America, 85*, 5274–5278.

Diaz, J. (1992, October). *Hispanic Children and AIDS: National Council of La Raza Center for Health Promotion Fact Sheet*. Washington, D.C.: National Council of La raza.

Diaz, T., Buehler, J., Castro, K., & Ward, J. (1993). AIDS trends among Hispanics in the United States. *American Journal of Public Health, 83*, 504–509.

DiClemente, R.J., Zorn, J., & Temoshok, L. (1986). Adolescents and AIDS: A survey of knowledge, beliefs, and attitudes about AIDS in San Francisco. *Journal of Public Health, 76*, 1443–1445.

Dillehay, T.D. & Meltzer, D.J. (1991). *The First Americans: Search and Research*. Boca Raton, Florida: CRC Press.

DiTomaso, N. & Hooijberg, R. (1996). Diversity and the demands of leadership. *Quarterly, 7*, 163–187.

Dodgen, C.F. & Shea, W.M. (2000). *Substance Use Disorders: Assessment and Treatment*. San Diego: Academic Press.

Doherty, M.C., Junge, B., Rathouz, P., Garfein, R.S., Riley, E., & Vlahov, D. (2000). The effect of a needle-exchange program on numbers of discarded needles: A 2-year follow-up. *American Journal of Public Health, 90*, 936–939.

Doll, R. & Hill, A.B. (1952). A study of the aetiology of carcinoma of the lung. *British Medical Journal, 2*, 1271–1285.

Dorsett, K.A. (1998). Note: *Kansas v. Hendricks*: Marking the beginning of a dangerous new era in civil commitment. *DePaul Law Review, 48*, 113–159.

Douglas, C.J., Kalman, C.M., & Kalman, T.P. (1985). Homophobia among physicians and nurses: An empirical study. *Hospital and Community Psychiatry, 36*, 1309–1311.

Douglass, F. (1968). *Narrative of the Life of Frederick Douglass, An American Slave, Written by Himself.* New York: New American Library. (Original work published 1845).

Dowdeswell, G.F. (1876). The coca leaf, observations on the properties and action of the leaf of the coca plant (Erythroxylon coca), made in the physiological laboratory of University College, *Lancet*, 631.

Dozier, E.P. (1966). Problem drinking among American Indians: The role of sociocultural deprivation. *Quarterly Journal of Studies on Alcohol, 27*, 72–87.

Drake, R.E. & Wallach, M.A. (1989). Substance abuse among the chronically mentally ill. *Hospital and Community Psychiatry, 40*, 1041–1046.

Dreifus, C. (1977). Sterilizing the poor. In C. Dreifus (Ed.). *Seizing Our Bodies: The Politics of Women's Health* (pp. 105–120). New York: Random House.

Driver, H.E. (1969). *Indians of North America* (2nd ed., rev.). Chicago, Illinois: University of Chicago Press.

Drug Court Clearinghouse & Technical Assistance Project, United States Department of Justice. (1998). *Looking at a Decade of Drug Courts.* [Sup. Docs. No. J1.2:C83/7].

DuBois, W.E.B. (1897). *The Conservation of Races. American Negro Academy, Occasional Paper no. 2.* Washington: American Negro Academy.

Durlacher, J. (2000). *Heroin: Its History and Lore.* London: Carlton Books.

Duszynski, K.R., Nieto, F.J., & Valente, C.M. (1995). Reported practices, attitudes, and confidence levels of primary care physicians regarding patients who abuse alcohol and other drugs. *Maryland Medical Journal, 44*, 439–446.

Dynes, W. (1987). *Homosexuality: A Research Guide.* New York: Garland.

Eberle, P.A. (1982). Alcohol abusers and non-abusers: A discriminant analysis of differences between 2 subgroups of batterers. *Journal of Health and Social Behavior, 23*, 260–271.

Edwards, A. & Thin, R.N. (1990). Sexually transmitted diseases in lesbians. *International Journal of STD and AIDS, 1*, 178–181.

Edwards, G. & Lader, M. (Eds.). (1994). *Addiction: Processes of Change.* New York: Oxford University Press.

Ehrlich, P.R., Bilderback, L., & Ehrlich, A.H. (1979). *The Golden Door: International Migration, Mexico, and the United States.* New York: Ballantine Books.

Einhorn, L. & Polgar, M. (1994). HIV-risk behavior among lesbians and bisexual women. *AIDS Education and Prevention, 6*, 514–523.

Eisenstadt, S.N. & Giesen, B. (1995). The construction of collective identity. *Archives of European Sociology, 36*, 72–192.

Elaine W. v. Joint Diseases North General Hospital. (1993). 613 N.E.2d 523 (N.Y. Ct. Appeals), *reversing* 580 N.Y.S.2d 246 (1992).

Elder, J.P., Campbell, N.R., Litrownik, A.J., Ayala, G.X., Slymen, D.J., Parra-Medina, D., & Lovato, C.Y. (2000). Predictors of cigarette and alcohol susceptibility and use among Hispanic migrant adolescents. *Preventive Medicine, 31*, 115–123.

Eldh, J. (1993). Construction of a neovagina with preservation of the glans penis as a clitoris in male transsexuals. *Plastic Reconstructive Surgery, 91*, 895–900.

Eliason, M., Donelan, C., & Randall, C. (1992). Lesbian stereotypes. *Health Care for Women International, 13*, 131–144.

Ellickson, P.L., McGiugan, K.A., Adam, V., Bell, R.M., & Hays, R.D. (1996). Teenagers and alcohol misuse in the United States: By any definition, it's a big problem. *Addiction, 91*, 1489–1503.

Ellis, H. (1895). Sexual inversion in women. *Alienist and Neurologist, 16*, 141–158.

El-Sadr, W. & Caps, L. (1992). The challenge of minority recruitment in clinical trials for AIDS. *Journal of the American Medical Association, 267*, 954–957.

Elster, J. (Ed.). (1999). *Addiction Entries and Exits*. New York: Russell Sage Foundation.

Emont, S.L., Dorell, S.M., Bishop, K., & McClain, R. (1995). The burden of smoking-attributable mortality among African-Americans—Indiana, 1990. *Addictive Behaviors, 20*, 563–569.

Engs, R.C., Hanson, D.J., Gliksman, L., & Smythe, C. (1990). Influence of religion and culture on drinking behaviours: A test of hypotheses between Canada and the USA. *British Journal of Addiction, 85*, 1475–1482.

Eskenazi, B., Pies, C., Newstetter, A., Shepard, C., & Pearson, K. (1989). HIV serology in artificially inseminated lesbians. *Journal of Acquired Immune Deficiency Syndromes, 2*, 187–193.

Evans, R.L. & Berent, I.M. (Eds.). (1992). *Drug Legalization: For and Against*. Chicago, Illinois: Open Court.

Evans, S. & Schaefer, S. (1987). Incest and chemically dependent women: Treatment implications. *Journal of Chemical Dependency Treatment, 1*, 141–172.

Ezra, D.B. (1993). Get off your butts: The employer's right to regulate employee smoking. *Tennessee Law Review, 60*, 905–955.

Faderman, L. (1985). The 'new gay' lesbians. *Journal of Homosexuality, 10*, 85–95.

Fahey, D.M. (1996). *Temperance and Racism: John Bull, Johnny Reb, and the Good Templars*. Lexington, Kentucky: University Press of Kentucky.

Falicov, C.J. (1998). *Latino Families in Therapy: A Guide to Multicultural Practice*. New York: Guilford.

Farrelly, M.C., Bray, J.W., Zarkin, G.A., & Wendling, B.W. (2001). The joint demand for cigarettes and marijuana: Evidence from national household surveys on drug abuse. *Journal of Health Economics, 20*, 51–68.

Fee, E. (1979). Nineteenth century craniology: The study of the female skull. *Bulletin of the History of Medicine, 53*, 415–433.

Feinberg, L. (1996). *Transgender Warriors*. Boston: Beacon Press.

Feinleib, M.R. (1989). *Report of the Secretary's Task Force on Youth Suicide*. Rockville, Maryland: U.S. Department of Health and Human Services.

Feldman, H.W. & Biernacki, P. (1988). The ethnography of sharing needles among intravenous drug users and implications for public policies and intervention strategies. In R.J. Battjes & R.W. Pickens (Eds.). (1988). *Needle Sharing Among Intravenous Drug Users: National and International Perspectives*. Washington, D.C: National Institute on Drug Abuse Research.

Fenichel, O. (1945). *On the Psychoanalytic Theory of Neurosis*. New York: W.W. Norton.

Fenton, J.J., Catalan, R., & Hargreaves, W.A. (1996). Effect of Proposition 187 on mental health service use in California: A case study. *Health Affairs, 15*, 182–190.

Ferguson v. Charleston. (2001). 121 S.Ct. 1281.

Fernandez, H. (1998). *Heroin*. Center City, Minnesota: Hazelden.

Ferrini, R. (2000). American College of Preventive Medicine public policy on needle-exchange programs to reduce drug-associated morbidity and mortality. *American Journal of Preventive Medicine, 18*, 173–175.

Ferris, D.G., Batish, S., Wright, T.C., Cushing, C., & Scott, E.H.J. (1996). A neglected lesbian health concern: Cervical neoplasia. *Journal of Family Practice, 43*, 581–584.

Fifeld, L. (1975). *On My Way to Nowhere: Alienated, Isolated, Drunk*. Los Angeles: Gay Community Services Center (unpublished). Cited in Bradford, J., Ryan, C., & Rothblum, E.D. (1994). National Lesbian Health Care Survey: Implications for mental health care. *Journal of Consulting and Clinical Psychology, 62*, 228–242.

Fisher, J.D. & Fisher, W.A. (2000). Theoretical approaches to individual-level change in HIV risk behavior. In J.L. Peterson & R.J. DiClemente (Eds.). *Handbook of HIV Prevention* (pp. 3–55). New York: Kluwer Academic/Plenum Publishing.

Flaskerud, J.H. (1986). The effects of culture-compatible intervention on the utilization of mental health services by minority clients. *Community Mental Health Journal, 22*, 127–141.

Flaskerud, J.H. & Soldevilla, E.Q. (1986). Filipino and Vietnamese clients: Utilizing an Asian mental health center. *Journal of Psychosocial Nursing, 24*, 32–36.

Food and Drug Act of June 30, 1906, 34 Stat. 768 (1906).

Food and Drug Administration (FDA) (1995a). Analysis Regarding the Food and Drug Administration's Jurisdiction Over Nicotine-Containing Cigarettes and Smokeless Tobacco Products. 60 Fed. Reg. 41,453–41,787.

Food and Drug Administration. (1996). Regulations Restricting the Sale and Distribution of Cigarettes and Smokeless Tobacco to Protect Children and Adolescents, 61 Fed. Reg. 44,396, codified at 21 C.F.R. parts 801, 803, 804, 807, 820, 897 (1997).

Foreyt, J.P., Jackson, A.S., Squires, W.G., Jr., Hartung, G.H., Murray, J.D., & Gotto, A.M., Jr. (1993). Psychological profile of college students who use smokeless tobacco. *Addictive Behaviors, 18*, 107–116.

Forsyth, B.W., Leventhal, J.M., Qi, K., Johnson, L., Schroeder, D., & Votto, N. (1998). Health care and hospitalizations of young children born to cocaine-using women. *Archives of Pediatric and Adolescent Medicine, 152*, 177–184.

Fossier, A.E. (1931). The marihuana menace. *New Orleans Medical and Surgical Journal 84*, 247. Cited in R.J. Bonnie & C.H. Whitebread II. (1999). *The Marijuana Conviction: A History of Marijuana Prohibition in the United States*. New York: Lindesmith Center.

Foster, G.M. (1985). How to get well in Tzintzuntzan. *Social Science and Medicine, 21*, 807–818.

Foster, G.M. (1984). How to stay well in Tzintzuntzan. *Social Science and Medicine, 19*, 523–533.

Foster, G.M. (1988). The validating role of humoral theory in traditional Spanish-American therapeutics. *American Ethnologist, 15*, 120–135.

Francis, L. (1996). *Native Time: A Historical Time Line of Native America*. New York: St. Martin's Griffin.

Francoeur, R.T., Perper, T., & Scherzer, N.A. (1991). *A Descriptive Dictionary and Atlas of Sexology*. New York: Greenwood Press.

Frank, D.A., Zuckerman, B.S., Amaro, H., Aboagye, K., Bauchner, H., Cabral, H., Fried, L., Hingson, R., Kayne, H., Levenson, S.M., et al. (1988). Cocaine use during pregnancy: Prevalence and correlates. *Pediatrics, 82*, 888–895.

Franks, A.L., Berg, C.J., Kane, M.A., Browne, B.B., Sikes, R. K., Elsea, W.R., & Burton, A. (1989). Hepatitis B virus infection among children born in the United States to Southeast Asian refugees. *New England Journal of Medicine, 321*, 1301–1305.

Fraumeni, J.F., Jr. & Mason, T.J. (1974). Cancer mortality among Chinese-Americans, 1950–1969. *Journal of the National Cancer Institute, 52*, 659–665.

French, L.A. (2000). *Addictions and Native Americans*. Westport, Connecticut: Praeger Publishers.

French, M.T. & Martin, R.F. (1996). The cost of drug abuse consequences: A summary of research findings. *Journal of Substance Abuse Treatment, 13*, 453–466.

French, S.A. & Perry, L.L. (1996). Smoking among adolescent girls: Prevalence and etiology. *Journal of the American Medical Women's Association, 51*, 25–28.

Freud, S. (1920). The psychogenesis of a case of homosexuality in a woman. In P. Rieff (Ed.) (1963). *Sexuality and the Psychology of Love* (pp. 133–59). New York: Collier. Chicago Press.

Freud, S. (1884). *Uber Coca*. Reprinted in R. Byck (Ed.). *Cocaine Papers by Sigmund Freud*. New York: Stonehill.

Friedman, B.C. (1988). *Male Homosexuality: A Contemporary Psychoanalytic Perspective*. New Haven: Yale University Press.

Frye, B.A. & D'Avanzo, C. (1994a). Cultural themes in family stress and violence among Cambodian refugee women in the inner city. *Advances in Nursing Science, 16*, 64–77.

Frye, B.A. & D'Avanzo, C. (1994b). Themes in managing culturally defined illness in the Cambodian refugee family. *Journal of Community Health Nursing, 11*, 89–98.

Fugita, S., Ito, K.L., Abe, J., & Takeuchi, D.T. (1991). Japanese Americans. In N. Mokuau (Ed.). *Handbook of Social Services for Asians and Pacific Islanders* (pp. 61–78). New York: Greenwood Press.

Furino, A. (Ed.). (1992). *Health Policy and the Hispanic*. Boulder, Colorado: Westview Press.

Furst, P.T. (1976). *Hallucinogens and Culture*. Novato, California: Chandler & Sharp Publishers, Inc.

Gadpaille, W. (1995). Homosexuality and homosexual activity. In H.I. Kaplan & B.J. Sadock (Eds.). *Comprehensive Textbook of Psychiatry*, vol. 1, 6th ed. (pp. 1321–1333). Baltimore: Williams and Wilkins.

Gaines, A.D. (1994). Race and racism. In W. Reich, Ed., *Encyclopedia of Bioethics*. New York: Macmillan.

Gallaher, M.M., Fleming, D.W., Berger, L.R., & Sewell, M. (1992). Pedestrian and hypothermia deaths among Native Americans in New Mexico. *Journal of the American Medical Association, 267*, 1345–1348.

Gallardo-Cooper, M. (1999). Latino perspectives. In S. Kromash (Chair). Cultural/Spiritual Diversity: A Social Worker's Guide to Sensitive Practice. Symposium conducted at the National Association of Social Workers, Melbourne, Florida. Cited in A.L. Santiago-Rivera, P. Arredondo, & M. Gallardo-Cooper. (2002). *Counseling Latinos and La Familia: A Practical Guide*. Thousand Oaks, California: Sage Publications.

Galloway, V.B. (1992). Toward a cultural reading of authentic texts. In *Languages for a Multicultural World in Transition* (pp. 87–121). Lincolnwood, Illinois: National Textbook.

Garber, M. (1992). *Vested Interests: Cross-Dressing and Cultural Anxiety*. New York: HarperCollins.

Garcia, J.L.A. (1992). African-American perspectives, cultural relativisim, and normative issues: Some conceptual questions. In H.E. Flack & E.D. Pellegrino (Eds.). *African-American Perspectives on Biomedical Ethics* (pp. 11–66). Washington, D.C.: Georgetown University Press.

Gardner-Loulan, J. (1983). It's a wonder we have sex at all. In J. Swallow (Ed.). *Out from Under: Sober Dykes and Our Friends*. San Francisco: Spinsters/Aunt Lute.

Garrett, J.T. & Garrett, M.W. The path of good medicine: Understanding and counseling Native American Indians. *Journal of Multicultural Counseling and Development, 22*, 134–144.

Gibson, P. (1989). Gay male and lesbian youth suicide. In *Report of the Secretary's Task Force on Youth Suicide*, Vol. 3 (pp. 110–142). Washington, D.C.: Department of Health and Human Services. [DHHS Pub. No. [ADM] 89-1623].

Gielen, A.C., O'Campo, P., Faden, R.R., & Eke, A. (1997). Women's disclosure of HIV status: Experiences of mistreatment and violence in an urban setting. *Women and Health, 25*, 19–31.

Gil, R.M. & Vazquez, C.I. (1996). *The Maria Paradox: How Latinas Can Merge Old World Traditions with New World Self-Esteem*. New York: Berkley Publishing.

Gill, D.G. (1932). Syphilis in the rural Negro: results of a study in Alabama. *Southern Medical Journal, 25*, 985–990.

Gilpin, E.A., White, M.M., Farkas, A.J., & Pierce, J.P. (1999). Home smoking restrictions: Which smokers have them and how are they associated with smoking behavior. *Nicotine and Tobacco Research, 1*, 153–162.

Gindorf, R. (1977). Wissenschaftliche Ideologien im Wandel: Die Angst von der Homo-sexualitat als intellektuelles Ereignis. In J.S. Hohmann (Ed.). *Der underdruckte Sexus* (pp. 129–144). Berlin: Andreas Achenbach Lollar. Cited in D.F. Greenberg. (1988). The Construction of Homosexuality. Chicago: University of Chicago Press.

Giovino, G.A., Schooley, M.W., Zhu, B.P., Chrisman, J.H., Tomar, S.L., Peddecord, J.P., et al. (1994). Surveillance for selected tobacco-use behaviors—United States, 1900–1994. *Morbidity and Mortality Weekly Report, 18*, 1–43.

Glaus, K.O. (1988). Alcoholism, chemical dependency and the lesbian client. *Women and Therapy, 8*, 131–144.

Gock, T.S. (1994). Acquired immunodeficiency syndrome. In N.W.S. Zane, D.T. Takeuchi, & K.N.J. Young (Eds.). *Confronting Critical Health Issues of Asian and Pacific Islander Americans* (pp. 247–265). Thousand Oaks, California: Sage Publications.

Godlewski, J. (1988). Transsexualism and anatomic sex: Ratio reversal in Poland. *Archives of Sexual Behavior, 17*, 547–548.

Gold, M., Gafni, A., Nelligan, P., & Millson, P. (1997). Needle-exchange programs: An economic evaluation of a local experience. *Canadian Medical Association, 157*, 255–262.

Golden, C. (1987). Diversity and variability in women's sexual identities. In the Boston Lesbian Psychologies Collective. (Eds.). *Lesbian Psychologies: Explorations and Challenges* (pp. 18–34). Urbana, Illinois: University of Illinois Press.

Goldkamp, J.S. (2000). The drug court response: Issues and implications for justice change. *Alabama Law Review, 63*, 923–959.

Golub, A.L. & Johnson, B.D. (1999). Some evidence of the latest war on drugs as a class war. Paper presented to the Society for the Study of Social Problems.

Gonsiorek, J.C. (1988). Mental health issues of gay and lesbian adolescents. *Journal of Adolescent Health Care, 9*, 114–122.

Gonzalez, A.J. (1966, March). La economia y el status politico. *Revista de Ciencias Sociales, 10*, 5–50.

Goode, E. (1999). *Drugs in American Society.* Boston: McGraw-Hill College.

Gootenberg, P. (1999). Introduction: Cocaine: The hidden histories. In P. Gootenberg (Ed.). *Cocaine: The Global Histories* (pp. 1–17). New York: Routledge.

Gordon, E.B. (1991). Transsexual healing: Medicaid funding of sex reassignment surgery. *Archives of Sexual Behavior, 20*, 61–79.

Gordon, D.R., Venturini, A., Del Tucco, M.R., Palli, D., & Paci, E. (1991). What healthy women think, feel, and do about cancer, prevention and breast cancer screening in Italy. *European Journal of Cancer, 27*, 913–917.

Gordon, L. (1976). *Woman's Body, Woman's Right: A Social History of Birth Control in America.* New York: Grossman.

Gould, S.J. (1981). *The Mismeasure of Man.* New York: W.W. Norton.

Gould-Martin, K. & Ngin, C. (1981). Chinese Americans. In A. Harwood (Ed.). *Ethnicity and Medical Care* (pp. 130–171). Cambridge, Massachusetts: Harvard University Press.

Grant, B.F. (1997). Prevalence and correlates of alcohol use and DSM-IV alcohol dependence in the United States: Results of the National Longitudinal Alcohol Epidemiology Survey. *Journal of Studies on Alcohol, 58*, 464–473.

Grant, I., Reed, R., & Adams, K.M. (1987). Diagnosis of intermediate-duration and subacute organic mental disorders in abstinent alcoholics. *Journal of Clinical Psychiatry, 48*, 319–323.

Gray v. Ohio, 4 Ohio 353 (1831).

Greenberg, D.F. (1988). *The Construction of Homosexuality.* Chicago: University of Chicago Press.

Greenberg, J.H., Turner, C.G., & Zegura, S.L. (1986). The settlement of the Americas: A comparison of the linguistic, dental, and genetic evidence. *Current Anthropology, 27*, 447–497.

Greene, B. (1994). Ethnic-minority lesbians and gay men: Mental health and treatment issues. *Journal of Consulting and Clinical Psychology, 62*, 243–251.

Greenwood, G.L., Relf, M.V., Huang, B., Pollack, L.M., Canchola, J.A., & Catania, J.A. (2002). Battering victimization among a probability-based sample of men who have sex with men. *American Journal of Public Health, 92*, 1964–1969.

Griesler, P.C., Kandel, D.B., & Davies, M. (2002). Ethnic differences in predictors of initiation and persistence of adolescent cigarette smoking in the National Longitudinal Survey of Youth. *Tobacco Research, 4*, 79–93.

Grinnell, G.B. (1905). Some Cheyenne plant medicines. *American Anthropologist, 7*, 38–43.

Grinspoon, L. & Bakalar, J. (1976). *Cocaine*. New York: Basic Books.

Grinspoon, L. & Bakalar, J.B. (1997). *Marihuana, The Forbidden Medicine*. New Haven: Yale University Press.

Grinspoon, L. & Bakalar, J.B. (1995). Marihuana as medicine: A plea for reconsideration. *Journal of the American Medical Association, 273*, 1875–1876.

Grossman, D.C., Milligan, B.C., & Deyo, R.A. (1991). Risk factors for suicide attempts among Navajo adolescents. *American Journal of Public Health, 81*, 870–874.

Gruskin, E.P., Hart, S., Gordon, N., & Ackerson, L. (2001). Patterns of cigarette smoking and alcohol use among lesbians and bisexual women enrolled in a large health maintenance organization. *American Journal of Public Health, 91*, 976–979.

Guendelman, S. & Abrams, B. (1994). Dietary, alcohol, and tobacco intake among Mexican-American women of childbearing age: results from HANES data. *American Journal of Health Promotion, 8*, 363–372.

Guendelman, S. & English, P. (1995). The effect of United States residence on birth outcomes among Mexican immigrants: An exploratory study. *American Journal of Epidemiology, 142*, 530–538.

Guinan, M.E. (1993). Black communities' belief in AIDS as "genocide": A barrier to overcome for HIV prevention. *Annals of Epidemiology, 3*, 193–195.

Gusfield, J.R. (1963). *Symbolic Crusade: Status, Politics and the American Temperance Movement*. Urbana: University of Illinois Press.

Gussow, Z. (1989). *Leprosy, Racism, and Public Health: Social Policy in Chronic Disease Control*. Boulder, Colorado: Westview Press.

Guttman, M.C. (1996). *The Meanings of Macho: Being a Man in Mexico City*. Berkeley, California: University of California Press.

Guydish, J., Bucardo, J., Yoing, M., Woods, W., Grinstead, O., & Clark, W. (1993). Evaluating needle exchange: Are there negative effects? *AIDS, 7*, 871–876.

Hagan, H., Des Jarlais, D.C., Friedman, S.R., Purchase, D., & Alter, M.J. (1995). Reduced risk of hepatitis B and hepatitis C among injection drug users in the Tacoma syringe exchange program. *American Journal of Public Health, 85*, 1531–1537.

Hage, J.J., Bloem, J.J.A.M., & Suliman, H.M. (1993). Review of the literature on techniques for phalloplasty with emphasis on the applicability in female-to-male transsexuals. *Journal of Urology, 150*, 1093–1098.

Hage, J.J., Bouman, F.G., de Graaf, F.H., & Bloem, J.J.A.M. (1993). Construction of the neophallus in female-to-male transsexuals: The Amsterdam experience. *Journal of Urology, 149*, 1463–1468.

Hage, J.J., Bout, C.A., Bloem, J.J.A.M., & Megens, J.A.J. (1993). Phalloplasty in female-to-male transsexuals: What do our patients ask for? *Annals of Plastic Surgery, 30*, 323–326.

Hahn, R.A. (1992). The state of federal health statistics on racial and ethnic groups. *Journal of the American Medical Association, 267*, 268–271.

Hall, J.M. (1993). Lesbians' experiences with alcohol problems: A critical ethnographic study of problematization, help seeking and recovery patterns. *Dissertation Abstracts International, 53*, 4590.

Haller, J.S. (1971). *Outcasts from Evolution: Scientific Attitudes of Racial Inferiority*. New York: McGraw-Hill.

Hamilton, J. (1999). All things considered: Study released supporting limited medical use of smokable marijuana. National Public Radio broadcast, Mar. 17.

Handelman, L. & Yeo, G. (1996). Using explanatory models to understand chronic symptoms of Cambodian refugees. *Clinical Research and Methods, 28*, 271–276.

Handlin, O. (1959). *The Newcomers: Negroes and Puerto Ricans in a Changing Metropolis*. Cambridge, Massachusetts: Harvard University Press.

Hann, H.W.L. (1994). Hepatitis B. In N.W.S. Zane, D.T. Takeuchi, & K.N.J. Young (Eds.). *Confronting Critical Health Issues of Asian and Pacific Islander Americans* (pp. 148–173). Thousand Oaks, California: Sage Publications.

Harris, N.V., Thiede, H., McGough, J.P., & Gordon, D. (1993). Risk factors for HIV infection among injection drug users: Results of blinded surveys in drug treatment centers, King County, Washington 1988–1991. *Journal of Acquired Immune Deficiency Syndromes, 6*, 1275–1282.

Harrison Act, 38 Stat. 785, ch. 1, Comp. Stat. 1916, 6287h.

Harrison, A.E. & Silenzio, V.M.B. (1996). Comprehensive care of lesbian and gay patients and families. *Models of Ambulatory Care, 23*, 31–46.

Hartman, D.E. (1995). *Neuropsychological Toxicology: Identification and Assessment of Human Neurotoxic Syndromes*. New York: Plenum Press.

Harwood, H.J., Napolitano, D.M., Kristiansen, L., & Collins, J. (1984). *Economic Costs to Society of Alcohol and Drug Abuse and Mental Illness: 1980*. Research Triangle Park, North Carolina: Research Triangle Institute.

Hatch, S. (1996). Women and Drug Treatment: Factors Influencing Women's Treatment Choices. Thesis, Department of Sociology, Georgia State University. Cited in C.E. Sterk, K. Dolan, & S. Hatch. (1999). Epidemiological indicators and ethnographic realities of female cocaine use. *Substance Use & Misuse, 34*, 2057–2072.

Hawkins, J.D., Catalano, R.F., & Miller, J.Y. (1992). Risk and protective factors for alcohol and other drug problems in adolescence and early adulthood: Implications for substance abuse prevention. *Psychology Bulletin, 112*, 64–105.

Hawkins, N., Day, S., & Suagee, M. (1993). *American Indian Women's Health Project*. Minneapolis, Minnesota: Minnesota Department of Human Services, Chemical Dependency Division. Cited in C.T. Lowery, American Indian perspectives on addiction and recovery. In P.L. Ewalt, E.M. Freedman, A.E. Fortune, D.L. Poole, & S.L. Witkin. (Eds.). *Multicultural Issues in Social Work: Practice and Research* (pp. 473–485). Washington, D.C.: NASW Press.

Hayes, M.E. & Bowery, L.E. (1932). Marihuana. *Journal of Criminal Law and Criminology, 23*, 1986-1094. Cited in R.J. Bonnie & C.H. Whitebread II. (1999). *The Marijuana Conviction: A History of Marijuana Prohibition in the United States*. New York: Lindesmith Center.

Haynes, S. (1993). Lesbian and breast cancer. Paper presented at Fenway Community Health Center. Cited in Roberts, S.J. & Sorenson, L. (1995). Lesbian health care: A review and recommendations for health promotion in primary care settings. *Nurse Practitioner, 20*, 42–47.

Hazen, H.H. (1914). Syphilis in the American Negro. *Journal of the American Medical Association, 63*, 463–466.

Heath, A.C., Meyer, J., Jardine, R., & Martin, N.G. (1991a). The inheritance of alcohol consumption patterns in a general population twin sample: II. Determinants of consumption frequency and quantity consumed. *Journal of Studies on Alcohol, 52*, 425–433.

Heath, A.C., Madden, P.A., Grant, J.D., McLaughlin, T.L., Todorov, A.A., & Bucholz, K.K. (1999). Resiliency factors protecting against teenage alcohol use and smoking: Influences of religion, religious involvement and values, and ethnicity in the Missouri Adolescent Female Twin Study. *Twin Research, 2*, 145–155.

Heath, A.C., Meyer, J., Jardine, R., & Martin, N.G. (1991b). The inheritance of alcohol consumption patterns in a general population twin sample: I. Multidimensional scaling of quantity/frequency data. *Journal of Studies on Alcohol, 52*, 345–352.

Heather, N. & Robertson, I. (2000). *Problem Drinking.* Oxford: Oxford University Press.

Heffernan, K. (1998). The nature and predictors of substance use among lesbians. *Addictive Behaviors, 23*, 517–528.

Heimer, R. (1998). Can syringe exchange serve as a conduit to substance abuse treatment? *Journal of Substance Abuse Treatment, 15*, 183–191.

Heizer, R.F. & Almquist, A.F. (1977). *The Other Californians: Prejudice and Discrimination under Spain, Mexico, and the United States to 1920.* Berkeley, California: University of California Press.

Heller, J.R., Jr. & Bruyere, P.T. (1946). Untreated syphilis in the male Negro. II. Mortality during 12 years of observation. *Journal of Venereal Disease Information, 27*, 34–38.

Heller, P. (1981). A quarrel over bisexuality. In G. Chapple & H.H. Schulte (Eds.). *The Turn of the Century: German Literature and Art, 1890–1915* (pp. 87–115). Bonn: Bouvier Verlag Herbert Grundmann.

Helm, J. (1980). Female infanticide, European diseases, and population levels among the MacKenzie Dene. *American Ethnologist, 7*, 259–285.

Helzer, J.E. & Burnam, A.M. (1991). Epidemiology of alcohol addiction: United States. In Norman S. Miller, Ed. *Comprehensive Handbook of Drug and Alcohol Addiction* (pp. 9–38). New York: Dekker.

Henderson, D.J., Boyd, C., & Mieczkowski, T. (1994). Gender, relationships, and crack cocaine: A content analysis. *Research in Nursing and Health, 17*, 265–272.

Henningfield, J.E. (1984). Behavioral pharmacology of cigarette smoking. *Advances in Behavioral Pharmacology, 4*, 131–210.

Hepburn, C. & Gutierrez, B. (1988). *Alive and Well: A Lesbian Health Guide.* Freedom, California: Crossing Press.

Herbst, A.L., Ulfelder, H., & Poskanzer, D.C. (1971). Adenocarcinoma of the vagina. Association of maternal stilbestrol therapy with tumor appearance in young women. *New England Journal of Medicine, 284*, 878–881.

Herd, D. (1997). Racial differences in women's drinking norms and drinking patterns: A national study. *Journal of Substance Abuse, 9*, 137–149.

Herdt, G. (1994). Third sexes and third genders. In G. Herdt (Ed.). *Third Sex, Third Gender: Beyond Sexual Dimorphism in Culture and History* (pp. 21–81). New York: Zone Books.

Heriot, A. (1975). *The Castrati in Opera.* New York: Da Capo Press.

Herning, R.I., Jones, R.T., Benowitz, R.L., et al. (1983). How a cigarette is smoked determines nicotine blood levels. *Clinical Pharmacology and Therapeutics, 33*, 84–90.

Hibbs, J.R. & Gunn, R.A. (1991). Public health intervention in a cocaine-related syphilis outbreak. *American Journal of Public Health, 81*, 1259–1262.

Hicks, D. (2000). The importance of specialized treatment programs for lesbian and gay patients. In J.R. Guss & J. Drescher (Eds.). *Addictions in the Gay and Lesbian Community* (pp. 81–94). New York: Haworth Press, Inc.

Hingson, R.W., Howland, J., Morelock, S., & Heeren, T. (1988). Legal interventions to reduce drunken driving and related fatalities among youthful drivers. *Alcohol, Drugs, and Driving, 4*, 87–98.

Hispanic Health Alliance. (1990). *Cross-Cultural Medicine: Clinical and Cultural Dimensions in Health Care Delivery to Hispanic Parents.* Chicago, Illinois: Crosscultural Pathways and the Hispanic Health Alliance.

Hitchcock, J.M. & Wilson, H.S. (1992). Personal risking: Lesbian self-disclosure of sexual orientation to professional health care providers. *Nursing Research, 41*, 178–183.

Hoffman, F. (1994).Cultural adaptations of Alcoholics Anonymous to Hispanic service populations. *Journal of the Addictions, 29*, 445–460.

Hoffman, M.B. (2000). The drug court scandal. *North Carolina Law Review, 78*, 1437–1518.

Hogan-Garcia, M. (2003). *The Four Skills of Cultural Diversity Competence: A Process for Understanding and Practice.* Pacific Grove, California: Brooks/Cole.

Hora, P.F., Schma, W.G., & Rsenthal, J.T.A. (1999). Therapeutic jurisprudence and the drug treatment court movement: Revolutionizing the criminal justice system's response to drug abuse. *Notre Dame Law Review, 74*, 439–533.

Howard, W.L. (1903). The Negro as a distinct ethnic factor in civilization. *Medicine (Detroit), 9*, 424.

Howard-Pitney, B. & Winkleby, M.A. (2002). Chewing tobacco: Who uses and who quits? Findings from NHANES III, 1988–1994. National Health and Nutrition Examination Survey III. *American Journal of Public Health, 92*, 250–256.

Hridlicka, A. (1932). Disease, medicine, and surgery among the American aborigines. *Journal of the American Medical Association, 99*, 1661–1666.

Hu, D.J. & Covell, R.M. (1986). Health care usage by Hispanic outpatients as a function of primary language. *Western Journal of Medicine, 144*, 490–493.

Hu, F.B., Hedeker, D., Flay, B.R., Sussman, S., Day, L.E., & Siddiqui, O. (1996). The patterns and predictors of smokeless tobacco onset among urban public school teenagers. *American Journal of Preventive Medicine, 12*, 22–28.

Hu, T.W., Bai, J., Keeler, T.E., Garnett, P.G., & Sung, H.Y. (1994). The impact of California Proposition 99, a major anti-smoking law, on cigarette consumption. *Journal of Health Policy, 15*, 26–36.

Hughes, T.L. & Wilsnack, S.C. (1997). Use of alcohol among lesbians: Research and clinical implications. *American Journal of Orthopsychiatry, 67*, 20–36.

Humphreys, L. (1970). *Tearoom Trade: Impersonal Sex in Public Places.* Chicago: Aldine.

Hunter, J. (1990). Violence against lesbian and gay male youths. *Journal of Interpersonal Violence, 5*, 295–300.

Hurmence, B. (Ed.). (1984). *My Folks Don't Want Me to Talk About Slavery: Twenty-One Oral Histories of Former North Carolina Slaves.* Winston-Salem, North Carolina: John F. Blair.

Hyland, A., Garten, S., Giovino, G.A., & Cummings, K.M. (2002). Mentholated cigarettes and smoking cessation: Findings from COIMMIT. Community Intervention Trial for Smoking Cessation. *Tobacco Control, 11*, 135–139.

In re A.W. (1990).569 A.2d 168 (D.C. App.).

In re Mental Health of K.K.B. (1980). 609 P.2d 747 (Okla.).

In re Philip Morris and Co. (1955). 51 F.T.C. 857.

Inciardi, J.A. (1988). Compulsory treatment in New York: A brief narrative history of misjudgment, mismanagements, and misrepresentation. *Journal of Drug Issues, 18*, 547.

Ingle, D.J. (1964). Racial differences and the future. *Science, 146*, 378.

Institute of Medicine (2001a). *Clearing the Smoke: Assessing the Science Base for Tobacco Harm Reduction.* Washington, D.C.: National Academy Press.

Institute of Medicine. (2001b). *Dispelling the Myths About Addiction: Strategies to Increase Understanding and Strengthen Research.* Washington, D.C.: National Academy Press.

Institute of Medicine. (1995). *Federal Regulation of Methadone Treatment.* Washington, D.C.: National Academy Press.

Institute of Medicine. (1999). *Marijuana and Medicine: Assessing the Science Base.* Washington, D.C.: National Academy Press.

Institute of Medicine. (1996). *Pathways of Addiction: Opportunities in Drug Abuse Research.* Washington, D.C.: National Academy Press.

Irwin, M., Fitzgerald, C., & Berg, W.P. (2000). The effect of the intensity of wireless telephone conversations on reaction time in a braking response. *Perceptual & Motor Skills, 90*, 1130–1134.

Isner, J.M., Ester, N.A., Thomson, P.D., Costanzo-Nordin, M.R., Subramanian, R., Miller, G., Katsas, G., Sweeney, K., & Sturner, W.Q. (1986). Acute cardiac events temporally related to cocaine abuse. *New England Journal of Medicine, 315*, 1438–1443.

Ja, D.Y. & Aoki, B. (1993). Substance abuse treatment: Cultural barriers in the Asian-American community. *Journal of Psychoactive Drugs, 25*, 61–71.

Jackson, J.C., Rhodes, L.A., Inui, T.S., & Buchwald, D. (1997). Hepatitis B among the Khmer: Issues of translation and concepts of illness. *Journal of General Internal Medicine, 12*, 292–298.

Jacobs, H. (1988). *Incidents in the Life of a Slave Girl*. New York: Oxford University Press.

Jacobson, P.D. & Wasserman, J. (1997). *Tobacco Control Laws: Implementation and Enforcement*. Santa Monica, California: Rand.

Jay, K. & Young, A. (1979). *The Gay Report: Lesbians and Gay Men Speak Out About Sexual Experiences and Lifestyles*, 2nd ed. New York: Summit Books.

Jenkins, C.N.H., Le, T., McPhee, S.J., & Stewart, S. (1996). Health care access and preventive care among Vietnamese immigrants: Do traditional beliefs and practices pose barriers? *Social Science and Medicine, 43*, 1049–1056.

Jenkins, C.N.H., McPhee, S.J., Bird, J.A., & Bonilla, N.T.H. (1990). Cancer risks and prevention practices among Vietnamese refugees. *Western Journal of Medicine, 153*, 34–39.

Jessor, R. & Jessor, S.L. (1977). Adolescent development and the onset of drinking: A longitudinal study. *Journal of Studies on Alcohol, 36*, 27–51.

Johansson, S.R. (1982). The demographic history of the native peoples of North America: A selective bibliography. *Yearbook of Physical Anthropology, 25*, 133–152.

Johnson v. State. (1992). 602 So. 2d 1288 (Fla.).

Johnson, A. (2002). Supporters ready to press plan for drug offenders. *Columbus Dispatch*, March 10, 1A.

Johnson, C.E. Jr. (1974). *Consistency of Reporting of Ethnic Origin in the Current Population Survey*. Washington, D.C.: Bureau of the Census [U.S. Department of Commerce Technical Paper No. 31].

Johnson, C.S. (1966). *Shadow of the Plantation*. Chicago: University of Chicago Press.

Johnson, F.A. & Marsella, A.J. (1978). Differential attitudes towards verbal behavior in students of Japanese and European ancestry. *Genetic Psychology Monographs, 97*, 43–56.

Johnson, F.A., Marsella, A.J., & Johnson, C.L. (1974). Social and psychological aspects of verbal behavior in Japanese-Americans. *American Journal of Psychiatry, 131*, 580–583.

Johnson, S.R., Guenther, S.M., Laube, D.W., & Keettel, W.C. (1981). Factors influencing lesbian gynecological care: A preliminary study. *American Journal of Obstetrics and Gynecology, 140*, 20–28.

Johnson, S.R. & Palermo, J.L. (1984). Gynecologic care for the lesbian. *Clinical Obstetrics and Gynecology, 27*, 624–730.

Johnson, S.R., Smith, E.M., & Guenther, S.M. (1987). Comparison of gynecologic health care problems between lesbians and bisexual women. *Journal of Reproductive Medicine, 32*, 805–811.

Johnston, L.D., O'Malley, P.M., & Bachman, J.G. (1988). *Illicit Drug Use, Smoking, and Drinking by America's High School Students, College Students, and Young Adults, 1975–1987*. Washington, D.C.: National Institute on Drug Abuse.

Jones, J. (1981). *Bad Blood: The Tuskegee Syphilis Experiment—A Tragedy of Race and Medicine*. New York: Free Press.

Jones, J.J. (1992). The Tuskegee legacy: AIDS and the black community. *Hastings Center Report, 22*, 38–40.

Jones, R.T. (1984). The pharmacology of cocaine. In J. Grabowski (Ed.). *Cocaine: Pharmacology, Effects, and Treatment of Abuse* (pp. 34–53). Rockville, Maryland: National Institute on Drug Abuse.

Jones, R.T., Benowitz, N.L., & Herning, R.I. (1981). Clinical relevance of cannabis tolerance and dependence. *Journal of Clinical Pharmacology, 21*, 143S–152S.

Joyce, T., Racone, A.D., McCalla, S., & Wehbeh, S. (1995). The impact of prenatal exposure to cocaine on newborn costs and length of stay. *Health Services Research, 30*, 341–358.

Kagan, R.A. & Nelson, W.P. (2001). The politics of tobacco regulation in the United States. In R.L. Rabin & S.D. Sugarman (Eds.). *Regulating Tobacco* (pp. 11–38). New York: Oxford University Press.

Kahn, E. (1987, Fall). Lesbians and AIDS: Let's go safe. *On Our Backs*, 12–14, 42–45.

Kalichman, S.C., Bekher, L., Cherry, C., Williams, E.A., & Allers, C.T. (1998). Risk for HIV infection and use of cocaine among indigent African American men. *American Journal of Health Behavior, 22*, 141–150.

Kampmeier, R.H. (1974). Final report on the "Tuskegee syphilis study." *Southern Medical Journal, 67*, 1349–1353.

Kandel, D.B., Chem, K., Warner, L.A., Kessler, R., & Grant, B. (1992). Prevalence and demographic correlates of symptoms of last year dependence on alcohol, nicotine, marijuana, and cocaine in the U.S. population. *Drug & Alcohol Dependence, 44*, 11–29.

Kandel, D.B. & Davies, M. (1992). Progression to regular marijuana involvement: Phenomenology and risk factors for near-daily use. In M. Glantz & R. Pickens (Eds.). *Vulnerability to Drug Abuse* (pp. 211–253). Washington, D.C.: American Psychological Association.

Kandel, D.B., Yamaguchi, K., & Chem, K. (1992). Stages of progression in drug involvement from adolescence to adulthood: Further evidence for the gateway theory. *Journal of Studies on Alcohol, 53*, 447–457.

Kane, S. (1993). National discourse and the dynamics of risk: Ethnography and AIDS intervention. *Human Organization, 52*, 224–228.

Kansas v. Hendricks. (1997). 521 U.S. 346.

Kanzaki, K. (1921). Is the Japanese menace in America a reality? *Annals of the American Academy of Political and Social Sciences*, 96–97.

Kaplan, E.H. & Heimer, R. (1992a). HIV prevalence among intravenous drug users: Model-based estimates from New Haven's legal needle exchange. *Journal of Acquired Immune Deficiency Syndromes, 5*, 163–169.

Kaplan, E.H. & Heimer, R. (1992b). A model-based estimate of HIV infectivity via needle sharing. *Journal of Acquired Immune Deficiency Syndromes, 5*, 1116–1118.

Kaplan, H.B. & Johnson, R.J. (1992). Relationships between illicit drug use and escalation of drug use: Moderating effects of gender and early adolescent experiences. In M.D. Glantz & R.W. Pickens (Eds.). *Vulnerability to Drug Abuse* (pp. 299–352). Washington, D.C.: American Psychological Association.

Kaplan, H.B., Martin, S.S., Johnson, R.J., & Robbins, C.A. (1996). Escalation of marijuana use: Application of a general theory of deviant behavior. *Journal of Health and Social Behaviors, 27*, 44–61.

Kaplan, L. (1986). *Working with Multiproblem Families*. Lexington, Massachusetts: Lexington Books.

Karan, L.D. & Rosecrans, J.A. (2000). Addictive capacity of nicotine. In M. Piasecki & P.A. Newhouse (Eds.). *Nicotine in Psychiatry: Psychopathology and Emerging Therapeutics* (pp. 83–107). Washington, D.C.: American Psychiatric Press, Inc.

Kay, M.A. (1977). Health and illness in a Mexican barrio. In E.A. Spencer (Ed.). *Ethnic Medicine in the Southwest* (pp. 96–166). Tucson, Arizona: University of Arizona Press.

Kay, M. & Yoder, M. (1987). Hot and cold in women's ethnotherapeutics: The American-Mexican West. *Social Science and Medicine, 25*, 347–355.

Keene, J. & Raynor, P. (1993). Addiction as 'soul sickness': The influence of client and therapist beliefs. *Addiction Research, 1*, 77–87.

Kelder, G.E., Jr. & Daynard, R.A. (1997). The role of litigation in the effective control of the sale and use of tobacco. *Stanford Law and Policy Review, 8*, 63–87.

Kellogg, J.H. (1895). *Ladies' Guide in Health and Disease.* Battle Creek, Michigan: Modern Medicine Publishing Co. Cited in C. Smith-Rosenberg. (1985). *Disorderly Conduct: Visions of Gender in Victorian America.* New York: Alfred A. Knopf, Inc.

Kelsey, J.L. (1979). A review of the epidemiology of human breast cancer. *Epidemiology Review, 1*, 74–109.

Kendler, K.S., Heath, A.C., Neale, M.C., Kessler, R.C., & Eaves, L.J. (1992). A population-based twin study of alcoholism in women. *Journal of the American Medical Association, 268*, 1877–1882.

Kennedy, D.M. (1970). *Birth Control in America: The Career of Margaret Sanger.* New Haven: Yale University Press.

Kerner, J.F., Breen, N., Tefft, M.C., & Silsby, J. (1998). Tobacco use among multi-ethnic Latino populations. *Ethnicity and Disease, 8*, 167–183.

Kessler, D. (1995). Statement. Regulation of Tobacco Products (Part 3). Hearings Before the Subcommittee on Health and the Environment of the Committee on Energy and Commerce. 103d Cong. 5.

Kessler, R.C., Crum, R.M., Warner, L.A., Nelson, C.B., Schulenberg, J., & Anthony, J.C. (1997). Lifetime co-occurrence of DSM-IIII-R alcohol abuse and dependence with other psychiatric disorders in the National Comorbidity Survey. *Archives of General Psychiatry, 54*, 313–321.

Kessler, R.C., Nelson, C.B., McGonagle, K.A., Edlund, M.J., Frank, R.G., & Leaf, P.J. (1996). The epidemiology of co-occurring addictive and mental disorders: Implications for prevention and service utilization. *American Journal of Orthopsychiatry, 66*, 17–30.

Khoury, E.L., Warheit, G.J., Zimmerman, R.S., Vega, W.A., & Gil, A.G. (1996). Gender and ethnic differences in the prevalence of alcohol, cigarette, and illicit drug use over time in a cohort of young Hispanic adolescents in south Florida. *Women and Health, 24*, 21–40.

Kilpatrick, D.G., Veronen, L.J., & Best, V.L. (1985). Factors predicting psychological distress among rape victims. In C.R. Figley (Ed.). *Trauma and Its Wake.* New York: Brunner/Mazel.

Kim, B.L.C. (1978). *The Asian-Americans: Changing Patterns, Changing Needs.* Montclair, New Jersey: Association of Korean Christian Scholars in America.

Kim, S. & Rew, W. (1994). Ethnic identity, role integration, quality of life, and depression in Korean-American women. *Archives of Psychiatric Nursing, 8*, 348–356.

Kinder, D.C. (1981). Bureaucratic cold warrior: Harry J. Anslinger and illicit narcotics traffic. *Pacific Historical Review, 50*, 169–191.

King, R.C. & Stansfield, W.D. (1990). *A Dictionary of Genetics.* London: Oxford University Press.

Kinsey, A.C., Wardell, B., & Martin, C. (1948). *Sexual Behavior in the Human Male.* Philadelphia: Saunders.

Kinsey, A.C., Wardell, B., Martin, C., & Gebhard, P. (1953). *Sexual Behavior in the Human Female.* Philadelphia: Saunders.

Kinzie, J.L., Naylor, P.H., Nathani, M.G., Peleman, R.R., Ehrinpreis, M.N., Lybik, M., Turner, J.R., Janisse, J.J., Massanari, M., & Mutchnick, M.G. (2001). African Americans with genotype 1 treated with interferon for chronic hepatitis C have a lower end of treatment response than Caucasians. *Journal of Viral Hepatitis, 8*, 264–269.

Kirch, D.G. (2000). Nicotine and major mental disorders. In M. Piasecki & P.A. Newhouse (Eds.). *Nicotine in Psychiatry: Psychopathology and Emerging Therapeutics* (pp. 111–130). Washington, D.C.: American Psychiatric Press, Inc.

Kitano, H.H. (1976). Japanese-American mental illness. In S.C. Plog & R.B. Edgerton (Eds.). *Changing Perspectives in Mental Illness* (pp. 256–284). New York: Holt, Rinehart, & Winston.

Klaus, P.A. & Rand, M.R. (1984). *Family Violence. Special Report by the Bureau of Justice Statistics.* Washington, D.C.: U.S. Department of Justice.

Klonoff, E.A. & Kandrine, H. (1999). Do blacks believe that HIV/AIDS is a government conspiracy against them? *Preventive Medicine, 28,* 451–457.

Knight, R.P. (1937). The dynamics and treatment of chronic alcohol addiction. *Bulletin of the Menninger Clinic, 1,* 233–250. Cited in Hall, J.M. (1993). Lesbians and alcohol: Patterns and paradoxes in medical notions and lesbians' beliefs. *Journal of Psychoactive Drugs, 25,* 109–119.

Koch, J., Kim, L.S., & Friedman, S.A. (1999). Gastrointestinal manifestations of HIV disease. In P.T. Cohen, M.A. Sande, & P.A. Volberding (Eds.). *The AIDS Knowledge Base: A Textbook on HIV Disease from the University of California, San Francisco and San Francisco General Hospital* (pp. 523–541). Philadelphia: Lippincott, Williams & Wilkins.

Kohls, L.R. (1984). *Survival Kit for Living Overseas.* Yarmouth, Maine: Intercultural Press.

Kolchin, P. (1993). *American Slavery 1619–1877.* New York: Hill and Wang.

Koob, G.F., Sanna, P.P., & Bloom, F.E. (1998). Neuroscience of addiction. *Neuron, 21,* 467–476.

Koss, M.P. (1988). Hidden rape: Sexual aggression and victimization in a national sample of students in higher education. In A.W. Burgess (Ed.). *Rape and Sexual Assault* (2: pp. 3–25). New York: Garland Publishing.

Koss, M.P. & Harvey, M. (1991). *The Rape Victim: Clinical and Community Approaches to Treatment.* Beverly Hills, California: Sage Publications.

Koutroulis, G. (2000). "The original tension" Negotiating abstinence in clinicians' accounts of harm reduction in nonresidential treatment of heroin withdrawal. *Journal of Substance Abuse Treatment, 19,* 89–98.

Krafft-Ebing, R.V. (1965). *Psychopathia Sexualis: A Medico-Forensic Study.* Trans. H.E. Wedeck. New York: G.P. Putnam's Sons. Orig. pub. 1886.

Kreiss, J.L. & Patterson, D.L. (1997). Psychosocial issues in primary care of lesbian, gay, bisexual, and transgender youth. *Journal of Pediatric Health Care, 11,* 166–274.

Krob, G., Braun, A., & Kuhnle, U. (1994). Hermaphroditism: Geographical distribution, clinical findings, chromosomes and gonadal histology. *European Journal of Pediatrics, 153,* 2–10.

Kuo, W.H. (1984). Prevalence of depression among Asian-Americans. *Journal of Nervous and Mental Disease, 172,* 449–457.

Kus, R.J. & Latcovich, M.A. (1995). Special interest groups in Alcoholics Anonymous: A focus on gay men's groups. In R.J. Kuss (Ed.). *Addiction and Recovery in Gay and Lesbian Persons* (pp. 67–82). New York: Haworth Press, Inc.

Kushner, R. (1975). *Why Me?* New York: Saunders.

La Fond, J.Q. (1999). The future of civil commitment after *Kansas v. Hendricks* and *Olmstead v. L.C.* Presented at the Mid-Year Meeting of the American College of Legal Medicine, Seattle, Washington, October 15.

Landes, R. (1963). Potawatomi medicine. *Transactions, Kansas Academy of Science, 66,* 553–599.

Lando, H.A., Haddock, C.K., Robinson, L.A., Klesges, R.C., & Talcott, G.W. (2000). Ethnic differences in patterns and correlates of age of initiation in a population of Air Force recruits. *Nicotine and Tobacco Research, 2,* 337–344.

Lang, S. (1996). There is more than just women and men: Gender variance in North American Indian cultures. In S.P. Ramet (Ed.). *Gender Reversals & Gender Cultures: Anthropological and Historical Perspectives* (pp. 183–196). London: Routledge.

Larson, E.J. *Sex, Race, and Science: Eugenics in the Deep South*. Baltimore: Johns Hopkins University Press.

LaScala, E.A., Johnson, F.W., & Greunewald, P.J. (2001). Neighborhood characteristics of alcohol-related pedestrian injury collisions: A geostatistical analysis. *Prevention Science*, 2, 123–134.

LaVeist, T.A. (1994). Beyond dummy variables and sample selection: What health service researchers ought to know about race as a variable. *Health Services Research, 29*, 1–16.

Lauderdale, D.S. & Goldberg, J. (1996). The expanded racial and ethnic codes in the Medicare data files: Their completeness of coverage and accuracy. *American Journal of Public Health, 86*, 712–716.

Lawrence, W. (1823). *Lectures on Physiology, Zoology, and the Natural History of Man, Delivered to the Royal College of Surgeons* [1819], 3rd ed. London: South. Cited in R.J.C. Young. (1995). *Colonial Desire: Hybridity in Theory, Culture, and Race*. London: Routledge.

Leacock, E.B. & Lurie, N.O. (Eds.). (1971). *North American Indians in Historical Perspective*. New York: Random House.

League of Nations, Advisory Committee on Traffic in Opium and Other Dangerous Drugs, June 1937. Cited in R.J. Bonnie & C.H. Whitebread II. (1999). *The Marijuana Conviction: A History of Marijuana Prohibition in the United States*. New York: Lindesmith Center.

Lederman, S.A. & Sierra, D. (1994). Characteristics of childbearing Hispanic women in New York City. In G. Lamberty & G. Coll (Eds.). *Puerto Rican Women and Children: Issues in Health, Growth, and Development* (pp. 85–102). New York: Plenum Press.

Lee, A.S. & Lee, E.S. (1977). The health of slaves and the health of freedmen: A Savannah study. *Phylon, 38*, 170–180.

Lee, D.A. & Fong, K. (1990, February/March). HIV/AIDS and the Asian and Pacific Islander community. *SIECUS Report*, 16–22.

Lee, L.P. (1938). The need for better housing in Chinatown. *Chinese Digest*.

Leichter, H.M. (1991). *Free to Be Foolish: Politics and Health Promotion in the United States and Great Britain*. Princeton, New Jersey: Princeton University Press.

Leifer, C. & Young, E.W. (1997). Homeless lesbians: Psychology of the hidden, the disenfranchised, and the forgotten. *Journal of Psychosocial Nursing, 35*, 28–33.

Lemmens, P.H., Vaeth, P.A.C., & Greenfield, T.K. (1999). Coverage of beverage alcohol issues in the print media in the United States, 1985–1991. *American Journal of Public Health, 89*, 1555–1560.

Levine, C. (1989). AIDS crisis sparks a quiet revolution. *Los Angeles Times, November 15*, B7.

Levine, C. (1980). Depo-Provera: Some ethical questions about a controversial contraceptive. In H.B. Holmes, B.B. Hoskins, & M. Gross. (Eds.). *Birth Control and Controlling Birth* (pp. 101–106). Clifton, New Jersey: Humana Press.

Levy, J.E. & Kunitz, S.J. (1974). *Indian Drinking: Navajo Practices and Anglo-American Theories*. New York: Wiley.

Lewis, A. (2000). Abroad at home: Breaking the silence. *New York Times*, July 29, A13.

Lewis, C.E., Saghir, M.T., & Robins, E. (1982). Drinking patterns in homosexual and heterosexual women. *Journal of Clinical Psychology, 43*, 277–279.

Lexau, B.J., Nelson, D., & Hatsukami, D.K. (1998). Comparing IV and non-IV cocaine users. Characteristics of a sample of cocaine users seeking to participate in research. *American Journal on Addictions, 7*, 262–271.

Li, H.Z. & Rosenblood, L. (1994). Exploring factors influencing alcohol consumption patterns among Chinese and Caucasians. *Journal of Studies on Alcohol, 55*, 427–433.

Liao, Y., Cooper, R.S., Cao, G., Durazo-Arvizu, R., Kaufman, J.S., Luke, A., & McGee, D.L. (1998). Mortality patterns among adult Hispanics: Findings from the NHIS, 1986–1990. *American Journal of Public Health, 88*, 227–232.

Lie, G. & Gentlewarrior, S. (1991). Intimate violence in lesbian relationships: Discussion of survey findings and practice implications. *Journal of Social Service Research, 15*, 41–59.

Lie, G., Schilit, R., Bush, J., Montagne, M., & Reyes, L. (1991). Lesbians in currently aggressive relationships: How frequently do they report aggressive past relationships? *Violence and Victims, 6*, 121–135.

Lieber, C.S. (1995). Medical disorders of alcoholism. *New England Journal of Medicine, 333*, 1058–1065.

Lillie, F. (1939). General biological introduction. In E. Allen (Ed.). *Sex and Internal Secretions: A Survey of Recent Research*, 2nd ed. Baltimore, Maryland: Williams and Wilkins.

Lin-Fu, J.S. (1988). Population characteristics and health care needs of Asian Pacific Americans. *Public Health Reports, 103*, 18–27.

Linsky, A. (1971). Theories of behavior and the image of the alcoholic in popular magazines, 1900–1960. *Public Opinion Quarterly, 34*, 573–581.

Lintner, B. (1999). *Burma in Revolt: Opium and Insurgency Since 1948*. Chiang Mai, Thailand: Silkworm Books.

Lipton, B. & Katz, M. (1989). Understanding the Hispanic market. *Medical Market Media, 24*, 9–10, 12, 18.

Littman, G. (1970). Alcoholism, illness, and social pathology among American Indians in transition. *American Journal of Public Health, 60*, 176–178.

Lockhart, L.L., White, B.A., Causby, V., & Isaac, A. (1994). Letting out the secret: Violence in lesbian relationships. *Journal of Interpersonal Violence, 9*, 469–492.

Logan, M.H. (1977). Anthropological research on the hot-cold theory of disease: Some methodological reflections. *Medical Anthropology, 1*, 87–108.

Logan, T.K., Leukefeld, C., & Farabee, D. (1998). Sexual and drug use behaviors among women crack users: Implications for prevention. *AIDS Education and Prevention, 10*, 327–340.

London, W.T. (1990). Prevention of hepatitis B and hepatocellular carcinoma in Asian residents in the United States. *Asian Journal of Clinical Science Monograms: Hepatitis B Virus Infections, 11*, 49–57.

Loue, S. (1996). Transsexualism in medicolegal limine: An examination and proposal for change. *Journal of Psychiatry and Law, Spring*, 27–51.

Loue, S., Lane, S.D., Lloyd, L.S., & Loh, L. (1999). Rephrasing the message: A new approach to HIV prevention in the United States Southeast Asian communities. *Journal of Health Care for the Poor and Underserved, 10*, 100–121.

Loue, S., Lloyd, L., & Loh, L. (1996). HIV prevention in U.S. Asian Pacific Islander communities: An innovative approach. *Journal of Health Care for the Poor and Underserved, 7*, 364–376.

Lucas, V.A. (1992). An investigation of the health care preferences of the lesbian population. *Health Care for Women International, 13*, 221–228.

Ludman, E.K., Newman, J.H., & Lynn, L.L. (1989). Blood-building foods in contemporary Chinese populations. *Journal of the American Dietetic Association, 89*, 1122–1124.

Lujan, C., DeBruyn, L.M., May, P.A., & Bird, M.E. (1989). Profile of abused and neglected American Indian children in the Southwest. *Child Abuse and Neglect, 13*, 449–461.

Luke, D., Esmundo, E., & Bloom, Y. (2000). Smoke signs: Patterns of tobacco billboard advertising in a metropolitan region. *Tobacco Control, 9*, 16–23.

Lum, O. (1995). Health status of Asians and Pacific Islanders. *Clinics in Geriatric Medicine, 11*, 53–67.

Lyman, S. (1971). Strangers in the city: The Chinese in the urban frontier. In F. Odo (Ed.). *Roots: An Asian American Reader*. Los Angeles, California: Continental Graphics.

MacCoun, R.P., Reuter, P., & Schelling, T. (1996). Assessing alternative drug control regimes. *Policy Analysis and Management, 15*, 330–352.

MacEwan, I. (1994). Differences in assessment and treatment approaches for homosexual clients. *Drug and Alcohol Review*, 13, 57–62.

MacKesy-Amiti, M.E. & Fendrick, M. (2000). Trends in inhalant use among high school students in Illinois: 1993–1995. *American Journal of Drug and Alcohol Abuse*, 26, 569–590.

Maddux, J.F. (1988). Clinical experience with civil commitment. In *Compulsory Treatment for Drug Abuse* (pp. 35–56). National Institute on Drug Abuse Research Monograph No. 86.

Mahoney, J., Arnold, R.C., Sterner, B.L., Harris, A., & Zwally, M.R. (1944). Penicillin treatment of early syphilis. II. *Journal of the American Medical Association*, 126, 63–67.

Maldonado, M. (1998). The HIV/AIDS epidemic among Latinos in the United States. *Update*, October, 1–7.

Mancall, P.C. (1995). *Deadly Medicine: Indians and Alcohol in Early America*. Ithaca, New York: Cornell University Press.

Manski, C.F. (2000). *Economic Analysis of Social Interactions*. Working Paper Series no. 7580 (National Bureau of Economic Research).

Marcell, A. (1994). Understanding ethnicity, identity formation, and risk behavior among adolescents of Mexican descent. *Journal of School Health*, 64, 323–327.

Margolis, R. (1994). Marijuana cannot be prescribed for therapeutic purposes. *Healthspan*, 3, 20.

Margulies, R.Z., Kessler, R.C., & Kandel, D.B. (1977). A longitudinal study of onset of drinking among high school students. *Journal of Studies on Alcohol*, 38, 897–912.

Marijuana Tax Act of 1937, Pub. L. No. 82-235, 65 Stat. 767 (1937), as amended by the Narcotic Control Act of 1956, Pub. L. No. 84-728, 70 Stat. 567.

Marin, G., Perez-Stables, E.J., & Marin, B.V. (1989). Cigarette smoking among San Francisco Hispanics: The role of acculturation and gender. *American Journal of Public Health*, 79, 196–199.

Markides, K.S., Ray, L.A., & Stroup-Benham, C.A. (1990). Acculturation and alcohol consumption in the Mexican American population of the southwestern United States: Findings from HHANES 1982–1984. *American Journal of Public Health*, 80, 20–26.

Marlatt, G.A. (1996). Harm reduction: Come as you are. *Addictive Behaviors*, 21, 779–788.

Marmor, M., Weiss, L.R., Lyden, M., Weiss, S.H., Saxinger, W.C., Spira, T.J., & Feorino, P.M. (1986). Possible female-to-female transmission of human immunodeficiency virus. *Annals of Internal Medicine*, 105, 969.

Marshall, M. & Oleson, A. (1994). In the pink: MADD and public health policy in the 1990s. *Journal of Public Health Policy*, Spring, 54–68.

Martin, D. & Lyon, P. (1972). *Lesbian/Woman*. New York: Bantam Books.

Martinez, C. & Martin, H.W. (1966). Folk diseases among urban-Mexican Americans. *Journal of the American Medical Association*, 196, 147–150.

Marzuk, P.M., Tardiff, K., Leon, A.C., Stajic, M., Morgan, E.B., & Mann, J.J. (1992). Prevalence of cocaine use among residents of New York City who committed suicide during a one-year period. *American Journal of Psychiatry*, 149, 371–375.

Marzuk, P.M., Tardiff, K., Leon, A.C., Stajic, M., Morgan, E.B., & Mann, J.J. (1990). Prevalence of recent cocaine use among motor vehicle fatalities in New York City. *Journal of the American Medical Association*, 263, 250–256.

Mason, J.L. (1994). Developing culturally competent organizations. *Focal Point*, 8, 1–8.

Massing, M. (1998). *The Fix*. New York: Simon and Schuster.

Matera, C., Warren, W.B., Moomjy, M., Fink, D.J., & Fox, H.E. (1990). Prevalence of use of cocaine and other substances in an obstetric population. *American Journal of Obstetrics and Gynecology*, 163, 797–801.

Mather, L. (1998). Theorizing about trial courts: Lawyers, policymaking, and tobacco litigation. *Law and Social Inquiry*, 23, 897–940.

Mathews, H.P. (1983). Context-specific variation in humoral classification. *American Anthropologist, 85,* 826–847.

Mathews, W.C., Booth, M.W., Turner, J.D., & Kessler, L. (1986). Physicians' attitudes towards homosexuality—A survey of a California medical society. *Western Journal of Medicine, 144,* 106–110.

Matthews, A. (1997). A guide to case conceptualization and treatment planning with minority group clients. *The Behavior Therapist, 20,* 35–39.

Mattison, J.B. (1886–87). Cocaine dosage and cocaine addiction. *Peoria Medical Monthly, 7,* 532–542, 571–581.

Mattson, S. (1995). Culturally sensitive prenatal care for Southeast Asians. *JOGNN, 24,* 335–341.

Mayeno, L. & Hirota, S.M. (1994). Access to health care. In N.W.S. Zane, D.T. Takeuchi, & K.N.J. Young (Eds.). *Confronting Critical Health Issues of Asian and Pacific Islander Americans* (pp. 347–375). Thousand Oaks, California: Sage Publications.

McCoy, A.W. (1991). *The Politics of Heroin: CIA Complicity in the Global Drug Trade.* Brooklyn, New York: Lawrence Hill Books.

McFarlane, J., Christoffel, K., Bateman, L., Miller, V., & Bullock, L. (1991). Assessing for abuse: Self-report versus nurse interview. *Public Health Nursing, 8,* 245–250.

McGlynn, K., London, W.T., Hann, H.W., & Sharrar, R.G. (1986). Prevention of primary hepatocellular carcinoma in Asian populations in the Delaware Valley. *Advances in Cancer Control: Health Care Planning and Research* (pp. 237–246). New York: Alan R. Liss.

McGowan, R. (1997). *Government Regulation of the Alcohol Industry: The Search for Revenue and the Common Good.* Westport, Connecticut: Quorum Books.

McGuire, H. & Lydston, G.F. (1893). Sexual crimes among southern Negroes; Scientifically considered. *Virginia Medical Monthly, 20,* 111. Quoted in J.S. Haller, Jr. (1971). *Outcasts from Evolution: Scientific Attitudes of Racial Inferiority 1859–1900.* Carbondale, Illinois: Southern Illinois University Press.

McKenney, N.R. & Bennett, C.E. (1994). Issues regarding data on race and ethnicity: The Census Bureau experience. *Public Health Reports, 109,* 16–25.

McKenzie, D. & Giesbrecht, N. (1981). Changing perceptions of the consequences of alcohol consumption in Ontario, 1950–1981. *Contemporary Drug Problems, 10,* 215–242.

McKirnan, D.J. & Peterson, P.L. (1989a). Alcohol and drug use among homosexual men and women: Epidemiology and population characteristics. *Addictive Behaviors, 14,* 545–553.

McKirnan, D.J. & Peterson, P.L. (1989b). Psychosocial and cultural issues in alcohol and drug abuse: An analysis of a homosexual community. *Addictive Behaviors, 14,* 555–563.

McLaughlin, L. (1982). *The Pill, John Rock, and the Catholic Church.* Boston: Little, Brown.

McNabb, M.E. (1984). Chewing nicotine gum for three months: What happens to plasma levels? *Canadian Medical Association Journal, 131,* 589–592.

McPherson, T.L. & Hersch, R.K. (2000). Brief substance use screening instruments for primary care settings: A review. *Journal of Substance Abuse Treatment, 18,* 193–202.

Mendoza, F.S. (1994). The health of Latino children in the United States. *Critical Health Issues for Children and Youth, 4,* 43–72.

Mercer v. Commonwealth of Virginia. (2000). 523 S.E.2d 213 (Va.).

Meredith, A.W., Abbott, D., & Adams, S. (1986). Family violence: Its relation to marital and parental satisfaction and family strengths. *Journal of Family Violence, 1,* 299–305.

Merikangas, K.R., Rounsaville, B.J., & Prusoff, B.A. (1992). Familial factors in vulnerability to substance abuse. In M.D. Glantz & R.W. Pickens (Eds.). *Vulnerability to Drug Abuse* (pp. 75–98). Washington, D.C.: American Psychological Association.

Mermelstein, R. (1999). Explanations of ethnic and gender differences in youth smoking: A multi-site, qualitative investigation. *Nicotine and Tobacco Research, 1,* S91–S98.

Merton, V. (1993). The exclusion of pregnant, pregnable, and once-pregnable people (a.k.a. women) from biomedical research. *American Journal of Law & Medicine, 19*, 369–451.

Messer, E. (1981). Hot-cold classification: Theoretical and practical implications of a Mexican study. *Social Science and Medicine, 15B*, 133–145.

Metler, R., Conway, G.A., & Stehr-Green, J. (1991). AIDS surveillance among American Indians and Alaska Natives. *American Journal of Public Health, 81*, 1469–1471.

Michigan Organization for Human Rights. (1991, August). The Michigan Lesbian Health Survey. Lansing, Michigan: Michigan Organization for Human Rights.

Miller, F.T., Busch, F., & Tanebaum, J.H. (1989). Drug abuse in schizophrenia and bipolar disorder. *American Journal of Drug and Alcohol Abuse, 15*, 291–295.

Miller, J.A. (1995). Caring for Cambodian refugees in the emergency department. *Journal of Emergency Nursing, 21*, 498–502.

Miller, N. (1995). *Out of the Past: Gay and Lesbian History from 1869 to the Present*. New York: Vintage.

Milman, D.H. & Su, E.H. (1973). Patterns of drug usage among university students. *Journal of the American College Health Association, 21*, 181–187.

Milorn, H.T. Jr. (1990). *Chemical Dependence: Diagnosis, Treatment, and Prevention*. New York: Springer-Verlag.

Mokuau, N. (1990). The impoverishment of native Hawaiians and the social work challenge. *Health & Social Work, 15*, 235–242.

Molloy, J.T. (1977). *The Woman's Dress for Success Book*. New York: Warner Books.

Montagu, A. (1964a). *Man's Most Dangerous Myth: The Fallacy of Race*, 4th rev. ed. Cleveland, Ohio: World.

Montagu, A.M.F. (1964b). Discussion and criticism on the race concept. *Current Anthropology, 5*, 317.

Monzon, O.T. & Carpellon, J.M.B. (1987). Female-to-female transmission of human immunodeficiency virus. *Lancet, 2*, 40–41.

Moore, J. (1994). The *chola* life course: Chicana heroin users and the barrio gang. *International Journal of the Addictions, 29*, 1115–1126.

Moore, J. & Devitt, M. (1989). The paradox of deviance in addicted Mexican American mothers. *Gender and Society, 3*, 53–70.

Moore, J.E. (1933). *The Modern Treatment of Syphilis*. Baltimore: Charles C. Thomas.

Moore, K.L. & Persaud, T.V.N. (1993). *The Developing Human: Clinically Oriented Embryology*, 5th ed. Philadelphia: W.B. Saunders.

Moore, L.J. & Boehnlein, J.K. (1991). Treating psychiatric disorders among Mien refugees from highland Laos. *Social Science and Medicine, 32*, 1029–1036.

Morais, H.M. (1967). *The History of the Negro in Medicine* (2nd ed.). New York: Publishers Co., Inc.

Morales, E. (1990). *Cadre Evaluation Report: (Year Three). Demonstration Project*. Funded by the Office of Substance Abuse Prevention, U.S. Department of Health. San Francisco, California: Community Substance Abuse Services, San Francisco Department of Health.

Morales, J. (1986). *Puerto Rican Poverty and Migration: We Just Had to Try Elsewhere*. New York: Praeger.

Morales, R. (1991). Alcohol abuse and Asian Americans. Paper presented at National Institute on Drug Abuse National Conference on Drug Abuse Research and Practice, Washington, D.C., Jan. 21. Cited in D.Y. Ja & B. Aoki. (1993). Substance abuse treatment: Cultural barriers in the Asian-American community. *Journal of Psychoactive Drugs, 25*, 61–71.

Morgan, J.P. & Zimmer, L. (1997). The social pharmacology of smokeable cocaine: Not all it's cracked up to be. In C. Reinarman & H.G. Levine (Eds.). *Crack in America: Demon Drugs and Social Justice* (pp. 131–170). Berkeley, California: University of California Press.

Morrow, S.K. & Hawxhurst, D.M. (1989). Lesbian partner abuse: Implications for therapists. *Journal of Counseling and Development, 68*, 58–62.

Morse, S.J. (1998). Fear of danger, flight from culpability. *Psychology, Public Policy & Law, 4*, 250–268.

Mroz, L.C. (1987). Smoking ban? What next? *Philip Morris Magazine*, Summer, 29.

Mulligan, K. & Schambelan, M. (1999). Wasting. In P.T. Cohen, M.A. Sande, & P.A. Volberding (Eds.). *AIDS Knowledge Base: A Textbook on HIV Disease from the University of California, San Francisco and San Francisco General Hospital* (pp. 403–13). Philadelphia: Lippincott, Williams & Wilkins.

Murdoch, R.O. (1999). Working and "drugging" in the city: Economies and substance use in a sample of working adults. *Substance Use and Misuse, 34*, 2115–2133.

Murdock, C.G. (1998). *Domesticating Drink: Women, Men, and Alcohol in America, 1870–1940*. Baltimore, Maryland: Johns Hopkins University Press.

Murray, M. & McMillan, C.L. (1993). Gender differences in perceptions of cancer. *Journal of Cancer Education, 8*, 53–62.

Murray, S.O. (1987a). Homosexual acts and selves in early modern Europe. *Journal of Homosexuality, 15*, 421–439.

Murray-Garcia, J.L., Selby, J.V., Schmittdiel, J., Grumbach, K., Quesenberry, C.P., Jr. (2000). Racial and ethnic differences in a patient survey: Patients' values, ratings and reports regarding physician primary care performance in a large health maintenance organization. *Medical Care, 38*, 300–310.

Musto, D.F. (1987). *The American Disease: Origins of Narcotic Control*. New York: Oxford University Press.

Nanda, S. (1994). Hijras: An alternative sex and gender role in India. In G. Herdt (Ed.), *Third Sex, Third Gender: Beyond Sexual Dimorphism in Culture and History* (pp. 373–417). New York: Zone Books.

Nanda, S. (1990). *Neither Man Nor Woman: The Hijras of India*. Belmont, California: Wadsworth Publishing Company.

Napoleon, H. (1991). Yuuvaraq: The Way of the Human Being. Fairbanks, Alaska: Center for Cross-Cultural Studies. Cited in C.T. Lowery, American Indian perspectives on addiction and recovery. In P.L. Ewalt, E.M. Freedman, A.E. Fortune, D.L. Poole, & S.L. Witkin. (Eds.). *Multicultural Issues in Social Work: Practice and Research* (pp. 473–485). Washington, D.C.: NASW Press.

Nast, H.J. & Pulido, L. (2000). Resisting corporate multiculturalism: Mapping faculty initiatives and institutional-student harassment in the classroom. *Professional Geographer, 52*, 722–737.

National Center on Addiction and Substance Abuse at Columbia University. (1998). *Behind Bars: Substance Abuse and America's Prison Population*. Available at http://www.casacolumbia.org/usrdoc/5745.pdf.

National Commission for the Protection of Human Subjects of Biomedical and Behavioral Research. (1978). The Belmont Report: Ethical Principles and Guidelines for the Protection of Human Subjects of Research. (DHEW Publication No. (OS) 78-0012). Washington, D.C.: Department of Health, Education, and Welfare.

National Gay and Lesbian Task Force. (1993, April). *Lesbian Health Issues and Recommendations*. Washington, D.C.: National Gay and Lesbian Task Force.

National Institute on Drug Abuse. (1992a). Annual Medical Examiner Data 1991: Data From the Drug Abuse Warning Network (DAWN) (Series 1, No. 11-b). Rockville, Maryland: National Academy Press.

National Institute on Drug Abuse. (2000). Commonly Abused Drugs. Available at http://www.drugabuse.gov.

National Institute on Drug Abuse. (1990). *National Household Survey on Drug Abuse*. Rockville, Maryland: National Academy Press.

National Institute on Drug Abuse. (1992b). *National Household Survey on Drug Abuse: Population Estimates 1991*. Rockville, Maryland: National Academy Press.

National Institute of Justice. (1996). *Evaluation of Drug Treatment in Local Corrections*. Washington, D.C.: United States Department of Justice, Office of Justice Programs, National Institute of Justice.

National Research Council. (2001). *Informing America's Policy on Illegal Drugs: What We Don't Know Keeps Hurting Us*. Washington, D.C.: National Academy Press.

National Research Council. (1999). *Pathological Gambling: A Critical Review*. Washington, D.C.: National Academy Press.

Nawakami, N., Haratani, T., Hemmi, T., & Araki, S. (1992). Prevalence and demographic correlates of alcohol-related problems in Japanese employees. *Social Psychiatry and Psychiatric Epidemiology, 27*, 198–202.

Neerhof, M.J., MacGregor, S.N., Retzky, S.S., & Sullivan, T.P. (1989). Cocaine abuse during pregnancy: Peripartum prevalence and perinatal outcome. *American Journal of Obstetrics and Gynecology, 161*, 633–638.

Nelson, J.A. (1997). Gay, lesbian, and bisexual adolescents: Providing esteem-enhancing care to a bettered population. *Nurse Practitioner, 22*, 94–109.

Neuberger, M.B. (1963). *Smoke Screen: Tobacco and the Public Welfare*. Englewood Cliffs, New Jersey: Prentice-Hall.

Nevada v. Encoe. (1994). 110 Nev. 1317.

Nicoloff, L.K. & Stiglitz, E.A. (1987). Lesbian alcoholism: Etiology, treatment, and recovery. In Boston Lesbian Psychologies Collective. (Ed.). *Lesbian Psychologies: Explorations and Challenges* (pp. 283–293). Urbana, Illinois: University of Illinois Press.

Nies, J. (1996). *Native American History: A Chronology of a Culture's Vast Achievements and Their Links to World Events*. New York: Ballantine Books.

Niesen, J. & Sandall, H. (1990). Alcohol and other drug abuse in a gay/lesbian population: Related to victimization? *Journal of Psychology & Human Sexuality, 3*, 151–168.

Noojin, R.O., Calloway, J.L., & Flower, A.H. (1945). Favorable response to penicillin therapy in a case of treatment-resistant syphilis. *North Carolina Medical Journal, January*, 34–37.

Nott, J.C. (1843). The mulatto a hybrid—Probable extermination of the two race if the whites and blacks are allowed to intermarry. *American Journal of the Medical Sciences, 6*, 252–256. Cited in R.J.C. Young. (1995). *Colonial Desire: Hybridity in Theory, Culture and Race*. London: Routledge.

Obeso, P. & Bordatto, O. (1979). Cultural implications in treating the Puerto Rican female. *American Journal of Drug and Alcohol Abuse, 6*, 345–353.

Obot, I.S., Hubbard, S., & Anthony, J.C. (1999). Level of education and injecting drug use among African Americans. *Drug and Alcohol Dependence, 55*, 177–182.

O'Brien, C.P. (1996). Drug addiction and drug abuse. In J.G. Hardman & L. Limbird (Eds.). *Goodman and Gilman's, The Pharmacologic Basis of Therapeutics* (pp. 557–577). New York: McGraw-Hill.

Oetting, E.R., Swaim, R.C., Edwards, R.W., & Beauvais, F. (1989). Indian and Anglo adolescent alcohol use and emotional distress: Path models. *American Journal of Alcohol and Drug Abuse, 15*, 153–172.

Office of National Drug Control Policy. (1999). *National Drug Control Strategy*. Washington, D.C.: Author.

Ogawa, D.M. (1971). *From Japs to Japanese: The Evolution of Japanese-American Stereotypes*. Berkeley, California: McCutchan.

Ogur, B. (1986). Long day's journey into night: Women and prescription drug abuse. *Women and Health, 11*, 99–115.

O'Neill, J.F. & Shalit, P. (1992). Health care of the gay male patient. *Primary Care, 19*, 191–201.

Ong, A. (1995). Making the biopolitical subject: Cambodian immigrants, refugee medicine, and cultural citizenship in California. *Social Science and Medicine, 40*, 1243–1257.

Onyekwuluje, A.B. (2000). Adult role models: Needed voices for adolescents, multiculturalism, diversity, and race relations. *The Urban Review, 32*, 67–85.

Oriel, K.A., Madlon-Kay, D.J., Govaker, D., & Mersy, D.J. (1996). Gay and lesbian physicians in training: Family practice program directors' attitudes and students' perceptions of bias. *Family Medicine, 28*, 720–725.

Osborne, A.C., Smart, R.G., Weber, T., & Birchmore-Timney, C. (2000). Who is using cannabis as medicine and why: An exploratory study. *Journal of Psychoactive Drugs, 32*, 435–443.

Osborne, N.G. & Feit, F.D. (1992). The use of race in medical research. *Journal of the American Medical Association, 267*, 275–279.

Osmond, D.H. (1999). Classification, staging, and surveillance of HIV. In P.T. Cohen, M.A. Sande, & P.A. Volberding (Eds.). *AIDS Knowledge Base: Textbook on HIV Disease from the University of California, San Francisco and San Francisco General Hospital* (pp. 3–12). Philadelphia: Lippincott, Williams & Wilkins.

Osmond, D.H. (1999). Epidemiology of HIV/AIDS in the United States. In P.T. Cohen, M.A. Sande, & P.A. Volberding (Eds.). *AIDS Knowledge Base Textbook on HIV Disease from the University of California, San Francisco and San Francisco General Hospital* (pp. 13–21). Philadelphia: Lippincott, Williams & Wilkins.

Osofsky, G. (1966). *Harlem: The Making of a Ghetto, Negro New York, 1890–1930*. New York: Harper and Row.

Osumi, M.D. (1982). Asians and California's anti-miscegenation laws. In N. Tsuchida (Ed.). *Asian and Pacific Islander Experiences: Women's Perspectives*. Minneapolis, Minnesota: Asian/Pacific American Learning Resource Center and General College, University of Minnesota.

Paglia, A. & Room, R. (1998). Alcohol and aggression: General population views about causation and responsibility. *Journal of Substance Abuse, 10*, 199–216.

Paisano, E.L. (1995). The American Indian, Eskimo, and Aleut population. In the Bureau of the Census, *Population Profile of the United States, 1995*. Washington, D.C.: U.S. Government Printing Office [Current Population Reports, Series 23-189].

Palinkas, L.A. & Pickwell, S.M. (1995). Acculturation as a risk factor for chronic disease among Cambodian refugees in the United States. *Social Science and Medicine, 40*, 1643–1653.

Paredes, A. (1976). The history of the concept of alcoholism. In R.E. Tarter & A.A. Sugerman (Eds.). *Alcoholism*. Reading, Massachusetts: Addison Wesley Publishing Company.

Parekh, B. (1995). Cultural pluralism and the limits of diversity. *Alternatives, 20*, 431–457.

Parker, V., Sussman, S., Crippens, D., Elder, P., & Scholl, D. (1998). The relation of ethnic identification with cigarette smoking among U.S. urban African American and Latino youth: A pilot study. *Ethnicity and Health, 3*, 135–143.

Pauley, I.B. (1968). The current status of the change of sex operation. *Journal of Nervous and Mental Disease, 147*, 460–471.

Paulsen, H.J. (1987). Tuberculosis in the Native American: Indigenous or introduced? *Review of Infectious Disease, 9*, 1180–1186.

Pedersen, P. (1991). Balance as a criterion for social services for Asian and Pacific Islander Americans. In N. Mokuau. (Ed.). *Handbook of Social Services for Asians and Pacific Islanders* (pp. 37–57). New York: Greenwood Press.

Peffer, G.A. (1986). Forbidden families: Emigration experiences of Chinese women under the Page Law, 1875–1882. *Journal of American Ethnic History, 6*, 28–46.

Pelham, T.L. & DeJong, A.R. (1992). Nationwide practices for screening and reporting prenatal cocaine abuse: A survey of teaching programs. *Child Abuse and Neglect, 16,* 763–770.

Penslar, R.L. (no date). Institutional Review Board Guidelines. Available at http://www.grants.nih.gov/grants/oprr/irb/irb.introduction.html.

People v. Hall. (1854). 4 Cal. 399.

People v. Morabito. (1992). 151 Misc. 2d 259 (N.Y. City Ct.).

People v. Newman. (1973). 298 N.E.2d 651, *cert. denied,* 414 U.S. 1163 (1973).

People v. Stewart. (1987). 16 Ms. 92 (San Diego Municipal Court, February 24).

Perez-Arce, P. (1994). Substance use patterns of Latinas: A commentary. *International Journal of the Addictions, 29,* 1189–1199.

Perez-Stable, E., Marin, G., & Marin, B. (1994). Behavioral risk factors: A comparison of Latinos and non-Latino whites in San Francisco. *American Journal of Public Health, 84,* 971–976.

Perkonigg, A., Lieb, R., Hofler, M., Schuster, P., Sonntag, H., & Wittchen, H.U. (1999). Patterns of cannabis use, abuse, and dependence over time: Incidence, progression, and stability in a sample of 1228 adolescents. *Addiction, 94,* 1663–1678.

Perrin, E.C. & Kulkin, H. (1996). Pediatric care for children whose parents are gay or lesbian. *Pediatrics, 97,* 629–635.

Perry, S.M. (1995). Lesbian alcohol and marijuana use: Correlates of HIV risk behaviors and abusive relationships. *Journal of Psychoactive Drugs, 27,* 413–419.

Pesare, P.J., Bauer, T.J., & Gleeson, G.A. (1950). Untreated syphilis in the male Negro: Observation of abnormalities over sixteen years. *American Journal of Syphilis, Gonorrhea, and Venereal Diseases, 34,* 201–213.

Piasecki, M. (2000). Smoking, nicotine, and mood. In M. Piasecki & P.A. Newhouse (Eds.). *Nicotine in Psychiatry: Psychopathology and Emerging Therapeutics* (pp. 131–147). Washington, D.C.: American Psychiatric Press, Inc.

Platt, J.J. (1986). *Heroin Addiction: Theory, Research and Treatment,* 2nd ed. Malabar, Florida: R.E. Krieger Publishing Co.

Platt, J.J. (1995). *Heroin Addiction: Theory, Research and Treatment,* Vol. 2. Malabar, Florida: R.E. Krieger Publishing Co.

Platt, J.J. (1995). *Heroin Addiction: Theory, Research and Treatment,* Vol. 3. Malabar, Florida: R.E. Krieger Publishing Co.

Platt, J.J. et al. (1998). Methadone maintenance treatment: Its development and effectiveness after 30 years. In J.A. Inciardi & L.D. Harrison. (Eds.). *Heroin in the Age of Crack Cocaine* (pp. 160–177). Thousand Oaks, California: Sage Publications.

Platzer, H. & James, T. (1997). Methodological issues conducting sensitive research on lesbian and gay men's experience of nursing care. *Journal of Advanced Nursing, 25,* 626–633.

Plitcha, S.B. & Weisman, C.S. (1995). Spouse or partner abuse, use of health services, and unmet need for medical care in U.S. women. *Journal of Women's Health, 4,* 45–54.

Poirier, S. (1990). Women's reproductive health. In R.D. Apple (Ed.). *Women, Health, and Medicine in America: A Historical Handbook* (pp. 217–245). New York: Garland Publishing, Inc.

Pope, T.M. (2000). Balancing public health against individual liberty: The ethics of smoking regulations. *University of Pittsburgh Law Review, 61,* 419–498.

Powell v. Texas. (1968). 392 U.S. 514.

Powers, H.W. (1915). Morphin and cocaine addiction with special reference to prognosis. *Illinois Medical Journal, 27,* 441–443.

Proctor, C.D. & Groze, V.K. (1994). Risk factors for suicide among gay, lesbian, and bisexual youth. *Social Work, 39,* 504–513.

Prince, E.E. Jr. (2000). *Long Green: The Rise and Fall of Tobacco in South Carolina.* Athens, Georgia: University of Georgia Press.

Prochaska, J.O. & Velicer, W.F. (1997). The transtheoretical model of health behavior change. *American Journal of Health Promotion, 12*, 38–48.

Public Health Cigarette Amendments of 1971. (1972). Hearing on S. 1454 Before the Consumer Subcommittee of the Senate Committee on Commerce, 92d Cong. 240.

Pure Food and Drug Act of 1906, Act of June 30, 1906, 34 Stat. 768.

Putnam, C. (1961). *Race and Reason.* Washington, D.C.: Public Affairs Press.

Quillian, D.D. (1906). Racial peculiarities: A cause of the prevalence of syphilis in Negroes. *American Journal of Dermatology & Genito-Urinary Disease, 10*, 277–279.

Quincy, K. (1988). *Hmong: History of a People.* Cheny, Washington: East Washington University Press.

Quinn, K. (2000). *Working Without Benefits: The Health Insurance Crisis Confronting Hispanic-Americans.* New York: Commonwealth Fund.

Quinones-Jenab, V. (2001). Preface. In V. Quinones-Jenab (Ed.). *The Biological Basis of Cocaine Addiction* (pp. vii–viii). New York: New York Academy of Sciences.

Rado, S. (1933). Fear of castration in women. *Psychoanalytic Quarterly, 2*, 425–475.

Rah, J.A. (2002). The removal of aliens who drink and drive: Felony DWI as a crime of violence under 18 U.S.C. 16(b). *Fordham Law Review, 70*, 2109–2169.

Ramakrishna, J. & Weiss, M.G. (1992). Health, illness, and immigration: East Indians in the United States. *Western Journal of Medicine, 157*, 265–270.

Ramirez, A.B. & Seipp, C. (1983). *Colonialism, Catholicism, and Contraception: A History of Birth Control in Puerto Rico.* Chapel Hill, North Carolina: University of North Carolina Press.

Randall, C.E. (1989). Lesbian phobia among BSN educators: A survey. *Journal of Nursing Education, 28*, 302–306.

Rankow, E.J. (1995). Lesbian health issues for the primary health care provider. *Journal of Family Practice, 40*, 486–493.

Rankow, E.J. (1997). Primary medical care of the gay or lesbian patient. *North Carolina Medical Journal, 58*, 92–96.

Ray, O.S. & Ksir, C. (1990). *Drugs, Society, and Human Behavior.* New York: McGaw-Hill.

Ray-Mazumder, S. (2001). Role of gender, insurance status and culture in attitudes and health behavior in a U.S. Chinese student population. *Ethnicity and Health, 6*, 197–209.

Raymond, C.A. (1988). Lesbians call for greater physician awareness, sensitivity to improve patient care. *Journal of the American Medical Association, 259*, 18.

Razzano, L.A., Hamilton, M.M., & Hughes, T.L. (2000). Mental health services utilization patterns among lesbians and homosexual women. Paper presented at the 108th Annual Meeting of the American Psychological Association, Washington, D.C. Cited in K.Y. Ritter and A.I. Terndrup. (2002). *Handbook of Affirmative Psychotherapy with Lesbians and Gay Men.* New York: Gulford Press.

Reagan, P. (1981). The interaction of health professionals and their lesbian clients. *Patient Counseling and Health Education, 3*, 21–25.

Reagan, R. (1988). Text of Reagan's remarks. Reprinted in *Pacific Citizen*, August 19–26, 5.

Reed, J. (1978). *From Private Vice to Public Virtue: The Birth Control Movement and American Society Since 1830.* New York: Basic Books.

Reid, W.H. & Wise, M.G. (1999). *DSM-IV Training Guide.* New York: Brunner/Mazel.

Reinarman, C. (1988). The social construction of an alcohol problem: The case of Mothers Against Drunk Drivers and social control in the 1980s. *Theory & Society, 17*, 91–120.

Reinarman, C. & Levine, H.G. (1997a). The crack attack: Politics and media in the crack scare. In C. Reinarman & H.G. Levine (Eds.). *Crack in America: Demon Drugs and Social Justice* (pp. 18–56). Berkeley, California: University of California Press.

Reinarman, C. & Levine, H.G. (1997b). Crack in context: America's latest demon drug. In C. Reinarman & H.G. Levine (Eds.). *Crack in America: Demon Drugs and Social Justice* (pp. 1–17). Berkeley, California: University of California Press.

Remafedi, G. (1990). Fundamental issues in the care of homosexual youth. *Medical Clinics of North America, 74*, 1169–1179.

Remafedi, G., Farrow, J.A., & Deisher, R.W. (1991). Risk factors for attempted suicide in gay and bisexual youth. *Pediatrics, 87*, 869–875.

Renard, R.D. (2001). *Opium Reduction in Thailand, 1970–2000: A Thirty-Year Journey*. Chaing Mai, Thailand: Silkworm Books.

Resick, P., Calhoun, K., Atkeson, B., & Ellis, E. (1981). Adjustment in victims of sexual assault. *Journal of Consulting and Clinical Psychology, 49*, 705–712.

Rice, D.P., Kelman, S., Miller, L., & Dunmeyer, S. (1991). Estimates of economic costs of alcohol and drug abuse and mental illness, 1985 and 1988. *Public Health Reports, 106*, 280–292.

Rice, D.P., Kelman, S., & Miller, L.S. (1991). Economic cost of drug abuse. In W.S. Cartwright & J.M. Kaple (Eds.). *Economic Costs, Cost-Effectiveness, Financing, and Community-Based Treatment* (pp. 10–32). Rockville, Maryland: United States Department of Health and Human Services.

Rice, R.J., Roberts, P.L., Handsfield, H.H., & Holmes, K.K. (1991). Sociodemographic distribution of gonorrhea incidence: Implications for prevention and behavioral research. *American Journal of Public Health, 81*, 1252–1258.

Rich, J.D., Macalino, G.E., McKenzie, M., Taylor, L.E., & Burris, S. (2001). Syringe prescription to prevent HIV infection in Rhode Island: A case study. *American Journal of Public Health, 91*, 699–700.

Richardson, T.L. (1997). Is menthol part of the puzzle? *Western Journal of Medicine, 166*, 189–194.

Richer, C.J. (2000). Fetal abuse law: Punitive approach and the honorable status of motherhood. *Syracuse Law Review, 50*, 1127–1149.

Riggs, P.D., Baker, S., Mikulich, S.K., Young, S.E., & Crowley, T.J. (1995). Depression in substance-dependent delinquents. *Journal of the American Academy of Child and Adolescent Psychiatry, 34*, 764–771.

Ritter, K.Y. & Terndrup, A.I. (2002). *Handbook of Affirmative Psychotherapy with Lesbians and Gay Men*. New York: Gulford Press.

Rivera Live: Whether marijuana use for medicinal purposes should be legalized. CNBC television broadcast, March 25, 1999.

Rivers, E., Schuman, S.H., Simpson, L., & Olansky, S. (1953). Twenty years of followup experience in a long-range medical study. *Public Health Reports, 68*, 391–195.

Rizk, B., Atterbury, J.L., & Groome, L.J. (1996). Reproductive risks of cocaine. *Human Reproduction Update, 2*, 43–55.

Roberts, M.H. (1925). The spinal fluid in the newborn. *Journal of the American Medical Association, 85*, 500–503.

Roberts, S.J. & Sorenson, L. (1994). Health promotion and early disease detection among lesbians: Results from the Boston Lesbian Health Project. Unpublished manuscript, cited in Roberts, S.J., Sorenson, L. (1995). Lesbian health care: A review and recommendations for health promotion in primary care settings. *Nurse Practitioner, 20*, 42–47.

Roberts, S.J. & Sorenson, L. (1995). Lesbian health care: A review and recommendations for health promotion in primary care settings. *Nurse Practitioner, 20*, 42–47.

Robertson, P. & Schachter, J. (1981). Failure to identify venereal disease in a lesbian population. *Sexually Transmitted Disease, 8*, 75–76.

Robins, L.N. (1966). *Deviant Children Grow Up: A Sociological and Psychiatric Study of Sociopathic Personality*. Baltimore, Maryland: Williams & Wilkins.

Robins, L.N. & McEvoy, L. (1990). Conduct problems as predictors of substance abuse. In L.N. Robins & M. Rutter (Eds.). *Straight and Devious Pathways from Childhood to Adulthood.* Cambridge, England: Cambridge University Press.

Robinson v. California. (1962). 370 U.S. 660.

Robinson, G. & Cohen, M. (1996). Gay, lesbian, and bisexual health care issues and medical curricula. *Canadian Medical Association Journal, 155,* 709–711.

Rodriguez, C.E. (1994). A summary of Puerto Rican migration to the United States. In G. Lamberty & C.G. Coll (Eds.). *Puerto Rican Women and Children: Issues in Health, Growth, and Development* (pp. 11–28). New York: Plenum Press.

Rodrigues-Trias, H. (1978). Sterilization of abuse. *Women's Health, 3,* 10–15.

Roe v. Wade, 410 U.S. 113 (1973).

Roldan, C.a., Aliabadi, D., & Crawford, M.H. (2001). Prevalence of heart disease in asymptomatic chronic cocaine users. *Cardiology, 95,* 25–30.

Rompalo, A. (1990). Sexually transmitted causes of gastrointestinal symptoms in homosexual men. *Medical Clinics of North America, 74,* 1633–1646.

Ron, M.A. (1983). The alcoholic brain: CT scan and psychological findings. *Psychological Medicine Monographs Supplement, 3,* 1–33.

Rorabaugh, W.J. (1979). *The Alcoholic Republic.* New York: Oxford University Press.

Roscoe, W. (1994). How to become a berdache: Toward a unified analysis of gender diversity. In G. Herdt (Ed.). *Third Sex, Third Gender: Beyond Sexual Dimorphism in Culture and History* (pp. 329–372). New York: Zone Books.

Roscoe, W. (1991). *The Zuni Man-Woman.* Albuquerque: University of New Mexico Press.

Rosen, D.H. (1974). *Lesbianism: A Study of Female Homosexuality.* Springfield, Illinois: Charles C. Thomas.

Rosengren, S.S., Longobucco, D.B., Bernstein, B.A., Fishman, S., Cooke, E., Boctor, F., & Lewis, S.C. (1993). Meconium testing for cocaine metabolite: Prevalence, perceptions, pitfalls. *American Journal of Obstetrics and Gynecology, 168,* 1449–1456.

Rothblum, E.D. (1994). "I only read about myself on bathroom walls": The need for research on the mental health of lesbians and gay men. *Journal of Consulting and Clinical Psychology, 62,* 213–220.

Rushton, J.P. (1988). Race differences in behavior: A review and evolutionary analysis. *Personality and Individual Differences, 9,* 1009–1024.

Russell, A., Voas, R.B., DeJong, W., & Chaloupka, M. (1995). MADD rates the states: A media advocacy event to advance the agenda against alcohol-impaired driving. *Public Health Reports, 110,* 240–245.

Ryan, C. & Bradford, J. (1988). The National Lesbian health Care Survey: An overview. In M. Shernoff & W.A. Scott (Eds.). *The Sourcebook on Lesbian/Gay Health Care,* 2nd ed. (pp. 30–40). Washington, D.C.: National Lesbian/Gay Health Foundation.

Sabatini, M.T., Patel, K., & Hirschman, R. (1984). Kaposi's sarcoma and T-cell lymphoma in an immunodeficient woman. *AIDS Research, 1,* 135–137.

Sadeghi, S.B., Sadeghi, A., Cosby, M., Olincy, A., & Robboy, S.J. (1989). Human papillovirus infection: Frequency and association with cervical neoplasia in a young population. *Acta Cytologica, 33,* 319–323.

Sadoff, M. Voiceover. *MAADVOCATE, 2,* 4.

Saghir, M.T. & Robins, E. (1973). *Male and Female Homosexuality: A Comprehensive Investigation.* Baltimore: Wilkins & Wilkins.

Samora, J. (1971). *Los Mojados: The Wetback Story.* Notre Dame, Indiana: University of Notre Dame Press.

Sanger, M. (1938). *Margaret Sanger: An Autobiography.* Elmsford, New York: Maxwell Reprint Company. 1970.

Santiago-Rivera, A.L., Arredondo, P., & Gallardo-Cooper, M. (2002). *Counseling Latinos and La Familia: A Practical Guide*. Thousand Oaks, California: Sage Publications.

Sapino, A., Pietribiasi, F., Godano, A., & Bussolati, G. (1992). Effect of long-term administration of androgens on breast tissues of female-to-male transsexuals. *Annals of the New York Academy of Science, 586*, 143–145.

Sasao, T. (1989). Patterns of substance use and health practices among Japanese Americans in southern California. Paper presented at the Third Annual Meeting of the Asian American Psychological Association, New Orleans. Cited in N. Zane & J.H. Kim. (1994). Substance use and abuse. In N.W.S. Zane, D.T. Takeuchi, & K.N.J. Young (Eds.). *Confronting Critical Health Issues of Asian and Pacific Islander Americans* (pp. 316–343). Thousand Oaks, California: Sage Publications.

Satel, S. (1997). Medical marijuana: Research, don't legalize. *Wall Street Journal*, Oct. 30, A22.

Sauer, W.H., Berlin, J.A., Strom, B.L., Miles, C., Carson, J.L., & Kimmel, S.E. (2002). Cigarette yield and the risk of myocardial infarction in smokers. *Archives of Internal Medicine, 162*, 300–306.

Saunders, J.M. & Valente, S.M. (1987). Suicide risk among gay men and lesbians: A review. *Death Studies, 11*, 1–23.

Savage, D.G. & Warren, J. (1996). U.S. threatens penalties if doctors prescribe pot drugs: Criminal charges, other sanctions are possible, officials warn California and Arizona physicians. *L.A. Times*, Dec. 31. A3.

Savin-Williams, R.C. (1989). *"And Then I Became Gay": Young Men's Stories*. New York: Routledge.

Savitt, T.L. (1985). Black health on the plantation: Masters, slaves, and physicians. In J.W. Leavitt & R.L. Numbers (Eds.). *Sickness and Health in America: Readings in the History of Medicine and Public Health* (2nd ed. rev., pp. 313–330). Madison, Wisconsin: University of Wisconsin Press.

Scacco, A. (Ed.). (1982). *Male Rape: A Casebook of Sexual Aggression*. New York: AMS Press.

Schaeffer, C.E. (1965). The Kutenai female berdache: Courier, guide, prophetess, and warrior. *Ethnohistory, 12*, 193–236.

Schatz, B. & O'Hanlan, K.A. (1994). *Anti-gay Discrimination in Medicine: Results of a National Survey of Lesbian, Gay, and Bisexual Physicians*. San Francisco, California: American Association of Physicians for Human Rights.

Scheper-Hughes, N. & Stewart, D. (1983). Curanderismo in Taos County, New Mexico—A possible case of anthropological romanticism? *Western Journal of Medicine, 139*, 875–884.

Schilit, R., Lie, G., & Montagne, M. (1990). Substance use as a correlate of violence in intimate lesbian relationships. *Journal of Homosexuality, 19*, 51–65.

Schinke, S.P., Moncher, M.S., Palleja, J., Zayas, L.H., & Schilling, R.F. (1988). Hispanic youth, substance abuse, and stress: Implications for prevention research. *International Journal of the Addictions, 23*, 809–826.

Schmidley, A.D. (2001). *Profile of the Foreign-Born Population of the United States: 2000*. Washington, D.C.: Government Printing Office [U.S. Census Bureau, Current Population Reports, Series P23-206].

Schmidt, G. (1984). Allies and persecutors: Science and medicine in the homosexuality issue. *Journal of Homosexuality, 10*, 127–140.

Schneider, M. (1989). Sappho was a right-on adolescent: Growing up lesbian. *Journal of Homosexuality, 17*, 111–130.

Schneider, S.G., Farberow, N.L., & Kruks, G.N. (1989). Suicidal behavior in adolescent and young gay men. *Suicide and Life-Threatening Behavior, 19*, 381–394.

Schoepf, B.G. (1991). Ethical, methodological, and political issues of AIDS research in Central Africa. *Social Science and Medicine, 33*, 749–763.

School of Public Health, University of California, Berkeley & Institute for Health Policy Studies, University of California, San Francisco. (1993). *The Public Health Impact of Needle Exchange Programs in the United States and Abroad: Summary, Conclusions, and Recommendations.* Authors.

Schreeder, M.T., Bender, T.R., McMahon, R.J., Moser, M.R., Murphy, B.L., Sheller, M.J., Heyward, W.L., Hall, D.B., & Maynard, J.E. (1983). Prevalence of hepatitis B in selected Alaskan Eskimo villages. *American Journal of Epidemiology, 118*, 543–549.

Schultes, R.E. (1972). An overview of hallucinogens in the western hemisphere. In P.T. Furst. (Ed.). *Flesh of the Gods: The Ritual Use of Hallucinogens* (pp. 3–54). New York: Praeger.

Schwartz, J. (1995). 1973 cigarette company memo proposed new brands for teens; RJR official cited need for "share of youth market." *Washington Post*, October 4, A2.

Schwartz, R.H. (1993). Syringe and needle exchange programs: Part I. *Southern Medical Journal, 86*, 318–322.

Scott, W.K., Sy, F.S., Jackson, K.L., Macera, C.A., & Harris, N.S. (1997). Survival after AIDS diagnosis in South Carolina, 1982–1992. *The Journal of the South Carolina Medical Association, 93*, 5–12.

Sears, J.T. (1991). *Growing Up Gay in the South: Race, Gender, and Journeys of the Spirit.* New York: Harrington Park Press.

Segen, J.C. (1992). *The Dictionary of Modern Medicine.* Park Ridge, New Jersey: Parthenon Publishing Group.

Seham, M. (1964). Discrimination against Negroes in hospitals. *New England Journal of Medicine, 271*, 940–943.

Selik, R.M., Castro, K.G., Pappaioanou, M., & Buehler, J.W. (1989). Birthplace and the risk of AIDS among Hispanics in the United States. *American Journal of Public Health, 79*, 836–839.

Sell, R.L. & Petrulio, C. (1996). Sampling homosexuals, bisexuals, gays, and lesbians for public health research: A review of the literature from 1990 to 1992. *Journal of Homosexuality, 30*, 31–47.

Semmes, C.E. (1996). *Racism, Health, and Post-Industrialism: A Theory of African-American Health.* Westport, Connecticut: Praeger.

Sengstock, M.C. (2001). Multicultural families—What makes them work? *Sociological Practice: A Journal of Clinical and Applied Sociology, 3*, 1–17.

Shai, D. & Rosenwaike, I. (1988). Violent deaths among Mexican-, Puerto Rican-, and Cuban-born migrants in the United States. *Social Science and Medicine, 26*, 269–276.

Shavers-Hornaday, V.L., Lynch, C.F., Burmeister, L.F., & Torner, J.C. (1997). Why are African Americans under-represented in medical research studies? Impediments to participation. *Ethnicity and Health, 2*, 31–45.

Shimada, J., Jackson, J.C., Goldstein, E., & Buchwald, D. (1995). "Strong medicine": Cambodian views of medicine and medical compliance. *Journal of General Internal Medicine, 10*, 369–374.

Shockley, W. (1968). Human quality problems and research taboos. In J.A. Pintus (Ed.). *New Concepts and Directions in Education.* Greenwich, Connecticut: Educational Records Bureau.

Shuckit, M.A. (2000). *Drug and Alcohol Abuse: A Clinical Guide to Diagnosis and Treatment.* New York: McGraw-Hill.

Shytle, R.D., Baker, M., Silver, A.A., Reid, B.M., & Sanberg, P.R. (2000). Smoking, nicotine, and movement disorders. In M. Piasecki & P.A. Newhouse (Eds.). *Nicotine in Psychiatry: Psychopathology and Emerging Therapeutics* (pp. 183–202). Washington, D.C.: American Psychiatric Press, Inc.

Siegel, D., Benowitz, N., Ernster, V.L., Grady, D.G., & Hauck, W.W. (1992). Smokeless tobacco, cardiovascular risk factors, and nicotine and cotinine levels in professional baseball players. *American Journal of Public Health, 82,* 417–421.

Siegel, D., Lazarus, N., Krasnovsky, F., Dubin, M., & Chesney, M. (1991). AIDS knowledge, attitudes and behavior among inner city, junior high school students. *Journal of School Health, 61,* 160–165.

Siegel, S. & Lowe, E. (1994). *Uncharted Lives: Understanding the Life Passages of Gay Men.* New York: Dutton.

Siegel, J.S. & Passel, J.S. (1979). *Coverage of the Hispanic Population of the United States in the 1970 Census.* Washington, D.C.: Bureau of the Census. [Current Population Reports, United States Department of Commerce Publication P23, No. 82].

Simkin, R.J. (1993). Unique health concerns of lesbians. *Canadian Journal of Obstetrics, Gynecology, & Women's Health Care, 5,* 516–522.

Sims, J.M. (1894). *The Story of My Life.* New York: D. Appleton.

Sinnika Dixon, A.L. (1999). The hidden community: Spatial dimensions of urban life. In D.A. Chekki (Ed.). *Research in Community Sociology, Vol. 9: Varieties of Community Sociology* (pp. 287–308). Greenwich, Connecticut: Jai Press.

Sivakumar, K., DeSilva, A.H., & Roy, R.B. (1989). *Trichomonas vaginalis* infection in a lesbian [letter]. *Genitourinary Medicine, 65,* 399–400.

Skene, A.J.C. (1889). *Education and Culture as Related to the Health and Diseases of Women.* Detroit: George S. Davis. Cited in C. Smith-Rosenberg. (1973). The cycle of femininity: Puberty to menopause in nineteenth century America. *Feminist Studies, 1,* 58–72. Reprinted in C. Smith-Rosenberg. (1985). *Disorderly Conduct: Visions of Gender in Victorian America.* New York: Alfred A. Knopf, Inc.

Slade, J. (2001). Marketing policies. In R.L. Rabin & S.D. Sugarman (Eds.). *Regulating Tobacco* (pp. 72–110). New York: Oxford University Press.

Sleeter, C.E. & Grant, C.A. (1987). An analysis of multicultural education in the United States. *Harvard Educational Review, 57,* 421–444.

Smeltzer, S.C. (1992). Women and AIDS: Sociopolitical issues. *Nursing Outlook, 40,* 152–157.

Smith, B. (1991). *Strategies for Courts to Cope with the Caseload Pressures of Drug Cases.* Chicago, Illinois: American Bar Association.

Smith, G. (1998). *Beer in America: The Early Years 1587–1840.* Boulder, Colorado: Brewers Publications.

Smith, J.E. & Krejci, J. (1991). Minorities join the majority: Eating disturbances among Hispanic and Native American youth. *International Journal of Eating Disorders, 10,* 179–186.

Smith, M.J. & Ryan, A.S. (1987). Chinese American families of children with developmental disabilities: An exploratory study of reactions to service providers. *Mental Retardation, 25,* 345–350.

Smith, V. (1988). Introduction. In H. Jacobs, *Incidents in the Life of a Slave Girl* (pp. xxvii–xl). New York: Oxford University Press.

Smith-Rosenberg, C. (1973). The cycle of femininity: Puberty to menopause in nineteenth century America. *Feminist Studies, 1,* 58–72. Reprinted in C. Smith-Rosenberg. (1985). *Disorderly Conduct: Visions of Gender in Victorian America.* New York: Alfred A. Knopf, Inc.

Smith-Rosenberg, C. (1985). *Disorderly Conduct: Visions of Gender in Victorian America.* New York: Oxford University Press.

Smith-Rosenberg, C. (1978). Sex as symbol in Victorian purity: An ethnohistorical analysis of Jacksonian America. *American Journal of Sociology, 134,* Supp. 212–247.

Snipp, C.M. (1986). Who are American Indians? Some observations about the perils and pitfalls of data for race and ethnicity. *Population Research Policy Review, 5,* 237–252.

Snyder, S.H. (1996). *Drugs and the Brain.* New York: Scientific American Books Inc.

Socarides, C.W. (1968). *The Overt Homosexual*. New York: Grune & Stratton.

Sokol, R.J., Miller, S.I., & Martier, S.S. (1981). *Preventing Alcohol Fetal Effects: A Practical Guide for OB/GYN Physicians and Nurses*. Rockville, Maryland: United States Department of Health and Human Services, Public Health Service, Alcohol, Drug Abuse, and Mental Health Administration, National Institute on Alcohol Abuse and Alcoholism.

Sorge, R. (1991). Harm reduction: A new approach to drug services. *HEALTH/PAC Bulletin, Winter*, 22–27.

Spickard, P.R. (1996). *Japanese Americans: The Formation and Transformation of an Ethnic Group*. New York: Twayne Publishers.

Spillane, J.F. (2000). *Cocaine: From Medical Marvel to Modern Menace in the United States, 1884–1920*. Baltimore, Maryland: Johns Hopkins University Press.

Stampp, M. (1956). *The Peculiar Institution: Slavery in the Ante-Bellum South*. New York: Vintage Books.

Stanley, E. (1931). Marihuana as a developer of criminals. *American Journal of Police Science, 2*, 256–257.

Stark, E. & Flitcraft, A. (1988). Violence among intimates: An epidemiological review. In V.B. Van Heselt, R.L. Morrison, A.S. Bellack, & M. Hersen (Eds.). *Handbook of Family Violence* (pp. 293–317). New York: Plenum Press.

State v. Deborah J.Z. (1999). 596 N.W.2d 490 (Wis. Ct. App.).

State v. Gethers. (1991). 585 So. 2d 1140 (Fla. Dist. Ct. App.).

State v. Gray. (1992). 62 Ohio St. 3d 514.

Stein, M., Tiefer, L., & Melman, A. (1990). Followup observations of operated male-to-female transsexuals. *Journal of Urology, 143*, 1188–1192.

Steinbrook, R. (1989). AIDS trials shortchange minorities and drug users. *Los Angeles Times, September 25*, 1–1.

Stekel, W. (1946). *The Homosexual Neurosis*. New York: Emerson Books.

Stepan, N.L. (1990). Race and gender: The role of analogy in science. In D.T. Goldberg (Ed.). *Anatomy of Racism* (pp. 38–57) Minneapolis: University of Minnesota Press.

Sterk C., Dolan, K., & Hatch, S. (1999). Epidemiological indicators and ethnographic realities of female cocaine use. *Substance Use & Misuse, 34*, 2057–2072.

Stermac, L., Sheridan, P.M., Davidson, A., & Dunn, S. (1996). Sexual assault of adult males. *Journal of Interpersonal Violence, 11*, 52–64.

Stevens, E. (1973). Machismo and marianismo. *Transaction Society, 10*, 57–63.

Stevens, P.E. (1993). Marginalized women's access to health care: A feminist narrative analysis. *Advances in Nursing Science, 16*, 39–56.

Stevens, P.E. (1994). Protective strategies of lesbian clients in health care environments. *Research in Nursing and Health, 17*, 217–229.

Stevens, P.E. (1995). Structural and interpersonal impact of heterosexual assumptions on lesbian health care clients. *Nursing Research, 44*, 25–30.

Stevens, P.E. & Hall, J.M. (1988). Stigma, health beliefs and experiences with health care in lesbian women. *Image: Journal of Nursing Scholarship, 20*, 69–73.

Stevens-Arroyo, A. & Diaz-Stevens, M. (1982). Puerto Ricans in the United States: A struggle for identity. In A.G. Dworkin & R.J. Dworkin (Eds.). *The Minority Report: An Introduction to Racial, Ethnic, and Gender Relations* (2nd ed.). New York: CBS Publishing, Holt, Rinehart, & Winston.

Steward, J. (1965). *The People of Puerto Rico*. Chicago, Illinois: University of Illinois Press.

Stitzer, M.L. & Chutuape, M.A. (1999). Other substance use disorders in methadone treatment: Prevalence, consequences, detection, and management. In E.C. Strain & M.L. Stitzer (Eds.). *Methadone Treatment for Opioid Dependence.* (pp. 86–117). Baltimore, Maryland: Johns Hopkins University Press.

Stolen, K.A. (1991). Gender, sexuality, and violence in Ecuador. *Ethnos, 56*, 82–100.

Stoller, K.B. & Bigelow, G.E. (1999). Regulatory, cost, and policy issues. In E.C. Strain & M.L. Stitzer (Eds.). *Methadone Treatment for Opioid Dependence*. (pp. 15–37). Baltimore, Maryland: Johns Hopkins University Press.

Stoller, R.J. (1964). A contribution to the study of gender identity. *Journal of the American Medical Association, 45*, 220–226.

Stoller, R.J. (1968). *Sex and Gender: On the Development of Masculinity and Femininity*. New York: Science House.

Storer, H.R. & Heard, F.F. (1865). *Criminal Abortion: Its Nature, Evidence, and Its Law*. Boston: Little, Brown, and Company.

Strang, J. & Farrell, M. (1992). Harm minimization for drug users. *British Medical Journal, 304*, 1127–1128.

Straus, M.A. & Gelles, R.J. (1990). *Physical Violence in American Families*. New Brunswick, New Jersey: Transaction Publishers.

Straus, M., Gelles, R., & Steinmetz, S. (1980). *Behind Closed Doors: Violence in the American Family*. New York: Doubleday.

Streatfield, D. (2001). *Cocaine [An Unauthorized Biography]*. New York: St. Martin's Press.

Strunin, L. (1991). Adolescents' perceptions of risk for HIV infection: Implications for future research. *Social Science and Medicine, 32*, 221–228.

Stryker, J. (1989). IV drug use and AIDS: Public policy and dirty needles. *Journal of Health Politics, Policy and Law, 14*, 719–740.

Substance Abuse and Mental Health Services Administration. (1995). *National Household Survey on Drug Abuse: Population Estimates 1994*. Rockville, Maryland: United States Department of Health and Human Services, Public Health Service, Substance Abuse and Mental Health Services Administration.

Substance Abuse and Mental Health Services Administration. (1998). *National Household Survey on Drug Abuse: Population Estimates 1997*. [DHHS Pub. No. (SMA) 98-3250]. Rockville, Maryland: Substance Abuse and Mental Health Services Administration.

Sue, S. & Morishima, J.K. (1982). *The Mental Health of Asian Americans*. San Francisco: Jossey-Bass.

Sugarman, J., Kass, N.E., Goodman, S.N., Perentesis, P., Fernandes, P., & Faden, R.R. (1998). What patients say about medical research. *IRB, 20*, 1–7.

Sullivan, C. (1991). Pathways to infection: AIDS vulnerability among the Navajo. *AIDS Education and Prevention, 3*, 241–257.

Swallow, J. (1983). Recovery: The story of an ACA. in J. Swallow (Ed.). *Out From Under: Sober Dykes and Our Friends*. San Francisco: Spinsters/Aunt Lute.

Sworts, V.D. & Riccitelli, C.N. (1997). Health education lessons learned: The H.A.P.I. kids program. *Journal of School Health, 67*, 283–285.

Szmuness, W., Stevens, C.E., Ikram, H., Much, M.J., Harley, E.J., & Hollinger, B. (1978). Prevalence of hepatitis B infection and hepatocellular carcinoma in Chinese-Americans. *Journal of Infectious Diseases, 137*, 822–829.

Tajfel, H. (1974). Social identity and intergroup behaviour. *Social Science Information, 13*, 65–93.

Tajfel, H. & Turner, J. (1986). The social identity theory of intergroup behaviour. In S. Worshel, Ed., *Psychology of Intergroup Relations*. Chicago: Nelson Hall.

Takada, E., Ford, J., & Lloyd, L.S. (1998). Asian Pacific Islander health. In S. Loue (Ed.). *Handbook of Immigrant Health* (pp. 303–327). New York: Plenum Press.

Takaki, R. (1989). *Strangers from a Different Shore*. New York: Penguin Books.

Talerman, A., Verp, M.S., Senekjian, E., Gilewski, T., & Vogelzang, N. (1990). True hermaphrodite with bilateral ovotestes, bilateral gonadoblastomas and the dysgerminomas, 46, XX/46,XY karotype, and a successful pregnancy. *Cancer, 66*, 2668–2671.

Tam, T.W., Weisner, C., & Mertens, J. (2000). Demographic characteristics, life context, and patterns of substance use among alcohol-dependent treatment clients in a health maintenance organization. *Alcoholism, Clinical and Experimental Research, 24*, 1803–1810.

Tart, C.T. (1971). *On Being Stoned: A Psychological Study of Marijuana Intoxication.* Palo Alto, California: Science and Behavior Books.

Tatum, B.D. (1993). Talking about race, learning about racism: The application of racial identity development theory in the classroom. *Harvard Educational Review, 62*, 1–24.

Taylor, C. (1994). Alcohol, drug, and tobacco dependence: Charting and comparing the likelihood and time-course of relapse and recovery. In G. Edwards & M. Lader (Eds.). *Addiction: Processes of Change* (pp. 13–31). Oxford, New York: Oxford University Press.

Taylor, E.J. (1988). *Dorland's Illustrated Medical Dictionary*, 27th ed. Philadelphia: W.S. Sanders Company.

Taylor, S.C. (1986). Evacuation and economic loss. In R. Daniels, S.C. Taylor, & H.H.L. Kitano (Eds.). *Japanese Americans: From Relocation to Redress* (pp. 163–167). Salt Lake City, Utah: University of Utah Press.

Tempelman, S. (1999). Constructions of cultural identity: Multiculturalism and exclusion. *Political Studies, 47*, 17–31.

Teske, R.H.C. & Parker, M.L. (1983). *Spouse Abuse in Texas: A Study of Women's Attitudes and Experiences.* Huntsville, Texas: Criminal Justice Center, Sam Houston State University.

Teufel, N.I. (1996). Nutrient characteristics of Southwest Native American pre-contact diets. *Journal of Nutritional and Environmental Medicine, 3*, 272–284.

Thaller, V., Buljan, D., Breitenfeld, D., Marusic, S., Breitenfeld, T., De-Syo, D., & Zoricic, Z. (1998). Anthropological aspects of alcohol consumption and alcohol related problems, *Colegium Anthropologicum, 22*, 603–611.

Therrien, M. & Ramirez, R.R. (2000). *The Hispanic Population in the United States: March 2000.* Washington, D.C.: United States Census Bureau [Current Population Reports, P20-535].

Thomas, S.B. & Quinn, S.C. (1993). The politics. In J. Stryker & M.D. Smith (Eds.). *Dimensions of HIV Prevention: Needle Exchange.* Menlo Park, California: Henry J. Kaiser Family Foundation.

Thomas, S.B. & Quinn, S.C. (1991). The Tuskegee syphilis study, 1932 to 1972: Implications for HIV education and AIDS risk education programs in the black community. *American Journal of Public Health, 81*, 1498–1504.

Thomassen, H.R., Edenberg, H.J., Crabb, D.W., Mai, X.L., Jerome, R.E., Li, T.K., Wang, S.P., Lin, Y.T., Lu, R.B., & Yin, S.J. (1991). Alcohol and aldehyde dehydrogenase genotypes and alcoholism in Chinese men. *American Journal of Human Genetics, 48*, 677–681.

Timpone, J.G., Wright, D.J., Li, N., Egorin, M.J., Enama, J.M., Galetto, G., & DATRI 004 Study Group. (1997). The safety and pharmacokinetics of single-agent and combination therapy with megestrol acetate and dronabinol for the treatment of HIV wasting syndrome: The DATRI 004 Study Group. *AIDS Research and Human Retroviruses, 13*, 305–315.

Tipton, F. (1886). The Negro problem from a medical standpoint. *The New York Medical Journal*, 569–572. Cited in C. Charatz-Litt. (1992). A chronicle of racism: The effects of the white medical community on black health. *Journal of the National Medical Association, 84*, 717–725.

Toleran, D.E. (1991). Pakikisama: Reaching the Filipino community with AIDS prevention. *MIRA, 5*, 1, 8–10.

Toomey, K.E., Oberschelp, A.G., & Greenspan, J.R. (1989). Sexually transmitted diseases and Native Americans: Trends in reported gonorrhea and syphilis morbidity. 1984–1988. *Public Health Reports, 104*, 566–572.

Townsend, M.H., Wallick, N.N., Pleak, R.R., & Cambre, K.M. (1997). Gay and lesbian issues in child and adolescent psychiatry training as reported by training directors. *Journal of the Academy of Child and Adolescent Psychiatry, 36,* 764–768.

Tran, T.V. (1993). Psychological traumas and depression in a sample of Vietnamese people in the United States. *Health and Social Work, 18,* 184–194.

Trevino, F.M., Bruhn, J.G., & Bunce, H. (1979). Utilization of community mental health services in a Texas-Mexico border city. *Social Science and Medicine, 13A,* 331–334.

Trevino, F.M. & Moss, A.J. (1983). Insurance coverage and physician visits among Hispanic and non-Hispanic people. In *Health, United States, 1983.* Washington, D.C.: Public Health Service [Publ. No. PHS 84-1232].

Trevino, F.M., Moyer, N.E., Burciaga Valdez, R., & Stroup-Benham, C.A. (1991). Health insurance coverage and utilization of health services by Mexican Americans, mainland Puerto Ricans, and Cuban Americans. *Journal of the American Medical Association, 265,* 233–237.

Trexler, R.C. (1995). *Sex and Conquest: Gendered Violence, Political Order, and the European Conquest of the Americas.* Ithaca, New York: Cornell University Press.

Trippet, S.E. & Bain, J. (1992). Reasons American lesbians fail to seek traditional health care. *Health Care for Women International, 13,* 145–153.

Trippet, S.E. & Bain, J. (1993). Physical health problems and concerns of lesbians. *Women & Health, 20,* 59–70.

Trotter, R.T. (1985). Folk medicine in the Southwest: Myths and medical facts. *Folk Medicine, 78,* 167–179.

Tucker, W.H. (1994). *The Science and Politics of Racial Research.* Urbana, Illinois: University of Chicago Press.

Turner, J.C., Hogg, M.A., Oakes, P.J., Reicher, S.D., & Weatherell, M.S. (1987). *Rediscovering the Social Group: A Self-Categorisation Theory.* Blackwell: Oxford.

Uba, L. (1992). Cultural barriers to health care for Southeast Asian refugees. *Public Health Reports, 107,* 544–548.

Ulrich, R.F. & Patten, B.M. (1991). The rise, decline, and fall of LSD. *Perspectives in Biology and Medicine, 3,* 561–578.

Unger, J.B., Palmer, P.H., Dent, C.W., Rohrbach, L.A., & Johnson, C.A. (2000). Ethnic differences in adolescent smoking prevalence in California: Are multi-ethnic at higher risk? *Tobacco Control, 2,* I19–I114.

United States v. 46 Cartons. (1953). 113 F. Supp. 336. (U.S. Dist.).

United States v. 354 Bulk Cartons. (1959). 178 F. Supp. 847. (U.S. Dist.).

United States v. Moore. (1973). 486 F.2d 1139 (D.C. Cir.).

United States v. Oakland Cannabis Buyers' Coop., 532 U.S. 483, reversing 190 F.3d 1109 (2001).

United States Bureau of the Census. (1988). *The Hispanic Population in the United States: March 1988.* Current Population Reports (Population Characteristics). Washington, D.C.: Government Printing Office [Series P-20, No. 438].

United States Bureau of the Census. (1990). *The Hispanic Population in the United States: March 1989.* Current Population Reports (Population Characteristics). Washington, D.C.: Government Printing Office [Series P-20, No. 444].

United States Bureau of the Census. (1993). *The Hispanic Population in the United States: March 1993.* Current Population Reports (Population Characteristics). Washington, D.C.: Government Printing Office.

United States Bureau of the Census. (1992). *Statistical Abstract of the United States, 1992.* Washington, D.C.: U.S. Bureau of the Census.

United States Department of Health and Human Services. (1996). *Health United States, 1995.* Washington, D.C.: U.S. Department of Health and Human Services [DHHS Publ. No. PHS 96-1232].

United States Department of Health and Human Services. (1997, January 8). Patterns: Patterns of drug use in 1994. Available at www.health.org/pubs/94hhs/patterns.htm.

United States Department of Health and Human Services. (1990). *Trends in Indian Health 1990.* Rockville, Maryland: USDHHS/PHS/Indian Health Service.

United States General Accounting Office. (1997). *Drug Courts: Overview of Growth, Characteristics, and Results.* [Sup. Docs. No. GA1.13:GCD-97-106].

United States General Accounting Office. (1991). *Women's Set-Aside Does Not Assure Drug Treatment for Pregnant Women.* [GAO/HRD-91-80, ADMS Block Grant].

United States General Accounting Office. (1994). *Young Children in Foster Care.* Washington, D.C. Author.

United States Preventive Services Task Force. (1989). *Guide to Clinical Preventive Devices: An Assessment of the Effectiveness of 169 Interventions.* Baltimore, Maryland: Williams and Wilkins.

United States Surgeon General. (2001). Women and Smoking: A Report of the Surgeon General. Available at http://www.cdc.gov/tobacco. Accessed 2/5/2003.

Uribe, V. & Harbeck, K.M. (1991). Addressing the needs of lesbian, gay, and bisexual youth: The origins of PROJECT 10 and school-based intervention. In K.M. Harbeck (Ed.). *Coming Out of the Classroom Closet: Gay and Lesbian Students, Teachers, and Curricula.* New York: Harrington Park Press.

Valdez, R.B., Morgenstern, H., Brown, E.R., Wyn, R., Wang, C., & Cumberland, W. (1993). Insuring Latinos against the costs of illness. *Journal of the American Medical Association, 269,* 233–237.

Valenta, L.J., Elias, A.N., & Domurat, E.S. (1992). Hormone pattern in pharmacologically feminized male transsexuals in the California state prison system. *Journal of the American Medical Association, 84,* 241–250.

van den Berghe, P.L. (1967). *Race and Racism: A Comparative Perspective.* New York: Wiley.

Van Etten, M.L. & Anthony, J.C. (1999). Comparative epidemiology of initial drug opportunities and transitions to first use: Marijuana, cocaine, hallucinogens, and heroin. *Drug and Alcohol Dependence, 54,* 117–125.

Van Evrie, J.H. (1861). *Negroes and Negro "Slavery."* New York.

Van Vliet, H.J. (1990). Deparation of drug markets and the normalization of drug problems in the Netherlands: An example for other nations? *Journal of Drug Issues, 20,* 463.

Vance, C.S. (1995). Social construction theory and sexuality. In M. Berger, B. Wallis, & S. Watson (Eds.). *Constructing Masculinity* (pp. 37–48). New York: Routledge.

Vasquez, M.J.T. (1994). Latinas. In L. Comas-Diaz & B. Greene (Eds.). *Women of Color: Integrating Ethnic and Gender Identities in Psychotherapy* (pp. 114–138). New York: Guilford Press.

Vaughan, P. (1970). *The Pill on Trial.* New York: Coward-McCann.

Vega, W. (1994). Latino outlook: Good health, uncertain prognosis. *Annual Review of Public Health, 15,* 39–67.

Vega, W.A., Gil, A., Warhelt, G., Apospori, E., & Zimmerman, R. (1993). The relationship of drug use to suicide ideation and attempts among African American, Hispanic, and white non-Hispanic male adolescents. *Suicide and Life Threatening Behavior, 23,* 110–119.

Vega, W.A., Kolody, B., Hwang, J., & Noble, A. (1993). Prevalence and magnitude of perinatal substance exposures in California. *New England Journal of Medicine, 329,* 850–854.

Verbrugge, L.M. (1990). Pathways of health and death. In R.D. Apple (Ed.). *Women, Health, and Medicine in America: A Historical Handbook* (pp. 41–79). New York: Garland Publishing, Inc.

Victor, M., Adams, R.D., & Collins, G.H. (1989). *The Wernicke-Korsakoff Syndrome and Neurologic Disorders Due to Alcoholism and Malnutrition*. Philadelphia, Pennsylvania: F.A. Davis Co.

Vogel, V.J. (1970). *American Indian Medicine*. Norman, Oklahoma: University of Oklahoma Press.

Vollmer, W.M., Hertert, S., & Allison, M.J. (1992). Recruiting children and their families for clinical trials: A case study. *Controlled Clinical Trials, 13*, 315–320.

von Krafft-Ebing, R. (1908). *Psychopathia Sexualis with Especial Reference to the Antipathic Sexual Instinct*. F.J. Rebman (Trans.). Brooklyn: Physicians and Surgeons Book Club.

Von Maffei, J., Beckett, W.S., Belanger, K., Triche, E., Zhang, H., Machung, J.F., & Leaderer, B.P. (2001). Risk factors for asthma prevalence among urban and nonurban African American children. *Asthma, 38*, 555–564.

Vonderlehr, R.A., Clark, T., Wenger, O.C., & Heller, J.R., Jr. (1936). Untreated syphilis in the male Negro: A comparative study of treated and untreated cases. *Venereal Disease Information, 17*, 260–265.

Wagenheim, K. & Jimenez de Wagenheim, O. (1994). *The Puerto Ricans: A Documentary History*. Princeton: Marcus Winer Publishers.

Waldner-Haugrud, L.K., Gratch, L.V., & Magruder, B. (1997). Victimization and perpetration rates of violence in gay and lesbian relationships: Gender issues explored. *Violence and Victims, 12*, 173–184.

Walinder, J. (1967). *Transsexualism: A Study of Forty-Three Cases*. trans. H. Fry. Stockholm: Scandinavian University Books.

Walker, W.O. II (Ed.). (1996). *Drugs in the Western Hemisphere: An Odyssey of Cultures in Conflict*. Wilmington, Delaware: Scholarly Resources Inc.

Wall, T.L., Horn, S.M., Johnson, M.L., Smith, T.L., & Carr, L.G. (2000). Hangover symptoms in Asian Americans with variations in the aldehyde dehydrogenase (ALDH2) gene. *Journal of Studies on Alcohol, 61*, 13–17.

Wallace, J.M., Jr., Forman, T.A., Guthrie, B.J., Bachman, J.G., O'Malley, P.M., & Johnston, L.D. (1999). The epidemiology of alcohol, tobacco, and other drug use among black youth. *Journal of Studies on Alcohol, 60*, 800–809.

Wallick, N.M., Cambre, K.M., & Townsend, M.H. (1992). How the topic of homosexuality is taught at U.S. medical schools. *Academic Medicine, 67*, 601–603.

Walpin, L. (1997). Combating heterosexism: Implications for Nursing. *Clinical Nurse Specialist, 11*, 126–132.

Walsh, S.L. & Strain, E.C. (1999). The pharmacology of methadone. In E.C. Strain & M.L. Stitzer (Eds.). *Methadone Treatment for Opioid Dependence*. (pp. 38–52). Baltimore, Maryland: Johns Hopkins University Press.

Walters, M.H. & Rector, W.G. (1986). Sexual transmission of hepatitis A in lesbians [letter]. *Journal of the American Medical Association, 256*, 594.

Warner, M. (1982). *Joan of Arc: The Image of Female Herosim*. New York: Vintage Books.

Weatherby, N.C., McCoy, H.V., Metsch, L.R., Bletzer, K.V., McCoy, C.B., & de la Rosa, M.R. (1999). Crack cocaine use in rural migrant populations: Living arrangements and social support. *Substance Use and Misuse, 34*, 685–706.

Weathers, B. (1980). *Alcoholism and the Lesbian Community: Needs Report*. Los Angeles: Alcoholism Center for Women. Cited in Hall, J.M. (1993). Lesbians and alcohol: Patterns and paradoxes in medical notions and lesbians' beliefs. *Journal of Psychoactive Drugs, 25*, 109–119.

Weathers, W.T., Crane, M.M., Sauvain, K.J., & Blackhurst, D.W. (1993). Cocaine use in women from a defined population: Prevalence at delivery and effects on growth in infants. *Pediatrics, 91*, 350–354.

Webb, J.A., Baer, P.E., McLaughlin, R.J., McKelvey, R.S., & Caid, C.D. (1991). Risk factors and their relation to initiation of alcohol use among early adolescents. *Journal of the American Academy of Child and Adolescent Psychiatry, 30*, 563–568.

Webster's Third New International Dictionary. (1993). Springfield, Massachusetts: Merriam-Webster.

Weed, F.J. (1990). Victim-activist role in the anti-drunk driving movement. *Sociology Quarterly, 31*, 459–473.

Weibel-Orlando, J. (1989). Hooked on healing: Anthropologists, alcohol and intervention. *Human Organization, 48*, 148–155.

Weijl, S. (1994). Theoretical and practical aspects of psychoanalytic therapy of problem drinkers. *Quarterly Journal of Studies on Alcohol, 5*, 200–211.

Weller, S.C. (1983). New data on intracultural variability: The hot-cold concept of medicine and illness. *Human Organization, 42*, 249–257.

Wells, K.B., Golding, J.M., Hough, R.L., Burnam, M.A., & Karno, M. (1989). Acculturation and the probability of use of health services by Mexican Americans. *Health Services Research, 24*, 237–257.

Westermeyer, J. (1982). *Poppies, Pipes, and People: Opium and Its Use in Laos*. Berkeley, California: University of California.

Wexler, D.B. & Schopp, R.F. (1992). Therapeutic jurisprudence: A new approach to mental health law. In D.S. Kagehiro & W.S. Laufer (Eds.). *Handbook of Psychology & Law* (pp. 361–373). New York: Springer-Verlag.

White, J.C. & Levinson, W. (1995). Lesbian health care: What a primary care physician needs to know. *Western Journal of Medicine, 162*, 463–466.

Wiecha, J.M. (1996). Differences in patterns of tobacco use in Vietnamese, African-American, Hispanic, and Caucasian adolescents in Worcester, Massachusetts. *American Journal of Preventive Medicine, 12*, 29–37.

Weitzner, K. & Hirsch, L.L. (1981). Diethylstilbesterol—medicolegal chronology. *Medical Trial Technique Quarterly, 28*, 145–170.

Wilbert, J. (1987). *Tobacco and Shamanism in South America*. New Haven, Connecticut: Yale University Press.

Wilkins, M.D. (1990). Solving the problem of prenatal substance abuse: An analysis of punitive and rehabilitative approaches. *Emory Law Journal, 39*, 1401–___.

Williams, D.R., LaVizzo-Mourey, R., & Warren, R.C. (1994). The concept of race and health status in America. *Public Health Reports, 109*, 26–41, citing G. King & D.R. Williams. Race and health: A multidimensional approach to African American health. In S. Levine, D.C. Walsh, B.C. Amick, & A.R. Tarlov. (Eds.). *Society and Health: Foundation for a Nation*. New York: Oxford University Press.

Williams, E.H. (1914, February 7). The drug habit menace in the South. *Medical Record, 85*, 247.

Williams, W.L. (1992). *The Spirit and the Flesh: Sexual Diversity in American Indian Culture*. Boston: Beacon Press.

Williams, R. (1986). Prevalence of hepatitis A virus antibody among Navajo schoolchildren. *American Journal of Public Health, 76*, 282–283.

Willowroot, A. (1983). Creativity, politics, and sobriety. In J. Swallow (Ed.). *Out from Under: Sober Dykes and Our Friends*. San Francisco: Spinsters/Aunt Lute.

Winick, B.J. (1997). The jurisprudence of therapeutic jurisprudence. *Psychology, Public Policy & Law, 3*, 184–209.

Winick, B.J. (1998). Sex offender law in the 1990s: A therapeutic jurisprudence analysis. *Psychology, Public Policy & Law, 4*, 505–578.

Wisconsin Statutes §§48.01, 48.02, 48.133, 48.205, 48.207, 48.345, 48.347, 48.355, 905.04 (1998).

Wise, A.J. & Bowman, S.L. (1997). Comparison of beginning counselors' responses to lesbian vs. heterosexual partner abuse. *Violence and Victims, 12*, 127–135.

Woodson, C.G. (1969). *A Century of Negro Migration.* New York: Russell and Russell.

Wren, C. (1999). Arizona finds cost savings in treating drug offenders. *New York Times*, April 21, A14.

Wu, C.T. (1972). *Chink! A Documentary History of Anti-Chinese Prejudice in America.* New York: World.

Yamaguchi, K. & Kandel, D.B. (1985). Dynamic relationships between premarital cohabitation and illicit drug use: A life history event analysis of role selection and role socialization. *American Sociological Review, 50*, 530–546.

Yamashiro, G. & Matsuoka, J.K. (1999). Help-seeking among Asian and Pacific Americans: A multiperspective analysis. In P.L. Ewalt, E.M. Freedman, A.E. Fortune, D.L. Poole, & S.L. Witkin. (Eds.). *Multicultural Issues in Social Work: Practice and Research* (pp. 458–472). Washington, D.C.: NASW Press.

Yarnold, B.M. (2000). Use of psychedelics among Miami's public school students, 1992. *Journal of Health and Social Policy, 12*, 71–79.

Yarnold, M. (1999). Cocaine use among Miami's public school students, 1992: Religion versus peers and availability. *Journal of Health and Social Policy, 11*, 69–84.

Ying, Y-W. (1990). Explanatory models of major depression and implications for help-seeking among immigrant Chinese-American women. *Culture, Medicine, and Psychiatry, 14*, 393–408.

Yinger, J.M. (1994). *Ethnicity: Source of Strength? Source of Conflict.* Albany, New York: State University of New York Press.

Young, A.M., Boyd, C., & Hubbell, A. (2000). Prostitution, drug use, and coping with psychological distress. *Journal of Drug Issues, 30*, 789–800.

Young, T., Palta, M., Dempsey, J., Skatrud, J., Weber, S., & Badr, S. (1993). The occurrence of sleep disordered breathing among middle-aged adults. *New England Journal of Medicine, 328*, 1230–1235.

Young, T.K. (1994). *The Health of Native Americans: Towards a Biocultural Epidemiology.* New York: Oxford University Press, Inc.

Youngberg v. Romeo. (1982). 457 U.S. 307.

Yu, E.S.H., Chen, E.H., Kim, K.K., & Abdulrahim, S. (2002). Smoking among Chinese Americans: Behavior, knowledge, and beliefs. *American Journal of Public Health, 92*, 1007–1012.

Zambrana, R.E., Scrimshaw, S.C.M., Collins, N., & Dunkel-Schetter, C. (1997). Prenatal health behaviors and psychosocial risk factors in pregnant women of Mexican origin: The role of acculturation. *American Journal of Public Health, 87*, 1022–1026.

Zavala-Martinez, I. (1994). Entremundos: The psychological dialectics of Puerto Rican migration and its implications for health. In G. Lamberty & C.G. Coll (Eds.), *Puerto Rican Women and Children: Issues in Health, Growth, and Development* (pp. 29–38). New York: Plenum.

Zeidenstein, L. (1990). Gynecological and childbearing needs of lesbians. *Journal of Nurse Midwifery, 35*, 10–18.

Zevin, S. & Benowitz, N.L. (2000). Pharmacokinetics and pharmacodynamics of nicotine. In M. Piasecki & P.A. Newhouse (Eds.). *Nicotine in Psychiatry: Psychopathology and Emerging Therapeutics* (pp. 37–57). Washington, D.C.: American Psychiatric Press, Inc.

Zúñiga, M.E. (1992). Families with Latino roots. In E.W. Lynch & M.J. Hanson (Eds.). *Developing Cross-Cultural Competence: A Guide for Working with Young Children and Their Families* (pp. 151–179). Baltimore, Maryland: Brooks.

8 U.S.C. §§1101, 1182, 1227.

42 U.S.C. §241(d).

21 Code of Federal Regulations §§897.14, 897.30, 897.32, 897.34 (1996).

29 Federal Register 8,325 (1964).

34 Federal Register 1,959 (1969).

60 Federal Register 41,453–41,683 (1995).

Index